WALDMAN'S

Atlas of Diagnostic Ultrasound of Painful Foot and Ankle Conditions

WALDMAN'S

Atlas of Diagnostic Ultrasound of Painful Foot and Ankle Conditions

STEVEN D. WALDMAN, MD, JD
Associate Dean - International Programs
Chair and Professor Department of Medical Humanities and Bioethics
University of Missouri-Kansas City School of Medicine
Kansas City, Missouri

Ultrasound Images by Michael Meng, DC, RMSK

Wolters Kluwer

Philadelphia • Baltimore • New York • London
Buenos Aires • Hong Kong • Sydney • Tokyo

Acquisitions Editor: Keith Donnellan
Product Development Editor: Nicole Dernoski
Editorial Assistant: Kathryn Leyendecker
Marketing Manager: Dan Dressler
Senior Production Project Manager: Alicia Jackson
Design Coordinator: Holly McLaughlin
Artist/Illustrator: Bernie Kida
Manufacturing Coordinator: Beth Welsh
Prepress Vendor: Aptara, Inc.

9 8 7 6 5 4 3 2 1

Printed in China

Library of Congress Cataloging-in-Publication Data

Names: Waldman, Steven D., author.
Title: Waldman's atlas of diagnostic ultrasound of painful foot and ankle conditions / Steven D. Waldman ; ultrasound images by Michael Meng.
Other titles: Atlas of diagnostic ultrasound of painful foot and ankle conditions
Description: Philadelphia : Wolters Kluwer, [2016]
Identifiers: LCCN 2016004242 | ISBN 9781496345462 (hardback)
Subjects: | MESH: Foot Diseases | Pain—diagnosis | Ultrasonography—methods
Classification: LCC RD563 | NLM WE 880 | DDC 617.5/8507543—dc23
LC record available at http://lccn.loc.gov/2016004242

LWW.com

CONTENTS

PREFACE

Diagnostic Ultrasonography in the Time of Point of Service Ultrasound

Now the time has come (Time)
There are things to realize (Time)
Time has come today (Time)
Time has come today (Time)

Time.......
Yeah

The Chambers Brothers 1966

While the efficacy and safety of ultrasonography as a diagnostic imaging modality for foot and ankle disease is well established, for some radiologists and nonradiologists alike, the utility of point-of-care ultrasonography and its role in quality patient care is less clear. Unlike the traditional diagnostic ultrasound examination performed in the radiology department by an ultrasound technician and subsequently interpreted by a radiologist at a time distant from the performance of the actual ultrasound examination, point-of-care ultrasonography differs from the traditional radiology department—based ultrasound evaluation paradigm in several fundamental and important ways:

1) Point-of-care ultrasound examination is most often performed to answer a straightforward binary question… does the patient have X pathology or not? For example, *does the patient have a Morton neuroma or not, does the patient have an intermetatarsal bursitis or not, does the patient have entrapment of the posterior tibial nerve at the ankle or not, etc.?* This answer will usually make or break the working clinical diagnosis made by the clinician when seeing a patient with foot and ankle pain… a clinical working diagnosis that was made from information gleaned from a thoughtfully performed targeted history and physical examination.

This is a very different clinical exercise than that undertaken by the radiologist and/or technician working within the sterile environment of the radiology department. This traditional radiology-based paradigm assumes that the person performing the ultrasound examination has not talked with or examined the patient in question and is thus limited to providing the treating physician the information obtained from the ultrasound examination in the form of a written report that is formulated in the clinical vacuum of the radiologist's reading room. This long accepted approach often yields an ultrasound report that is by necessity limited to what is normal and what is abnormal within a specific anatomic region rather than a report that includes what is really needed… concise clinical diagnosis. Sometimes this traditional approach suffices, but often the "sterile" ultrasound report the treating clinician receives back from the radiologist (not uncommonly some days after he or she initially examines the patient) often raises more questions than it answers. Until recently, we have accepted the limitations embedded in this traditional imaging paradigm as a matter of course and for the most part have attributed these limitations to shortcomings inherent to the imaging modality itself rather than a flaw in the actual process embedded in the traditional paradigm.

2) In contradistinction to the ultrasound report that is the product of the traditional imaging paradigm, the point-of-service ultrasound examination is most commonly performed by the clinician who is actually treating the patient. This is the person who is armed with "up close and personal" information about the patient that was obtained from a carefully taken history and physical examination rather than by an ultrasound technician/radiologist who is tasked with obtaining ultrasound images in a standardized fashion to insure that the entire anatomic region is adequately imaged… a process that is more often than not driven by anatomic rather than disease- and/or diagnosis-driven considerations. This is not to say that trained ultrasound technicians/radiologists are not highly skilled at taking proper images, but it is to say that an ultrasound examination that is performed by the clinician that is actually treating the patient will more often yield a targeted ultrasound examination that is driven by information obtained in the course of the history and physical examination.

Since more than any other imaging modality, ultrasound is user dependent, any additional information that can help the person performing and interpreting the ultrasound examination separate clinically relevant pathology from pathology that is not contributing to the patient's current complaint is priceless. The ultrasound examination performed by the treating clinician will more often focus on the pathology associated with the working clinical diagnosis rather than the anatomic region per se. This clinical information will often increase the diagnostic accuracy of the examination and this information can be further enhanced by performing dynamic real-time scanning of the suspected pathology, for example, triggering of a digit and subluxation of a tendon at the time that the patient is being examined. Instead of the traditional use of ultrasound as an adjunct to physical diagnosis, point-of-care ultrasound actually becomes part of it!

Furthermore, the treating physician often has specialized clinical knowledge of the common and uncommon conditions encountered in their daily clinical practice that may be utilized to help guide the targeted point-of-care ultrasound examination… knowledge that even the most skilled ultrasound technician or radiologist may not have or may not think of when working in the clinical vacuum of the radiology department. This specialized knowledge is most beneficial to the patient when ultrasound is incorporated by the treating physician into the "laying on of the hands" as he or she formulates a clinical diagnosis.

While all would agree that a faster and more accurate diagnosis would be a desirable outcome, some would be quick to say that the radiologist interpreted ultrasound examination is the gold standard when it comes to ultrasound and nonradiologists should steer clear of using ultrasound in the diagnosis of painful conditions. While this statement might seem logical on the surface… for after all, radiologists have specific prescribed training in the interpretation of ultrasound images… recent scientific studies comparing the accuracy of point-of-care ultrasound interpretations made by treating clinicians with reports rendered by radiologists do not prove this out. When comparing nonradiologists' interpretation of point-of-care ultrasounds with radiologists' interpretation of technician-obtained images, the nonradiologists did just as well, with nonradiologists scoring very high in both sensitivity and specificity of ultrasound diagnosis. That is not to say that lack of experience in performing ultrasound evaluation, lack of clinical knowledge, and/or the use of poor-quality ultrasound equipment will not harm the patient regardless of who performs and interprets the examinations…. but it suggests that point-of-care ultrasonography fits into contemporary clinical practice.

Thus it seems that in fact "*the time* ***has*** *come today*" to embrace this paradigm shift toward point-of-care ultrasonography in the care of our patients. *Ultrasound Diagnosis of Painful Conditions of the Foot and Ankle—A Comprehensive Atlas* attempts to do this by providing a ready reference for all who would like to use ultrasonography to evaluate and treat their patients. I have included almost 534 classic ultrasound images and anatomic drawings of common and uncommon pathologic conditions encountered in clinical practice. I have also provided the reader with important clinical correlates and physical diagnostic tests that will help guide the clinician toward the correct clinical diagnosis. I hope you enjoy reading and using this text as much as I enjoyed writing it.

Steven D. Waldman, MD, JD
2016

CHAPTER 1

Arthritis and Other Abnormalities of the Ankle Joint

ANATOMIC CONSIDERATIONS

The ankle joint, which is also known as the tibiotalar or tibiocrual joint, is a synovial hinge-type joint that allows dorsiflexion and plantar flexion. The joint is composed of three bones: the tibia, the fibula, and the talus (Fig. 1.1). The tibia and fibula articulate with the talus at the ankle joint. The articular surface is dome shaped and is referred to as the mortise (Fig. 1.2). The articular surfaces are covered with hyaline cartilage, which are susceptible to arthritis. The joint is completely surrounded by a dense capsule that provides support to the joint. The majority of strength to the ankle joint is provided by the major ligaments which include the deltoid, anterior talofibular, calcaneofibular, and posterior talofibular ligaments (Fig. 1.3). The joint capsule is lined with a synovial membrane that attaches to the articular cartilage and may give rise to bursae. The tibiotalar joint is innervated by the deep peroneal and tibial nerves. In addition to arthritis, the joint is susceptible to the development of tendinitis, bursitis, fractures, and disruption of the ligaments, cartilage, and tendons.

CLINICAL CORRELATES

The ankle joint's articular cartilage is susceptible to damage, which will result in arthritis with its associated pain and functional disability if left untreated (Fig. 1.4). Osteoarthritis of the

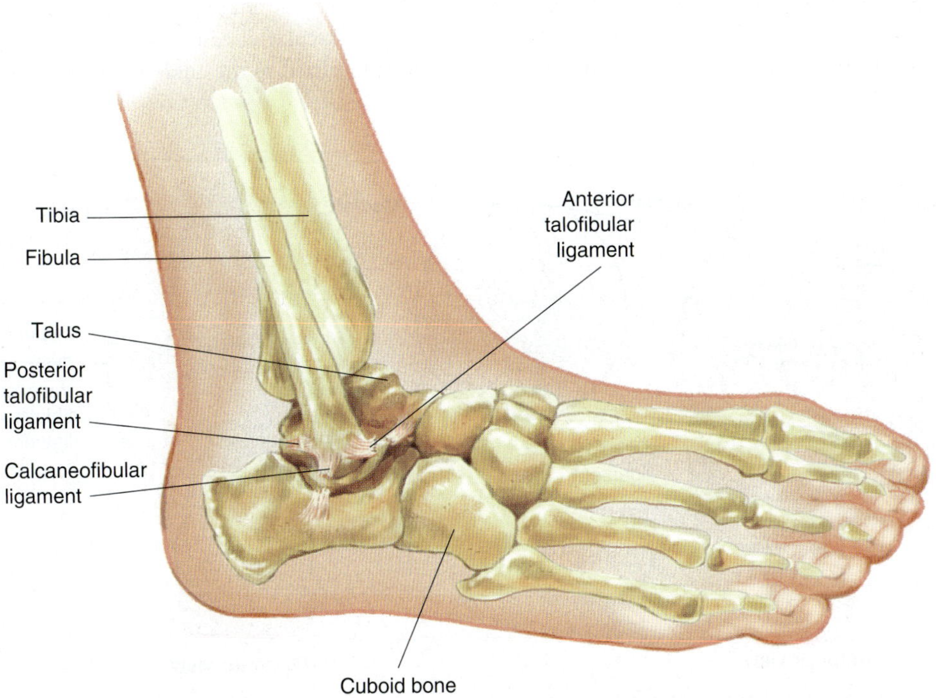

FIGURE 1.1 The articulations of the ankle joint.

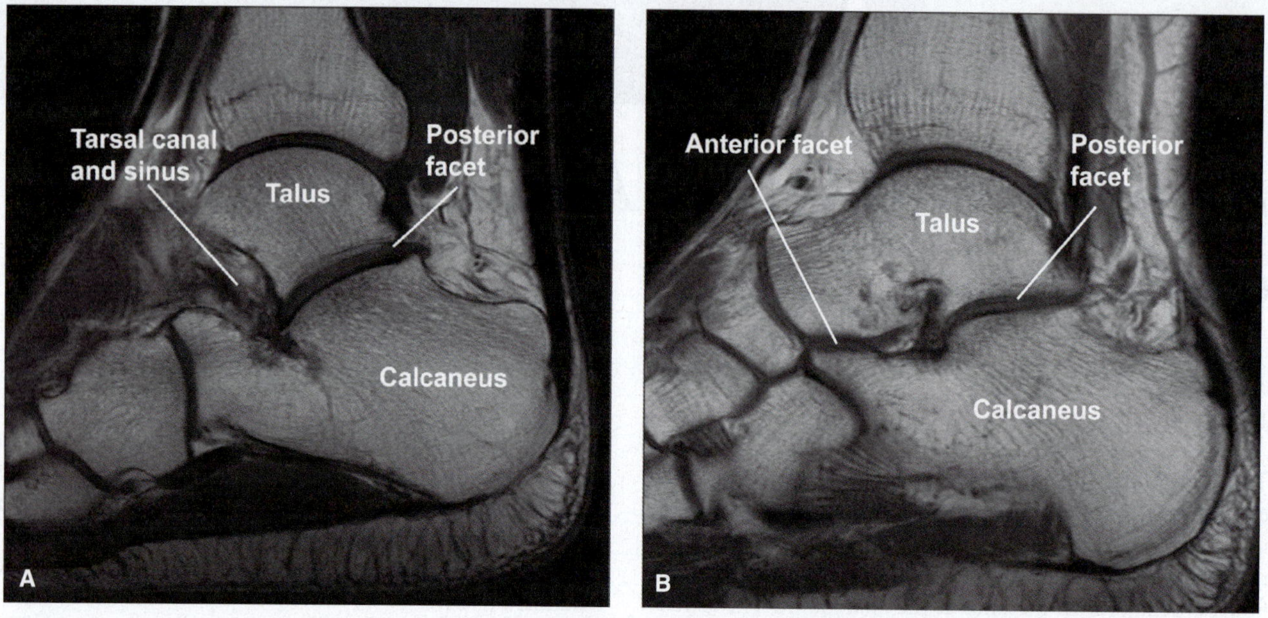

FIGURE 1.2 **A,B:** The articular surface of the tibiotalar joint is dome shaped. (From Berquist TH. Fractures/dislocations. In: *Imaging of the Foot and Ankle*. 3rd ed. Philadelphia, PA, Lippincott Williams & Wilkins; 2011:279.)

joint is the most common form of arthritis that results in ankle joint pain and functional disability, with rheumatoid arthritis and posttraumatic arthritis also causing arthritis of the ankle joint. The ankle joint is the most commonly injured joint in the human body, with sports injuries from basketball, football, tennis, and cross country running being frequent causes of pain and functional disability. Less common causes of arthritis-induced ankle joint pain include the collagen vascular diseases, infection, villonodular synovitis, and Lyme disease (Fig. 1.5). Acute infectious arthritis of the ankle joint is best treated with early diagnosis, with culture and sensitivity of the synovial fluid, and prompt initiation of antibiotic therapy. The collagen vascular diseases generally manifest as a polyarthropathy rather than a monoarthropathy limited to the ankle joint, although ankle pain secondary to the collagen vascular diseases responds exceedingly well to ultrasound-guided intra-articular injection of the ankle joint.

Patients with ankle joint pain secondary to arthritis and collagen vascular disease related joint pain complain of pain that is localized to the ankle joint and distal lower extremity.

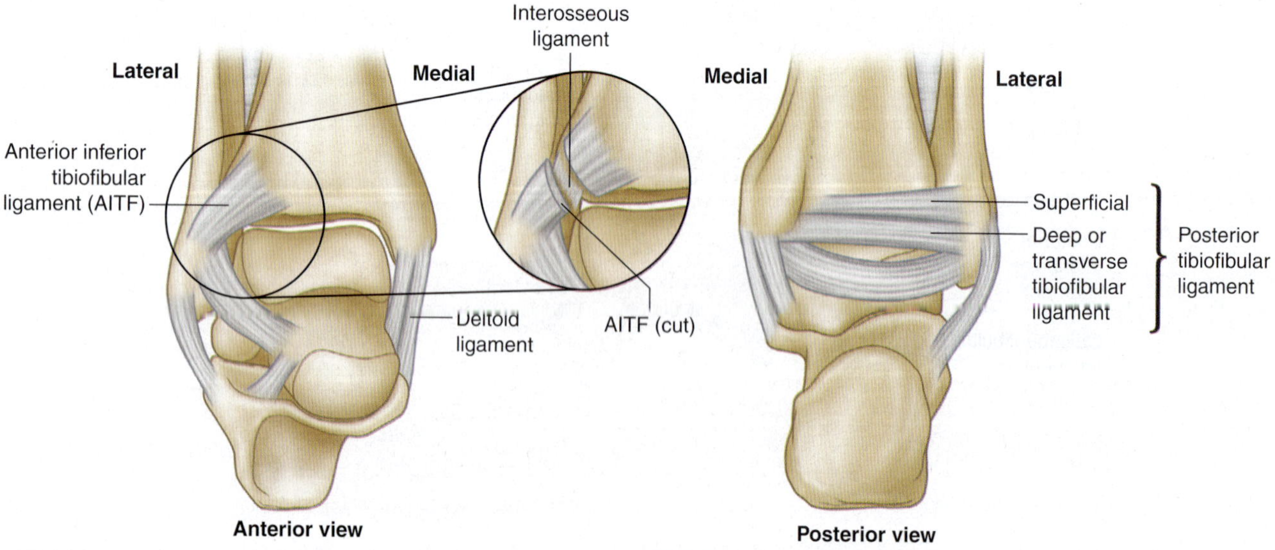

FIGURE 1.3 The ankle joint is completely surrounded by a dense capsule that provides support to the joint. Most of the strength of the ankle joint is provided by the deltoid, anterior talofibular, calcaneofibular, and posterior talofibular ligaments. (From Patel A, Horton G. Anatomy of the foot and ankle. In: Altcheck DW, DiGiovanni CW, eds. *Foot and Ankle Sports Medicine*. Philadelphia, PA: Lippincott Williams & Wilkins; 2013:1–10.)

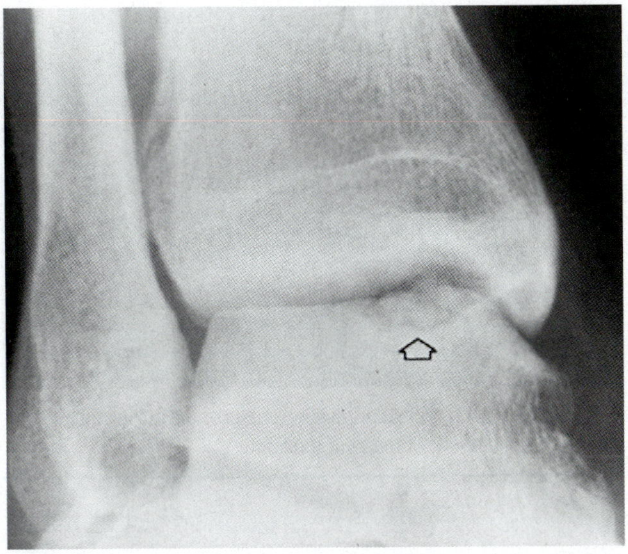

FIGURE 1.4 Osteochondral defect (*arrow*) at the ankle. (From Eisenberg R. *Clinical Imaging: An Atlas of Differential Diagnosis*. 5th ed. Philadelphia, PA: Lippincott Williams & Wilkins; 2010:1057.)

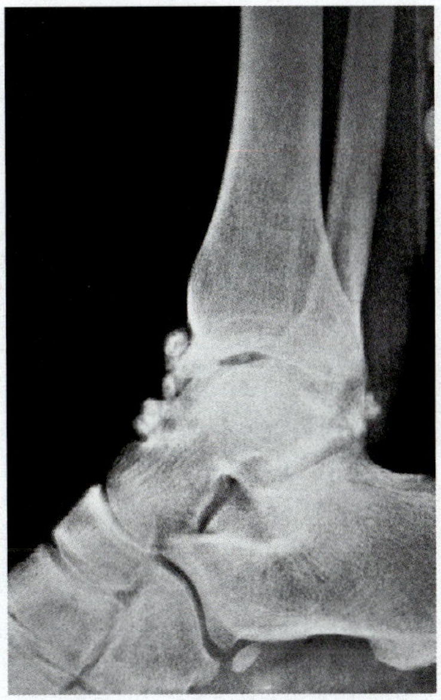

FIGURE 1.6 Lateral radiograph demonstrating joint mice which are causing ankle pain.

Activity, especially involving dorsiflexion of the ankle joint makes the pain worse, with rest and heat providing some relief. The pain is constant and characterized as aching. Sleep disturbance is common with awakening when the patient rolls over onto the affected ankle. Some patients complain of a grating, catching, or popping sensation with range of motion of the joint, and crepitus may be appreciated on physical examination.

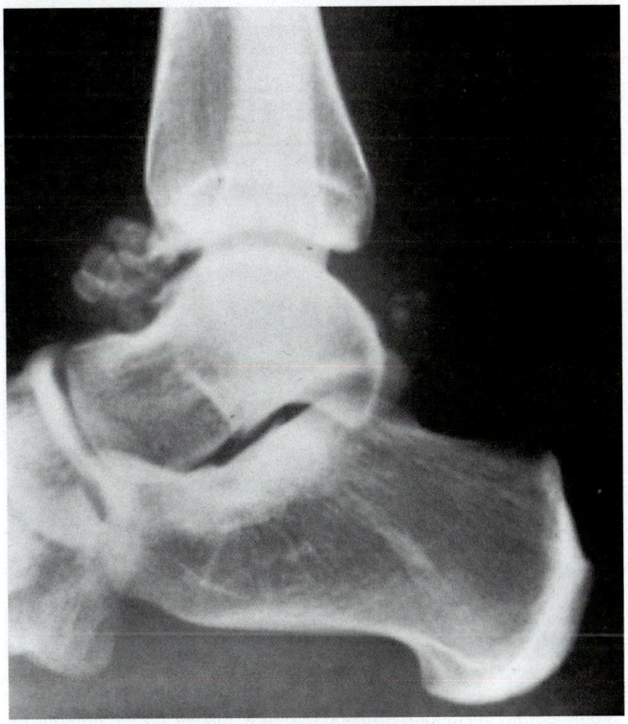

FIGURE 1.5 Synovial osteochondromatosis of the ankle. (From Eisenberg R. *Clinical Imaging: An Atlas of Differential Diagnosis*. 5th ed. Philadelphia, PA: *Lippincott Williams & Wilkins*; 2010:1057.)

Functional disability often accompanies the pain associated with many pathologic conditions of the ankle joint. Patients will often notice increasing difficulty in performing their activities of daily living and tasks that require walking, climbing stairs, and walking on uneven surfaces are particularly problematic. If the pathologic process responsible for the patient's pain symptomatology is not adequately treated, the patient's functional disability may worsen and muscle wasting may occur.

Plain radiographs are indicated in all patients who present with ankle pain as not only intrinsic ankle disease as well as other regional pathology may be perceived as ankle pain by the patient (Fig. 1.6). Based on the patient's clinical presentation, additional testing may be indicated, including complete blood cell count, sedimentation rate, and antinuclear antibody testing. MRI, CT, or ultrasound of the ankle joint is indicated if the diagnosis is unclear as well as to identify other coexistent pathology (Fig. 1.7).

ULTRASOUND TECHNIQUE

To perform evaluation of the ankle joint, the patient is placed in the supine position with the affected lower extremity flexed at the knee so that the foot rests comfortably on the examination table. A high-frequency linear ultrasound transducer is placed in the longitudinal plane over the anterior aspect of the ankle joint (Fig. 1.8). An ultrasound survey scan is obtained which demonstrates the V-shaped anterior tibiotalar joint (Fig. 1.9). After the joint space is identified, color Doppler imaging is used to identify major vessels including the dorsalis

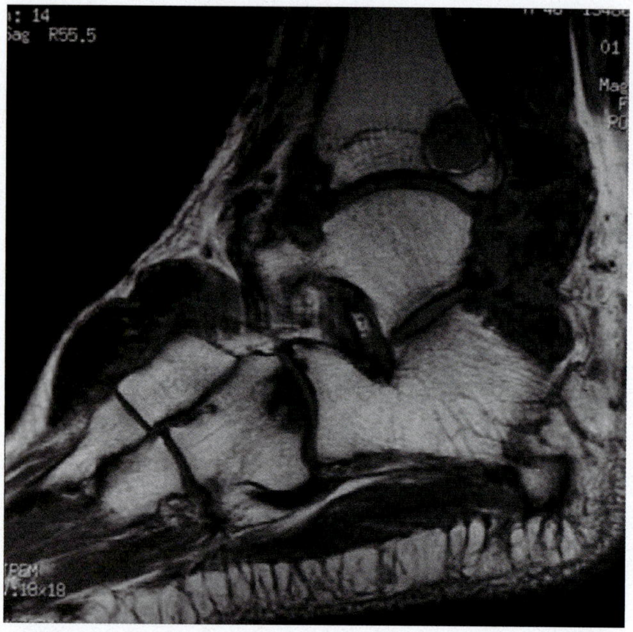

FIGURE 1.7 Pigmented villonodular synovitis. Sagittal T1-weighted magnetic resonance image showing lumpy synovial thickening of very low signal intensity due to hemosiderin. There are bone erosions and an extension into adjacent tendon sheaths. (From Schatz J, Soper J, McCormack S, et al. Imaging of tumors in the ankle and foot. *Top Magn Reson Imaging* 2010;21(1):37–50.)

pedis artery which frequently runs over the superior aspect of the joint (Fig. 1.10).

After the joint space and major vessels are identified, the joint is evaluated for the presence of arthritis, synovitis, effusion, crystal deposition, and abnormal masses including ganglion cysts (Figs. 1.11 to 1.19). If there is history of trauma, the adjacent bone is imaged to identify periosteal defect and bleeding (Figs. 1.20 to 1.23).

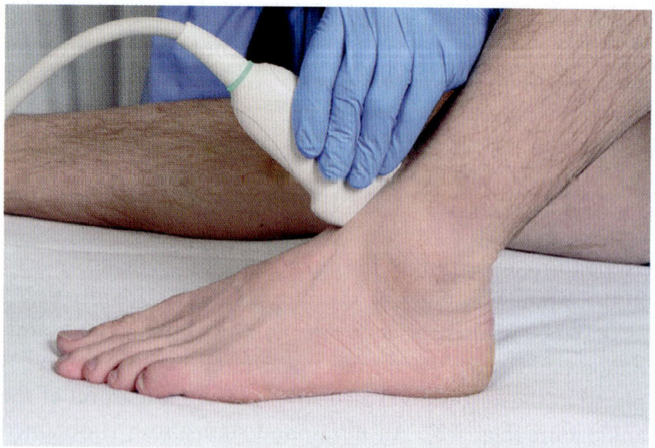

FIGURE 1.8 Correct longitudinal position for ultrasound transducer for ultrasound evaluation of the ankle joint.

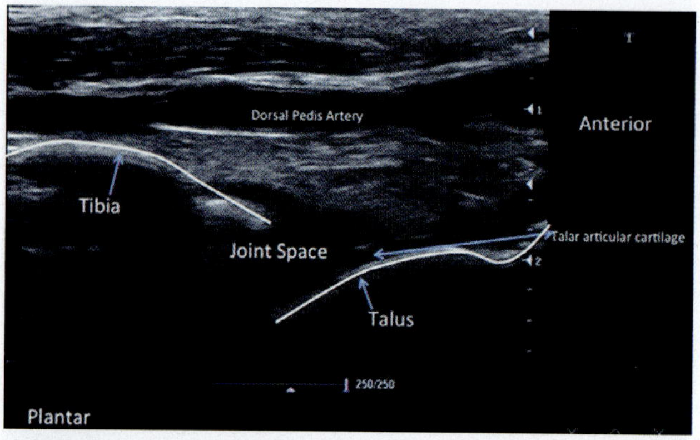

FIGURE 1.9 Longitudinal ultrasound image of the ankle joint demonstrating characteristic V shape of the joint.

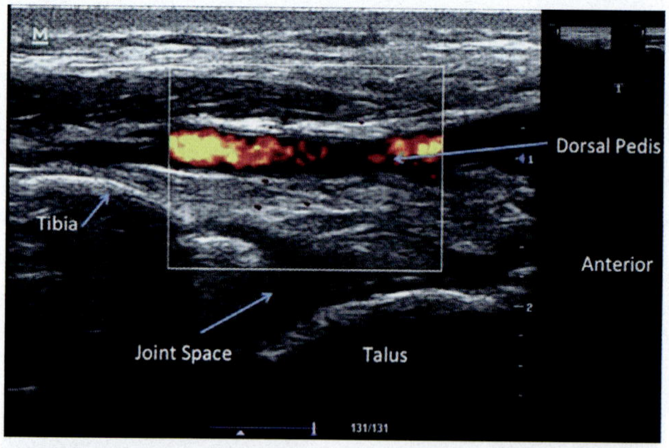

FIGURE 1.10 Longitudinal color Doppler image demonstrating the dorsalis pedis artery overlying the tibiotalar joint.

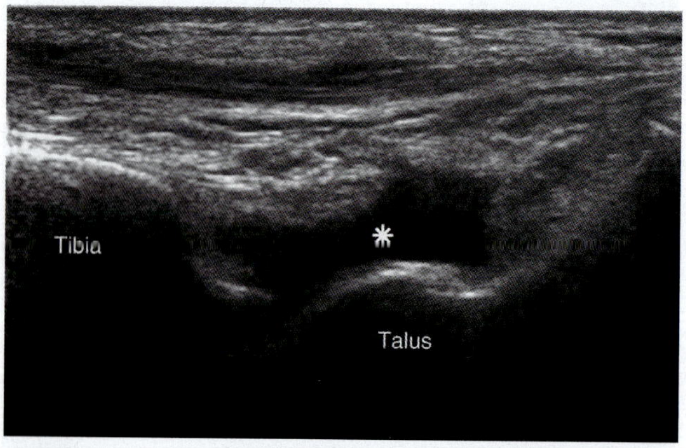

FIGURE 1.11 Longitudinal ultrasound anterior aspect of ankle. There is a moderate ankle joint effusion (*asterisk*) displacing the anterior fat pad. (From Lee R, Griffith J. Foot and ankle. In: Beggs I, ed. *Musculoskeletal Ultrasound*. Philadelphia, PA: Lippincott Williams & Wilkins; 2014:170.)

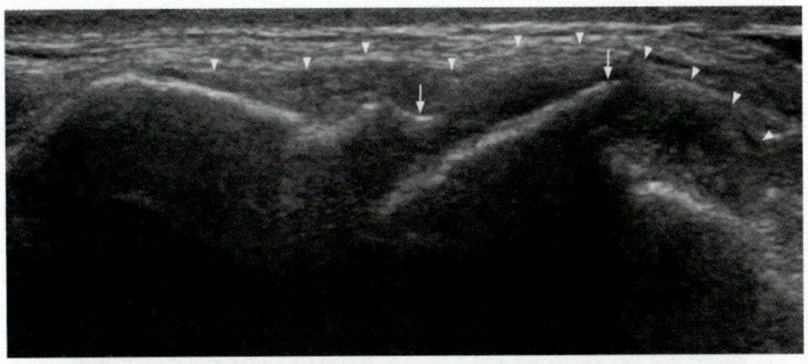

FIGURE 1.12 Longitudinal ultrasound anterolateral aspect of ankle showing quite severe osteoarthrosis with joint space narrowing, marginal osteophytosis (*arrows*), together with moderate capsular thickening (*arrowheads*). (From Lee R, Griffith J. Foot and ankle. In: Beggs I, ed. *Musculoskeletal Ultrasound*. Philadelphia, PA: Lippincott Williams & Wilkins; 2014:170.)

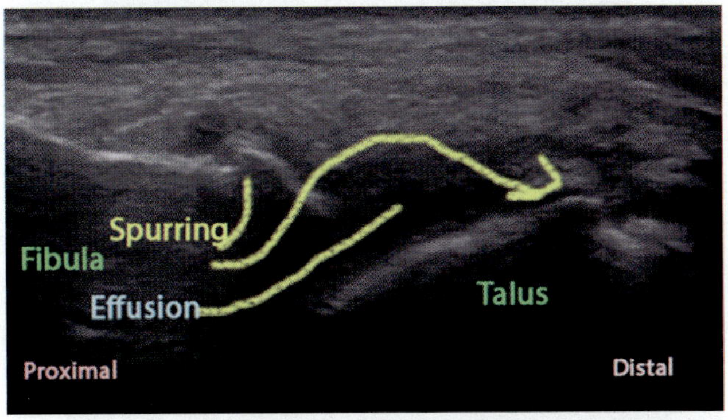

FIGURE 1.13 Longitudinal ultrasound image of the lateral ankle demonstrating significant osteoarthritis of the ankle joint. Note the osteophytic spurring and effusion.

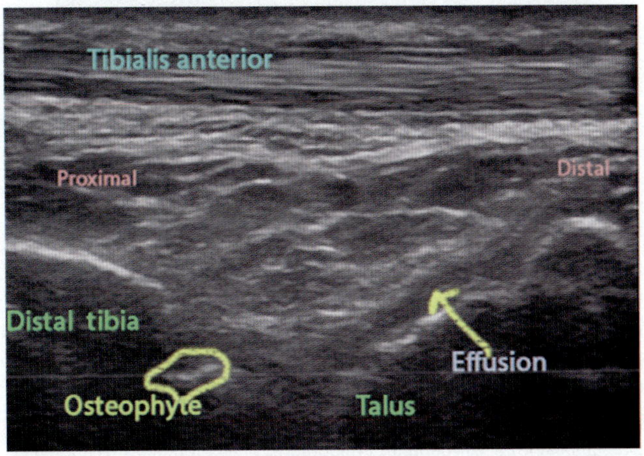

FIGURE 1.14 Longitudinal ultrasound image of the ankle demonstrating findings consistent with osteoarthritis. Note the osteophyte formation and effusion.

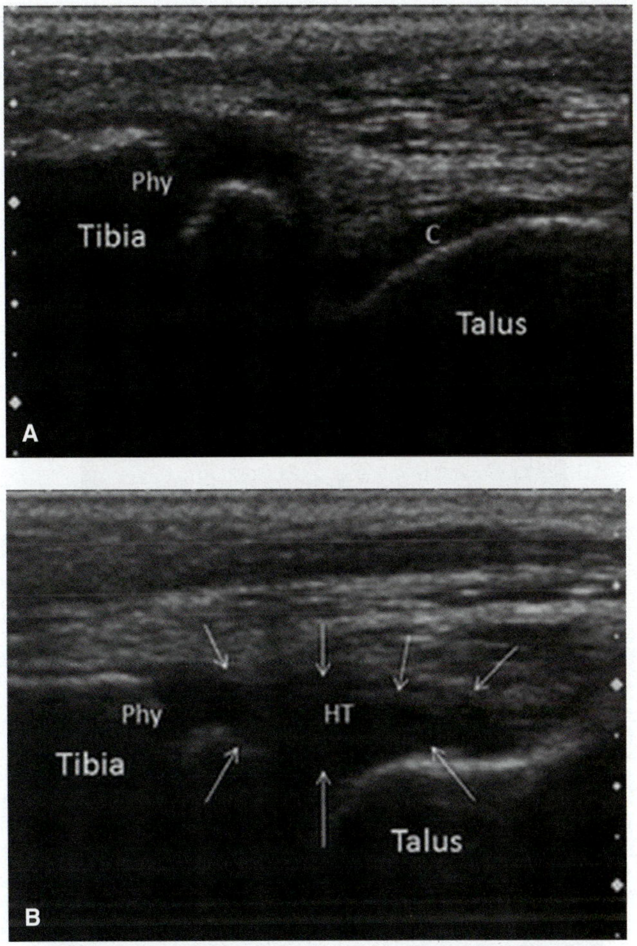

FIGURE 1.15 Ultrasound examination of the ankle of the ankle demonstrating hemarthrosis. Note the difference between the healthy ankle **(A)** and the contralateral ankle showing an acute hemarthrosis **(B)**. Phy, physis; C, cartilage; HT, hemarthrosis. (From Querol F, Rodriguez-Merchan EC. The role of ultrasonography in the diagnosis of the musculoskeletal problems of haemophilia. *Haemophilia* 2012;18(3):e215–e226.)

CLINICAL PEARLS

Bursitis, ligamentous strains and sprains, tendinopathy, osteoarthritis, synovitis, avascular necrosis, and impingement syndromes may coexist with ankle joint disease and may contribute to the patient's pain symptomatology (Fig. 1.24). Ultrasound guidance is useful for needle placement for both injection and joint aspiration if careful attention is paid to the regional anatomy (Fig. 1.25).

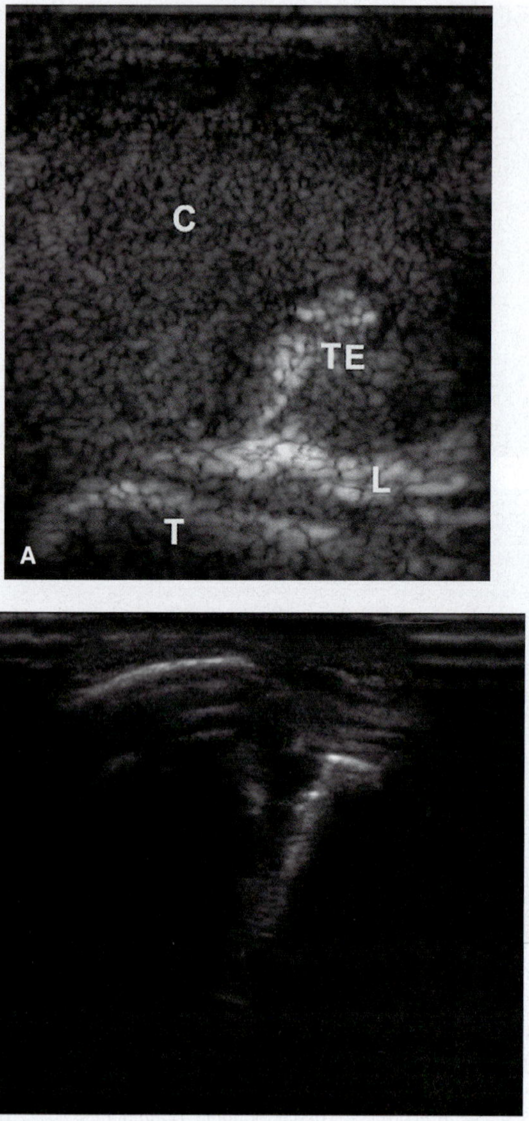

FIGURE 1.16 **A:** Transverse ultrasound image demonstrating crustal arthropathy of the ankle joint. **B:** The same fracture with the probe placed in the transverse plane. C, hypoechoic crystal mass; T, tibia; TE, tibialis anterior tendon; L, medial collateral ligament. (From Balint PV, Kane D, Sturrock RD. Case number 26: massive cholesterol crystal deposition: unusual location in rheumatoid arthritis. *Ann Rheum Dis* 2003;62(6):512.)

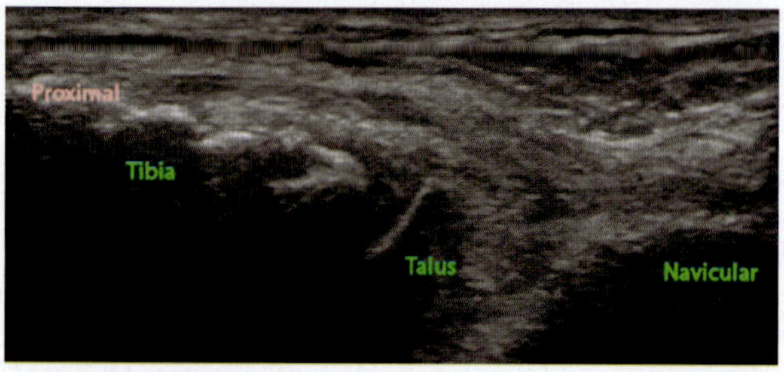

FIGURE 1.17 Longitudinal ultrasound image demonstrating avascular necrosis involving the tibiotalar joint. Note the shape and narrowing of the talus.

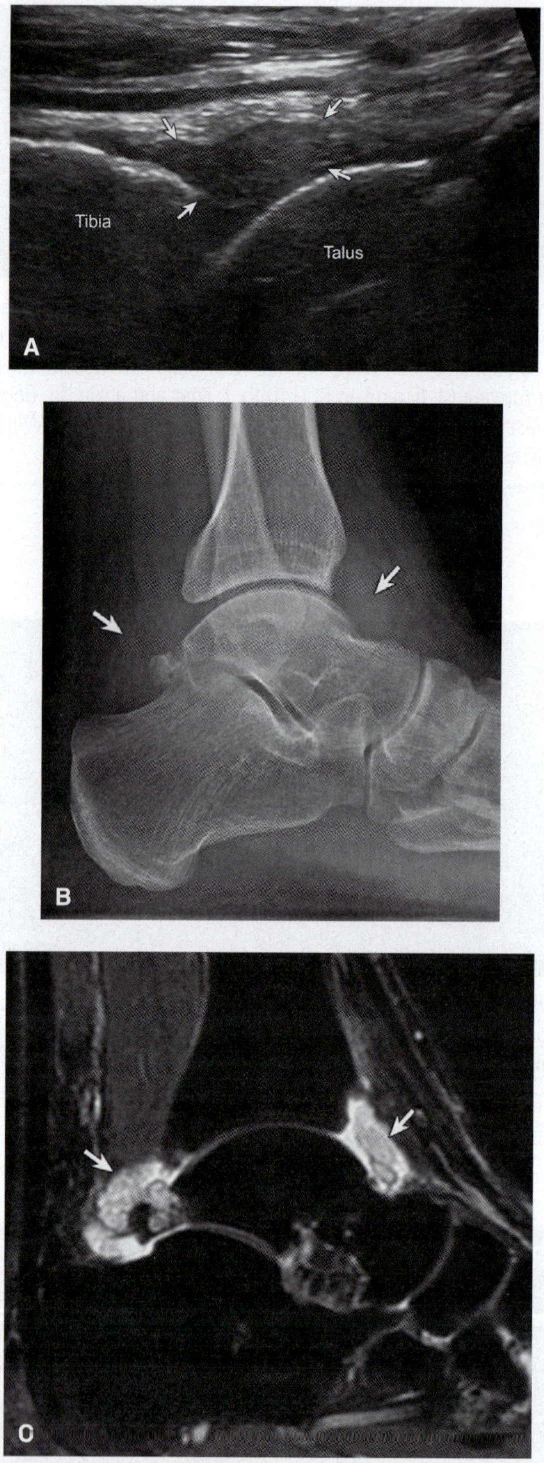

FIGURE 1.18 Synovial chondromatosis. **A:** Ultrasound image in the sagittal plane over the dorsal ankle shows hypoechoic distention of the anterior ankle joint recess (*arrows*). Involvement of both the anterior and posterior ankle joint recesses (*arrows*) are shown on radiography **(B)** and sagittal fluid-sensitive MR image **(C)** (pathologically proven). (From Jacobson JA, Fessell DP. Soft tissue masses. In: Beggs I, ed. *Musculoskeletal Ultrasound*. Philadelphia, PA: Lippincott Williams & Wilkins; 2014:215.)

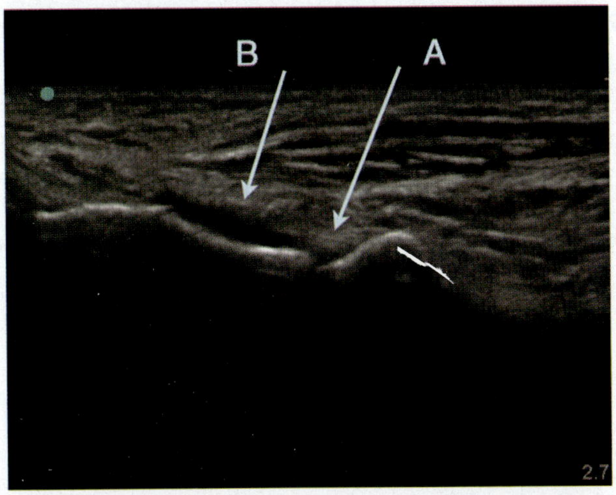

FIGURE 1.19 Obvious fracture of distal fibula above lateral malleoli. Note the stepoff in the cortex (*arrow A*) and periosteal bleeding (*arrow B*). (From Hedelin H, Goksor L-A, Karlsson J, et al. Ultrasound-assisted triage of ankle trauma can decrease the need for radiographic imaging. *Am J Emerg Med* 2013;31(12):1686–1689.)

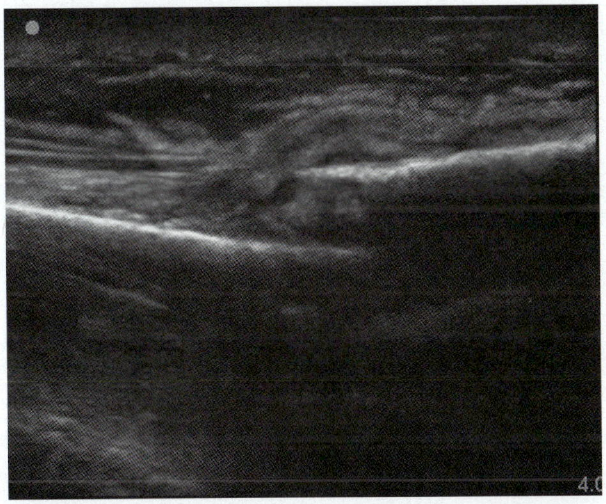

FIGURE 1.20 Severely displaced fracture of fibula as seen on ultrasound image. (From Hedelin H, Goksor LA, Karlsson J, et al. Ultrasound-assisted triage of ankle trauma can decrease the need for radiographic imaging. *Am J Emerg Med* 2013;31(12):1686–1689.)

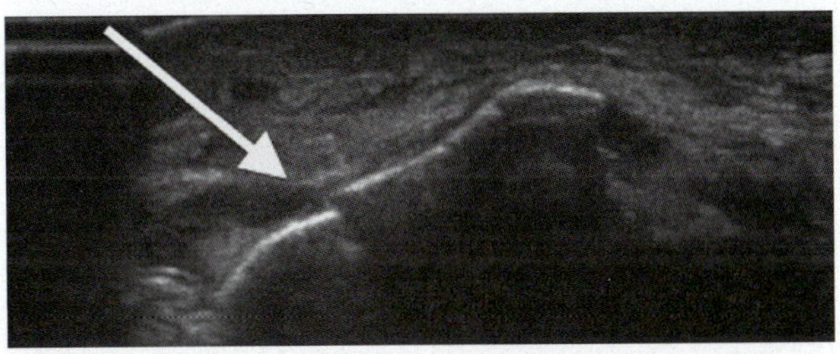

FIGURE 1.21 A fracture with little displacement as seen on ultrasound. Note the stepoff in the cortex (*arrow*). (From Hedelin H, Goksor LA, Karlsson J, et al. Ultrasound-assisted triage of ankle trauma can decrease the need for radiographic imaging. *Am J Emerg Med* 2013;31(12):1686–1689.)

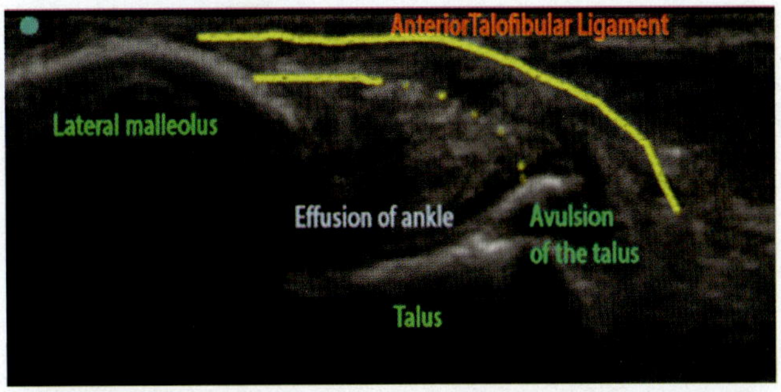

FIGURE 1.22 Transverse ultrasound image of the anterior talofibular ligament demonstrating an avulsion fracture of the talus. Note the effusion within the lateral ankle joint.

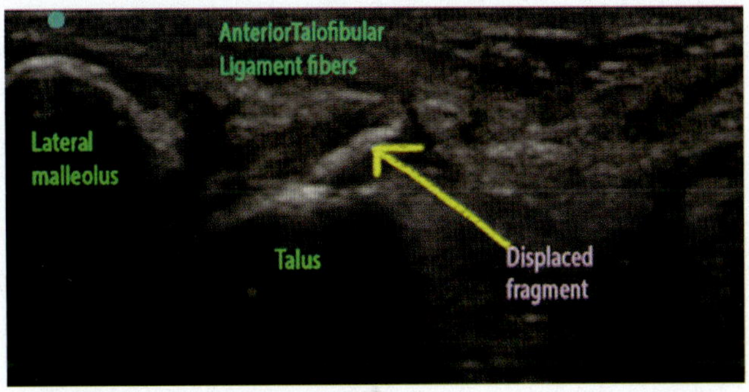

FIGURE 1.23 Transverse ultrasound image demonstrating a displaced avulsion fracture of the talus in a patient with a severe sprain of the anterior talofibular ligament.

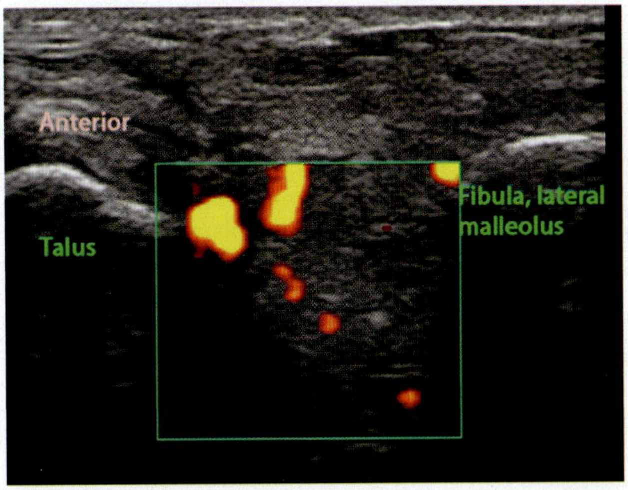

FIGURE 1.24 Color Doppler image of a severe sprain of the anterior talofibular ligament.

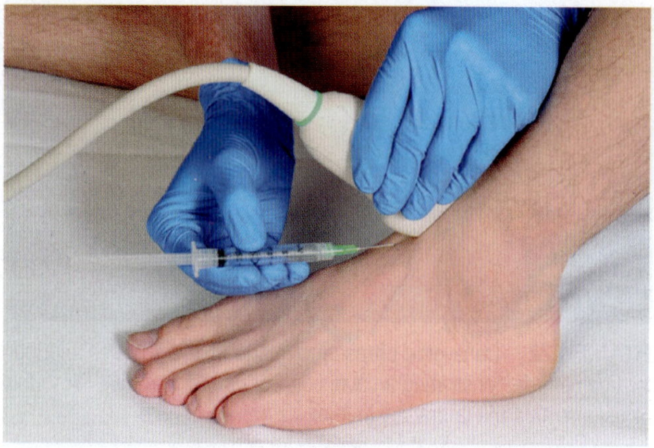

FIGURE 1.25 Correct in-plane needle placement for ultrasound-guided ankle joint injection.

Suggested Readings

Erickson SJ. Sonography of the foot and ankle. *Foot Ankle Clin* 2000;5:29–48.

Waldman SD. Functional anatomy of the ankle and foot. In: *Pain Review.* Philadelphia, PA: Saunders; 2009:155–156.

Waldman SD. Intra-articular injection of the ankle joint. In: *Pain Review.* Philadelphia, PA: Saunders; 2009:590–591.

Waldman SD. Intra-articular injection of the ankle joint. In: *Atlas of Pain Management Injection Techniques.* 3rd ed. Philadelphia, PA: Saunders; 2012:410–412.

Waldman SD, Campbell RSD. Anatomy: special imaging considerations of the ankle and foot. In: *Imaging of Pain.* Philadelphia, PA: Saunders; 2011:417–419.

Ward ST, Williams PL, Purkayastha S. Intra-articular corticosteroid injections in the foot and ankle: a prospective 1-year follow-up investigation. *J Foot Ankle Surg* 2008;47(2):138–144.

CHAPTER 2

Arthritis and Other Abnormalities of the Subtalar Joint

ANATOMIC CONSIDERATIONS

The subtalar joint, (which is also known as the talocalcaneal joint) is a condyloid synovial plane-type articulation between the talus and calcaneus which allows eversion and inversion of the ankle (Figs. 2.1 and 2.2). The articular surfaces are covered with hyaline cartilage, which are susceptible to arthritis. The joint is completely surrounded by a dense capsule that provides support to the joint. The majority of strength to the subtalar joint is provided by the medial and lateral talocalcaneal ligaments and the interosseous ligament (Fig. 2.3). The joint capsule is lined with a synovial membrane that attaches to the articular cartilage and may give rise to bursae. In addition to arthritis, the tibiofibular joint is susceptible to the development of tendinitis, bursitis, and disruption of the ligaments, cartilage, and tendons.

CLINICAL CORRELATES

The subtalar joint, which is also known as the talocalcaneal joint, is a condyloid synovial plane-type articulation between the talus and calcaneus which allows eversion and inversion of the ankle (Fig. 2.1). The joint's articular cartilage is susceptible to damage, which left untreated, will result in arthritis with its associated pain and functional disability (Fig. 2.4). Osteoarthritis of the joint is the most common form of arthritis that results in subtalar joint pain and functional disability, with rheumatoid arthritis and post-traumatic arthritis also causing arthritis of the subtalar joint. The joint is commonly injured, with sports injuries from basketball, football, tennis, and cross country running being frequent causes of pain and functional disability. Less common causes of arthritis-induced subtalar joint pain include the collagen vascular diseases, infection,

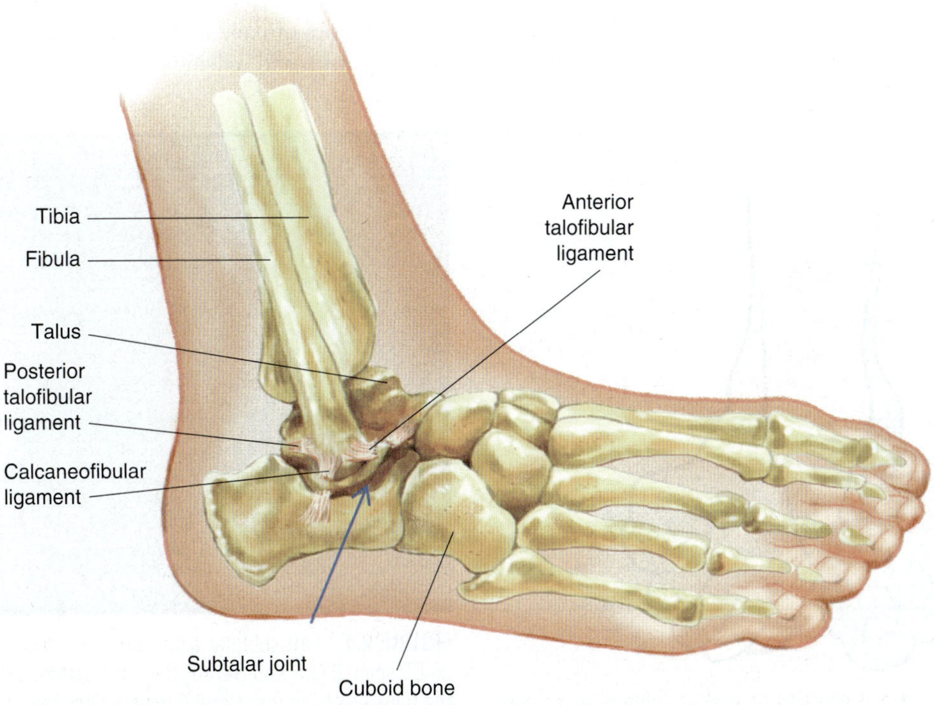

FIGURE 2.1 The subtalar joint. (Anatomical Chart Company.)

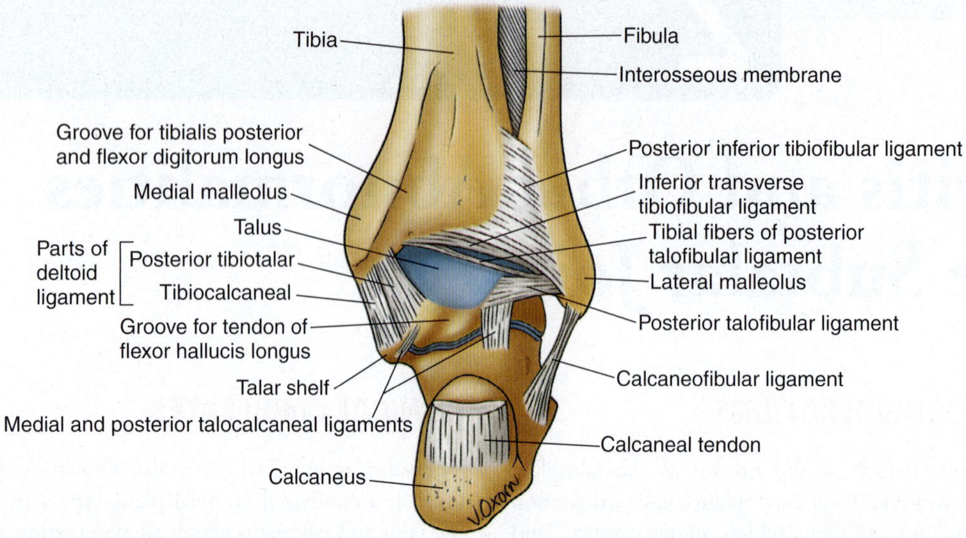

FIGURE 2.2 Most of the strength of the subtalar joint is provided by the medial and lateral talocalcaneal ligaments and the interosseous ligament.

synovial cysts, villonodular synovitis, tumors, and Lyme disease (Fig. 2.5). Acute infectious arthritis of the subtalar joint is best treated with early diagnosis, with culture and sensitivity of the synovial fluid and prompt initiation of antibiotic therapy (Fig. 2.6). The collagen vascular diseases generally manifest as a polyarthropathy rather than a monoarthropathy limited to the subtalar joint, although subtalar pain secondary to the collagen vascular diseases responds exceedingly well to ultrasound-guided intra-articular injection of the subtalar joint.

Patients with subtalar joint pain secondary to arthritis and collagen vascular disease related joint pain complain of pain that is localized deep within the heel. Activity, especially involving inversion of the joint makes the pain worse, with rest and heat providing some relief. The pain is constant and characterized as aching. Sleep disturbance is common with awakening when the patient rolls over onto the affected subtalar joint. Some patients complain of a grating, catching, or popping sensation with range of motion of the joint, and crepitus may be appreciated on physical examination.

Functional disability often accompanies the pain associated with the many pathologic conditions of the subtalar joint. Patients will often notice increasing difficulty in performing their activities of daily living and tasks that require walking, climbing stairs, and walking on uneven surfaces are particularly

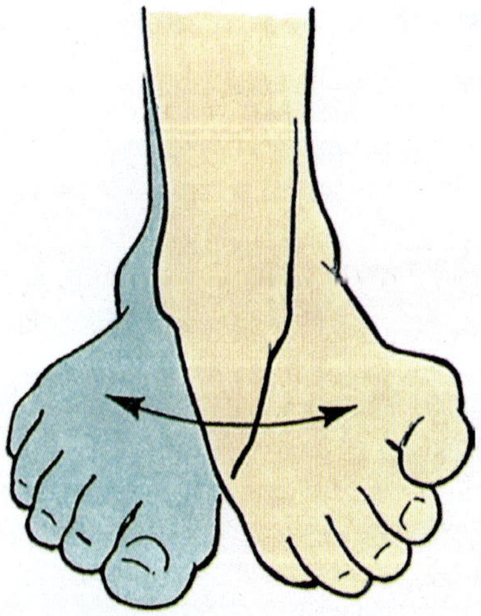

FIGURE 2.3 Inversion and eversion of foot at subtalar and transverse tarsal joints.

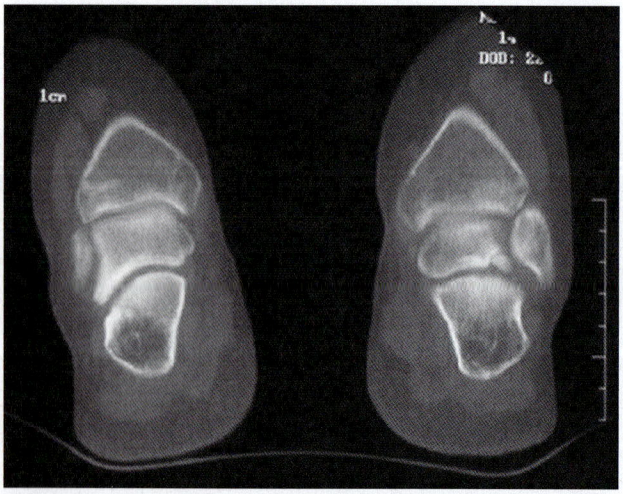

FIGURE 2.4 Left subtalar osteochondritis dissecans lesion as seen on CT scan. (From Kadakia AP, Sarkar J. Osteochondritis dissecans of the talus involving the subtalar joint: a case report. *J Foot Ankle Surg* 2007;46(6):488–492.)

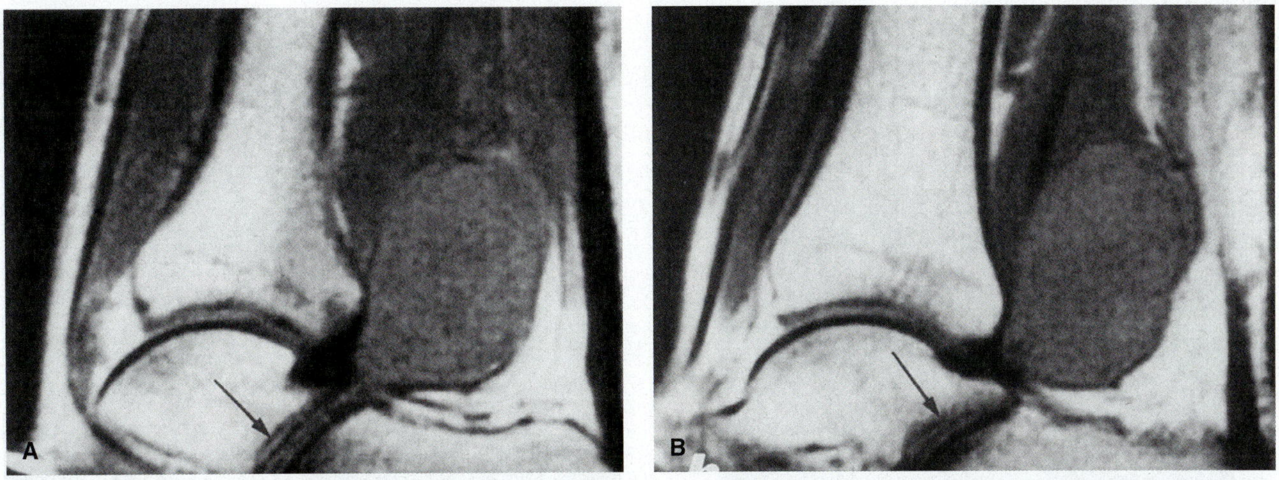

FIGURE 2.5 **A,B:** Sagittal T1-weighted magnetic resonance images. Note the extra-articular mass consistent with nodular synovitis involving the left ankle and extending into the subtalar joint space by a thin peduncle (*arrow*). (From Villani C, Tucci G, Di Mille M, et al. Extra-articular localized nodular synovitis (giant cell tumor of tendon sheath origin) attached to the subtalar joint. *Foot Ankle Int* 1996;17(7):413–416.)

problematic. If the pathologic process responsible for the patient's pain symptomatology is not adequately treated, the patient's functional disability may worsen and muscle wasting may occur.

Plain radiographs are indicated in all patients who present with subtalar pain as not only intrinsic subtalar disease as well as other regional pathology may be perceived as subtalar pain by the patient (Fig. 2.7). Based on the patient's clinical presentation, additional testing may be indicated, including complete blood cell count, sedimentation rate, and antinuclear antibody testing. MRI, CT, or ultrasound of the subtalar joint is indicated if avascular necrosis or meniscal tear is suspected or if the diagnosis is unclear (Fig. 2.8).

ULTRASOUND TECHNIQUE

To perform ultrasound evaluation of the subtalar joint, the patient is then placed in the curled up lateral position with

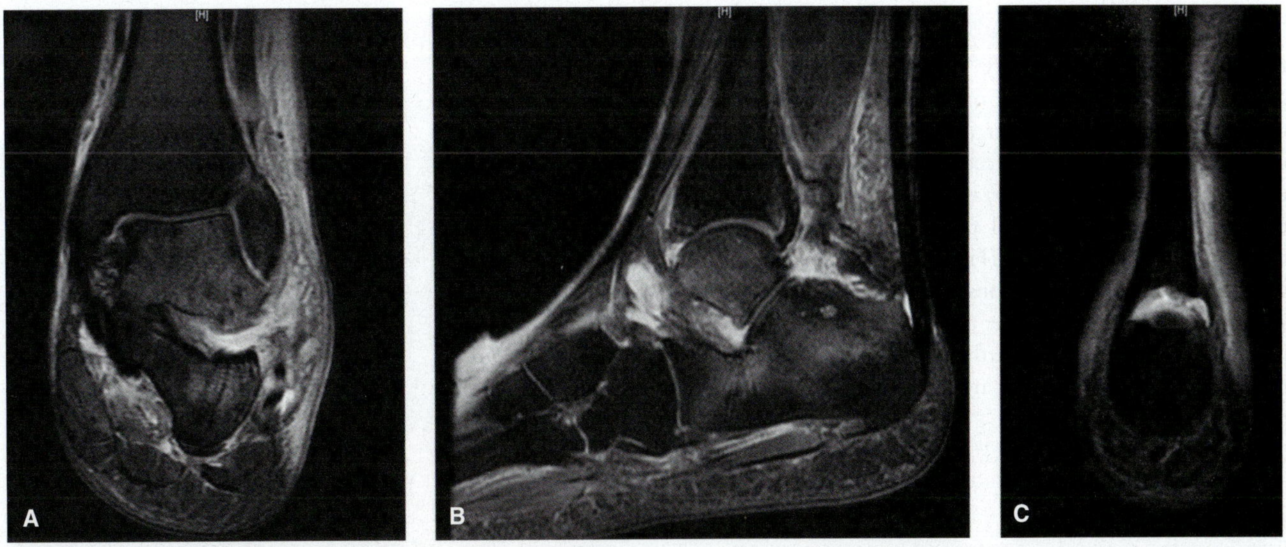

FIGURE 2.6 T2-weighted magnetic resonance images. **A:** Coronal image of a septic subtalar joint illustrating increased signal uptake in subtalar joint and bone marrow edema of talus and calcaneus. **B:** Sagittal image illustrating collection/abscess within sinus tarsi and anterior and posterior synovitis/septic arthritis (as indicated by increased signal intensity within and periarticular to the subtalar joint). **C:** Coronal image taken 5 days after admission and after arthroscopic washout showing posterior joint capsular involvement with increased signal intensity on this sequence. (From Wynes J, Harris W, Hadfield RA, et al. Subtalar joint septic arthritis in a patient with hypogammaglobulinemia. *J Foot Ankle Surg* 2013;52(2):242–248.)

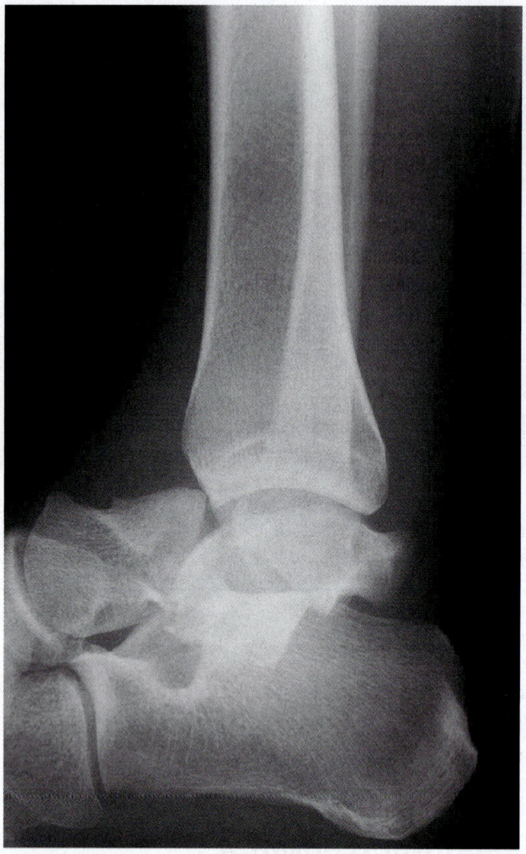

FIGURE 2.7 Lateral radiograph demonstrating joint mice which are causing subtalar pain. (From Bucholz RW, Heckman JD. *Rockwood & Green's Fractures in Adults.* 5th ed. Philadelphia, PA: Lippincott Williams & Wilkins; 2001.)

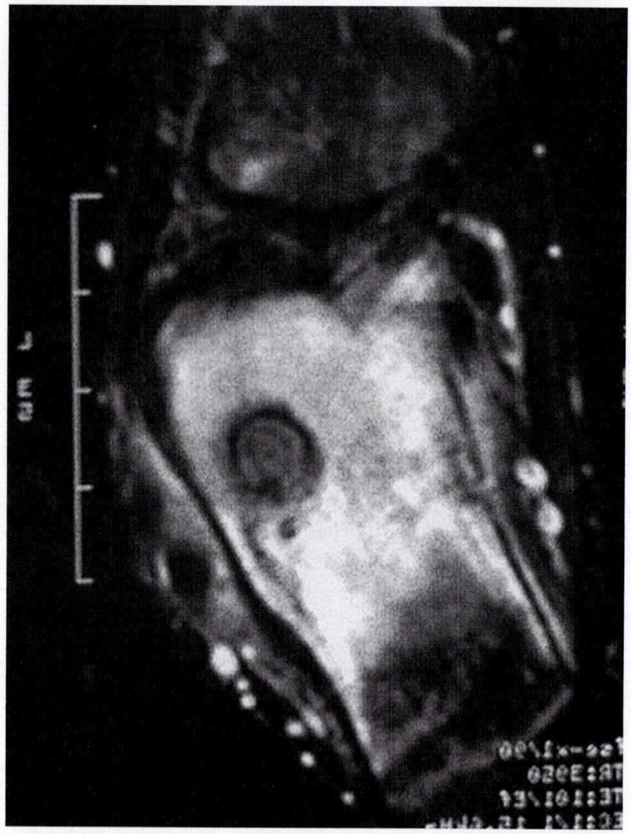

FIGURE 2.8 Heavily T2-weighted axial magnetic resonance image of left foot demonstrating an osteoid osteoma. Note the ring of decreased signal intensity, or the bull's eye appearance, typical of osteoid osteoma. (From Morris GB, Goldman FD. Osteoid osteoma causing subtalar joint arthralgia: a case report. *J Foot Ankle Surg* 2003;42(2):90–94.)

the affected lower extremity with the lateral side facing down with the ankle placed on a rolled-up towel to accentuate eversion of the subtalar joint. A high-frequency linear ultrasound transducer is placed over the lateral ankle with the cranial aspect of the ultrasound transducer oriented in the coronal plane. This will place the transducer over the middle of the subtalar joint (Fig. 2.9). An ultrasound survey scan is obtained which demonstrates the middle facet of the subtalar joint (Fig. 2.10). After the joint space is identified, the joint is for the presence of arthritis, synovitis, effusion, crystal deposition, and abnormal masses including ganglion cysts (Figs. 2.11 and 2.12).

CLINICAL PEARLS

Bursitis, ligamentous strains and sprains, tendinopathy, osteoarthritis, synovitis, avascular necrosis, and impingement syndromes may coexist with subtalar joint disease and may contribute to the patient's pain symptoms. The use of multiple imaging modalities may help clarify the diagnosis and identify occult pathology (Fig. 2.13).

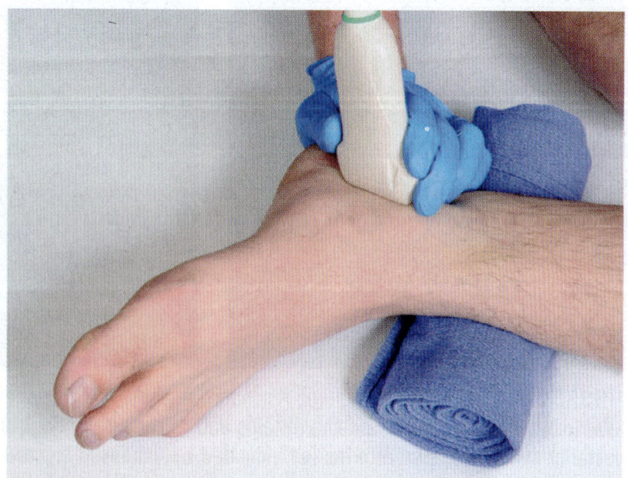

FIGURE 2.9 Correct longitudinal position for ultrasound transducer for ultrasound evaluation of the subtalar joint.

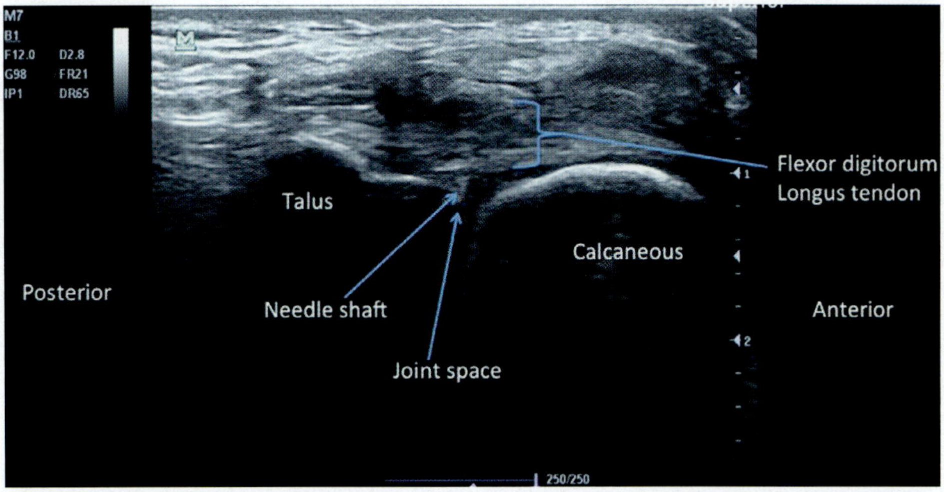

FIGURE 2.10 Longitudinal ultrasound image of the subtalar joint demonstrating characteristic V shape of the joint.

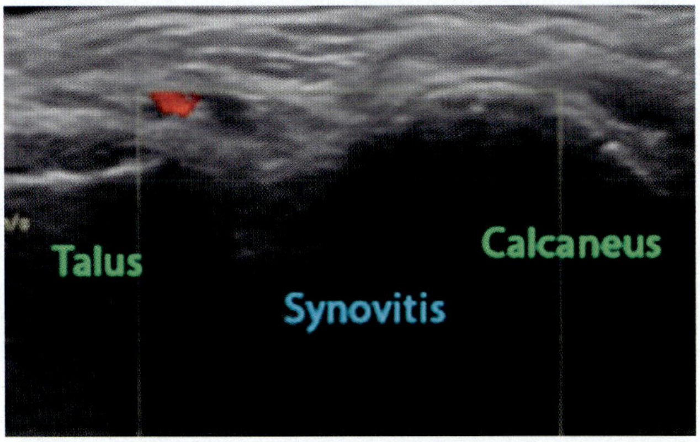

FIGURE 2.11 Lateral longitudinal ultrasound image demonstrating arthritis and synovitis of the subtalar joint in a patient with active rheumatoid arthritis.

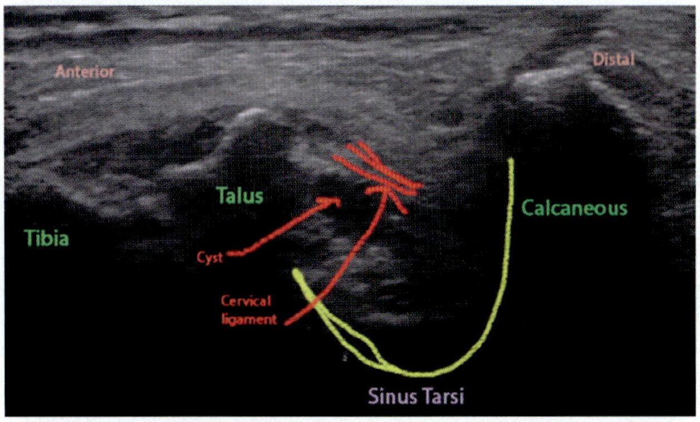

FIGURE 2.12 Lateral longitudinal ultrasound image of the ankle demonstrating a cyst within the subtalar joint in a patient with ankle pain.

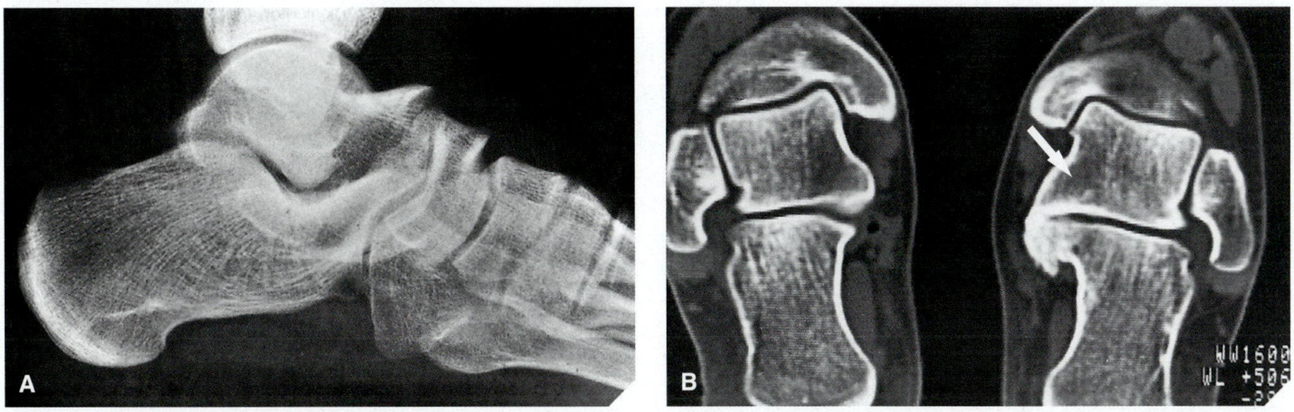

FIGURE 2.13 A 25-year-old man presented with pain in his left foot that was particularly pronounced after prolonged walking or standing. **A:** Lateral radiograph of the left foot shows sclerotic changes in the middle facet of the subtalar joint, narrowing of the posterior talocalcaneal joint space, and a prominent talar beak—features suggesting tarsal coalition. **B:** Coronal CT section clearly demonstrates narrowing of the middle facet joint space and an osseous bridge (*arrow*). The normal right foot is shown for comparison. (From Greenspan A. Anomalies of the upper and lower limbs. In: *Orthopedic Imaging: A Practical Approach.* 5th ed. Philadelphia, PA: Lippincott Williams & Wilkins; 2011:926.)

Suggested Readings

Henning T, Finnoff JT, Smith J. Sonographically guided posterior subtalar joint injections: anatomic study and validation of 3 approaches. *PM R* 2009; 1(10):925–931.

Waldman SD. Functional anatomy of the ankle and foot. In: *Pain Review.* Philadelphia, PA: Saunders; 2009:155–156.

Waldman SD. Intra-articular Injection of the subtalar joint. In: *Atlas of Pain Management Injection Techniques.* 3rd ed. Philadelphia, PA: Saunders; 2012:413–415.

Waldman SD, Campbell RSD. Anatomy: special imaging considerations of the ankle and foot. In: *Imaging of Pain.* Philadelphia, PA: Saunders; 2011:417–419.

Ward ST, Williams PL, Purkayastha S. Intra-articular corticosteroid injections in the foot and ankle: a prospective 1-year follow-up investigation. *J Foot Ankle Surg* 2008;47(2):138–144.

CHAPTER 3

Arthritis and Other Abnormalities of the Talonavicular Joint

ANATOMIC CONSIDERATIONS

The talonavicular joint, which together with the calcaneonavicular joint make up Chopart's joint, which represents the posterior border of the midfoot (Fig. 3.1). The talonavicular joint comprises articulation of the talus and the navicular bone (Fig. 3.2). The articular surfaces are covered with hyaline cartilage, which are susceptible to arthritis. Most of the strength of the talonavicular joint is provided by the talonavicular and plantar calcaneonavicular ligaments (Fig. 3.3). The joint capsule is lined with a synovial membrane that attaches to the articular cartilage and may give rise to bursae. In addition to arthritis, the tibiofibular joint is susceptible to the development of tendinitis, bursitis, and disruption of the ligaments, cartilage, and overlying tendons.

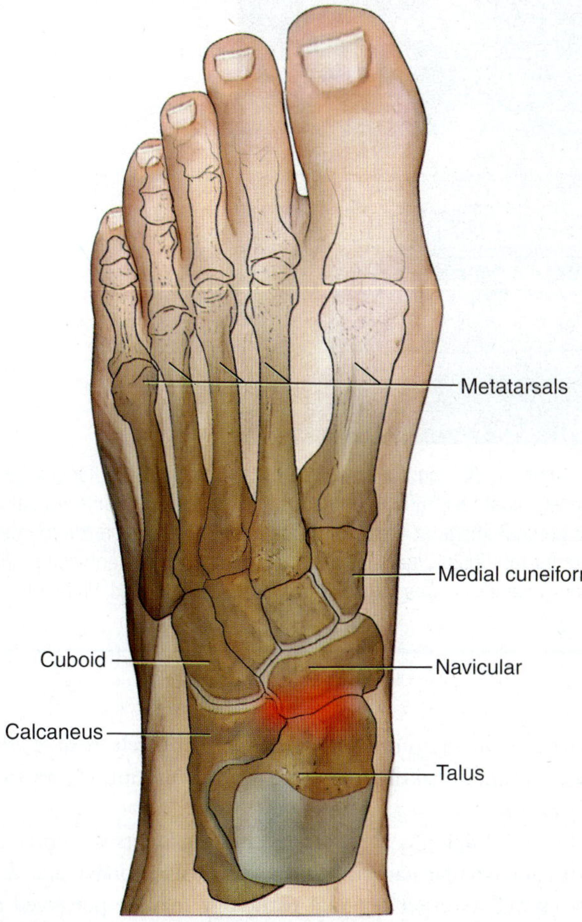

FIGURE 3.1 The articulations of the talonavicular joint.

CLINICAL CORRELATES

The talonavicular joint, which together with the calcaneonavicular joint make up Chopart's (also known as the transmetatarsal joint) joint, which represents the posterior border of the midfoot (Fig. 3.1). The talonavicular joint comprises the articulation of the talus and the navicular bone. The joint's articular cartilage is susceptible to damage, which left untreated will result in arthritis with its associated pain and functional disability. Osteoarthritis of the joint is the most common form of arthritis that results in talonavicular joint pain and functional disability, with rheumatoid arthritis and posttraumatic arthritis also causing arthritis of the talonavicular joint (Fig. 3.4). The joint is susceptible to strains and sprains due to the stresses placed on the midfoot especially when engaging in high-impact activities such as running on hard surfaces with inadequate footwear (Fig. 3.5). Less common causes of arthritis-induced talonavicular joint pain include the collagen vascular diseases, infection, villonodular synovitis, and Lyme disease. Acute infectious arthritis of the talonavicular joint is best treated with early diagnosis, with culture and sensitivity of the synovial fluid and prompt initiation of antibiotic therapy. The collagen vascular diseases generally manifest as a polyarthropathy rather than a monoarthropathy limited to the talonavicular joint, although talonavicular pain secondary to the collagen vascular diseases responds exceedingly well to ultrasound-guided intra-articular injection of the talonavicular joint.

Patients with talonavicular joint pain secondary to arthritis and collagen vascular disease related joint pain complain of pain that is localized to the anterior ankle and midfoot. Activity, especially involving inversion and eversion of the talonavicular joint makes the pain worse, with rest and heat providing some relief. The pain is constant and characterized as aching. Sleep disturbance is common with awakening when the patient rolls over onto the affected talonavicular joint. Some patients complain of a grating, catching, or popping sensation with

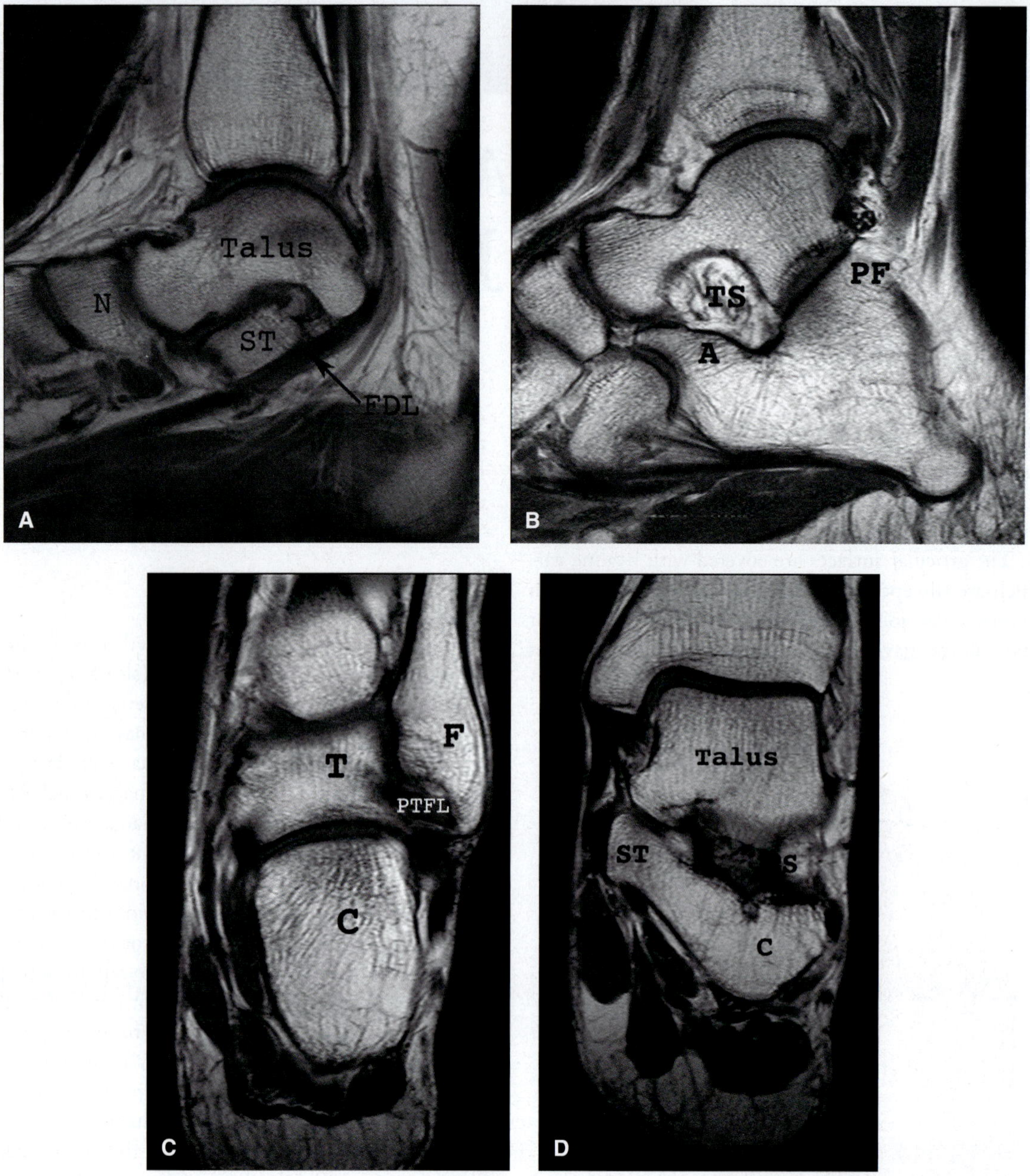

FIGURE 3.2 T1-weighted MR images demonstrating hindfoot and midfoot anatomy. **A:** Sagittal image at the flexor digitorum longus level (FDL). **B:** Sagittal image at talonavicular level demonstrating the posterior talocalcaneal facet (PF), the tarsal sinus (TS), and the anterior calcaneal process (A). **C:** Coronal image at the level of the lateral ankle mortise. **D:** Coronal image at the level of the posterior medial ankle mortise. N, navicular; ST, sustentaculum tali; C, calcaneus; T, talus; F, fibula; PTFL, posterior talofibular ligament; TS, tarsal sinus; ST, sustentaculum tali; DL, deltoid ligament. (From Berquist TH. Anatomy, normal variants, and basic biomechanics. In: *Imaging of the Foot and Ankle*. 3rd ed. Philadelphia, PA: Lippincott Williams & Wilkins; 2011:1–46.)

range of motion of the joint, and crepitus may be appreciated on physical examination.

Functional disability often accompanies the pain associated with the many pathologic conditions of the talonavicular joint. Patients will often notice increasing difficulty in performing their activities of daily living and tasks that require walking, climbing stairs, and walking on uneven surfaces are particularly problematic. If the pathologic process responsible for the patient's pain symptomatology is not adequately treated, the patient's functional disability may worsen and muscle wasting may occur.

Plain radiographs are indicated in all patients who present with talonavicular pain as not only intrinsic talonavicular disease as well as other regional pathology may be perceived as talonavicular pain by the patient (Figs. 3.4 and 3.6). Based on the patient's clinical presentation, additional testing may be

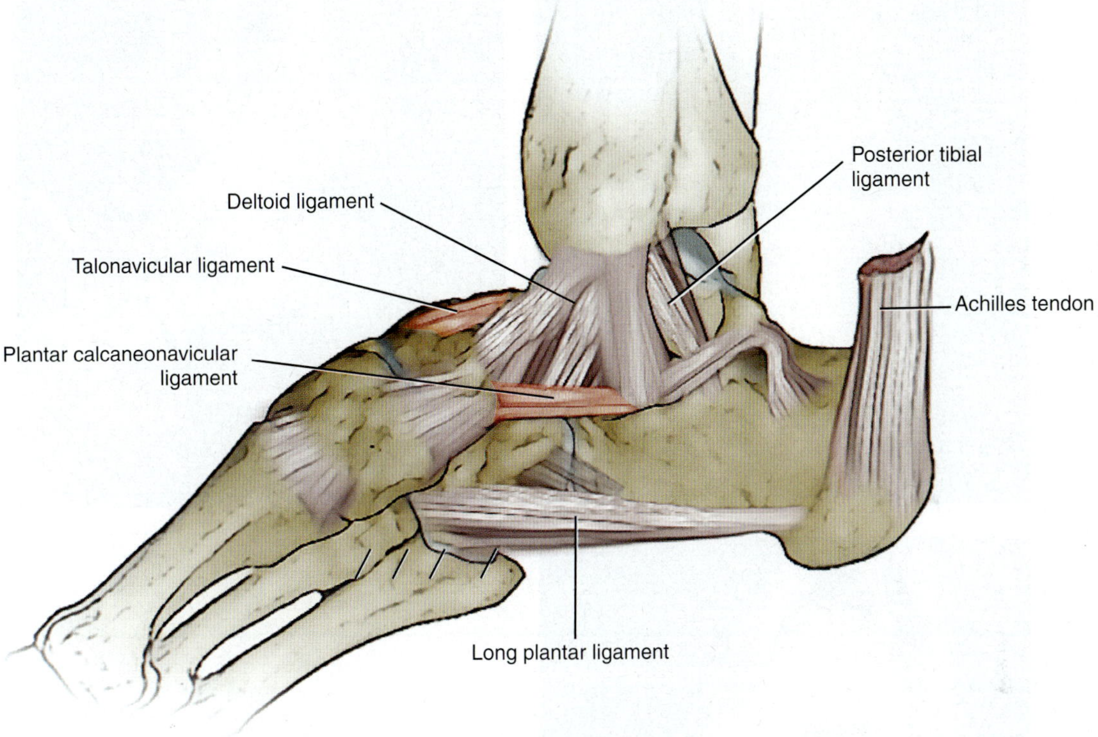

FIGURE 3.3 The articulations of the talonavicular joint.

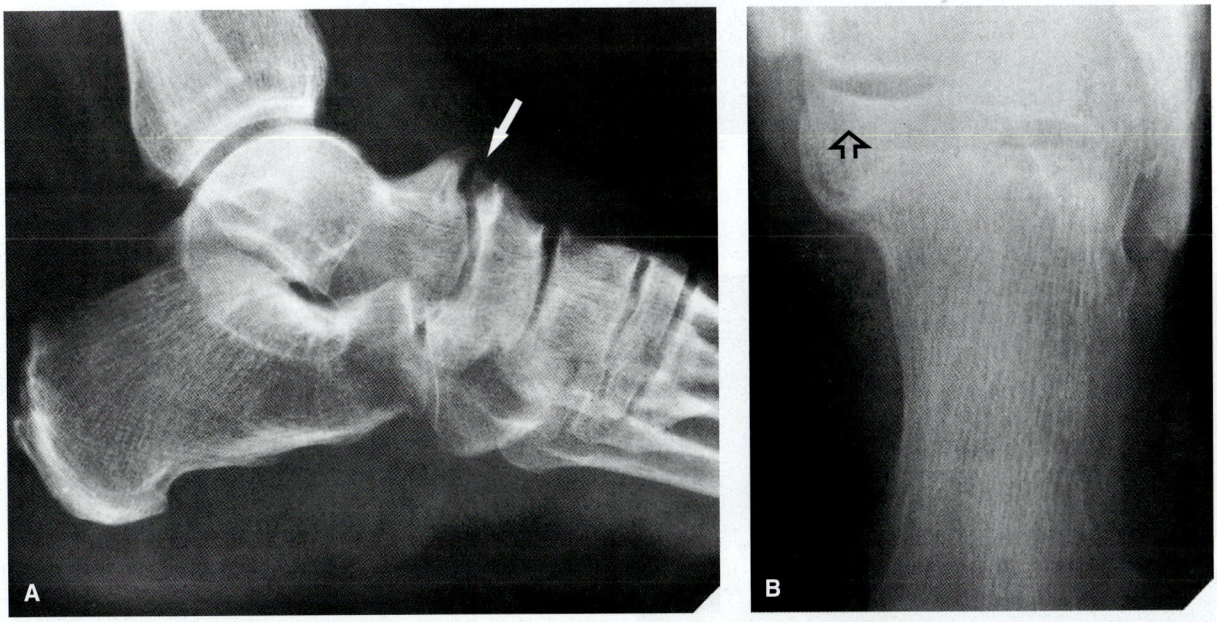

FIGURE 3.4 Talonavicular osteoarthritis. **A:** Lateral radiograph of the foot of a 61-year-old woman demonstrates a talar beak and degenerative changes in the talonavicular joint (*arrow*). The middle and posterior facets of the subtalar joint appear normal. **B:** A Harris–Beath view shows normal middle facet of subtalar joint (*open arrow*) and no evidence of tarsal coalition. (From Greenspan A. Anomalies of the upper and lower limbs. In: *Orthopedic Imaging: A Practical Approach.* 5th ed. Philadelphia, PA: Lippincott Williams & Wilkins; 2011:927.)

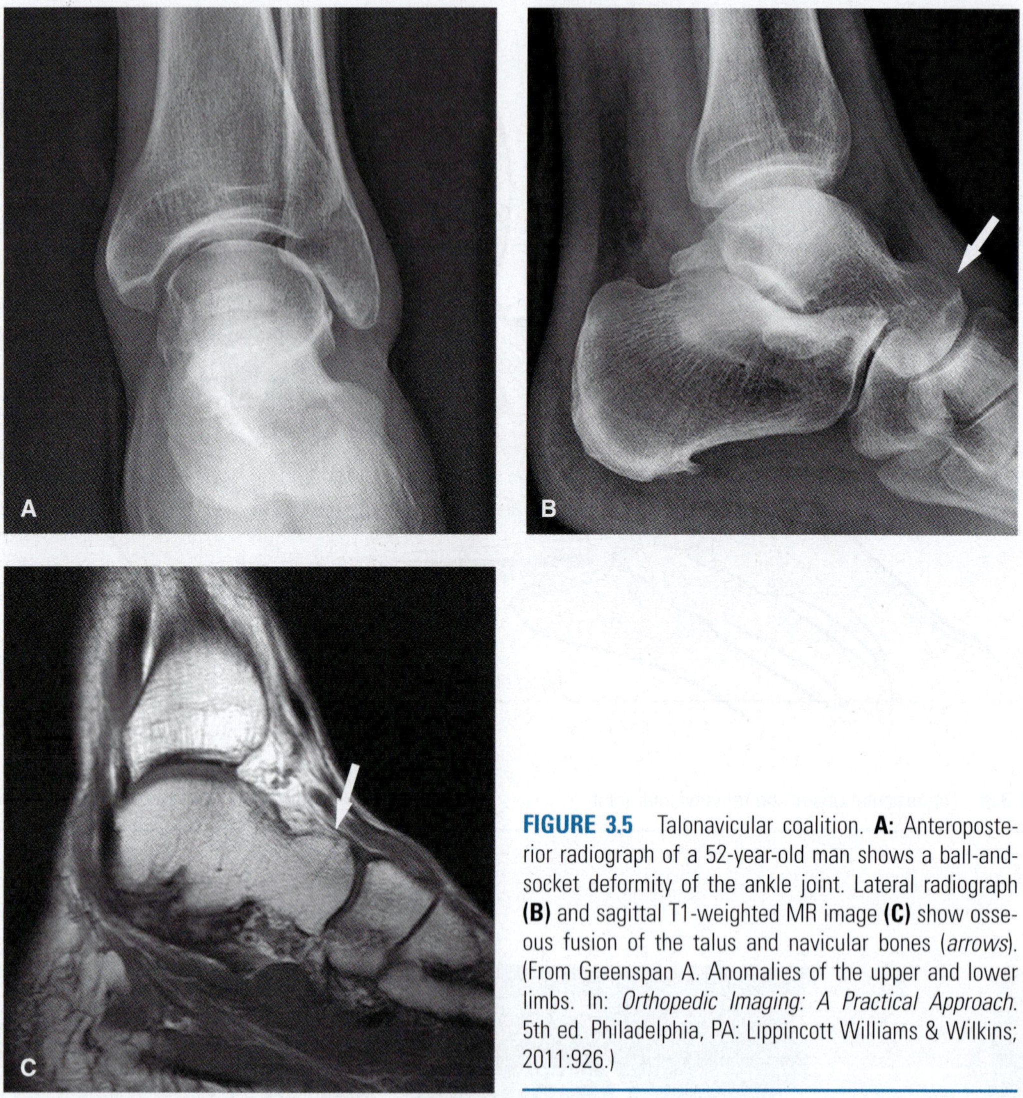

FIGURE 3.5 Talonavicular coalition. **A:** Anteroposterior radiograph of a 52-year-old man shows a ball-and-socket deformity of the ankle joint. Lateral radiograph **(B)** and sagittal T1-weighted MR image **(C)** show osseous fusion of the talus and navicular bones (*arrows*). (From Greenspan A. Anomalies of the upper and lower limbs. In: *Orthopedic Imaging: A Practical Approach.* 5th ed. Philadelphia, PA: Lippincott Williams & Wilkins; 2011:926.)

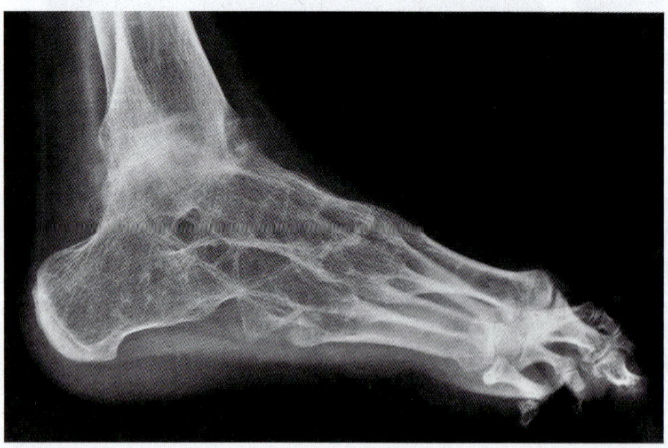

FIGURE 3.6 Radiograph of 25-year-old woman with polyarticular arthritis. (From Chew FS, Mulcahy H, Ha AS. Ankle and foot. In: *Musculoskeletal Imaging: A Teaching File.* 3rd ed. Philadelphia, PA: Lippincott Williams & Wilkins; 2012:509.)

indicated, including complete blood cell count, sedimentation rate, and antinuclear antibody testing. MRI, CT, or ultrasound of the talonavicular joint is indicated if avascular necrosis or meniscal tear is suspected or if the diagnosis is unclear (Fig. 3.7).

ULTRASOUND TECHNIQUE

To perform ultrasound evaluation of the talonavicular joint, the patient is then placed in the supine position with the affected lower extremity flexed at the knee so that the foot rests comfortably on the examination table. A high-frequency linear ultrasound transducer is placed in the longitudinal plane over the anteromedial aspect of the ankle which will position the transducer over the talonavicular joint (Fig. 3.8). An ultrasound survey scan is obtained which demonstrates the V-shaped anterior talonavicular

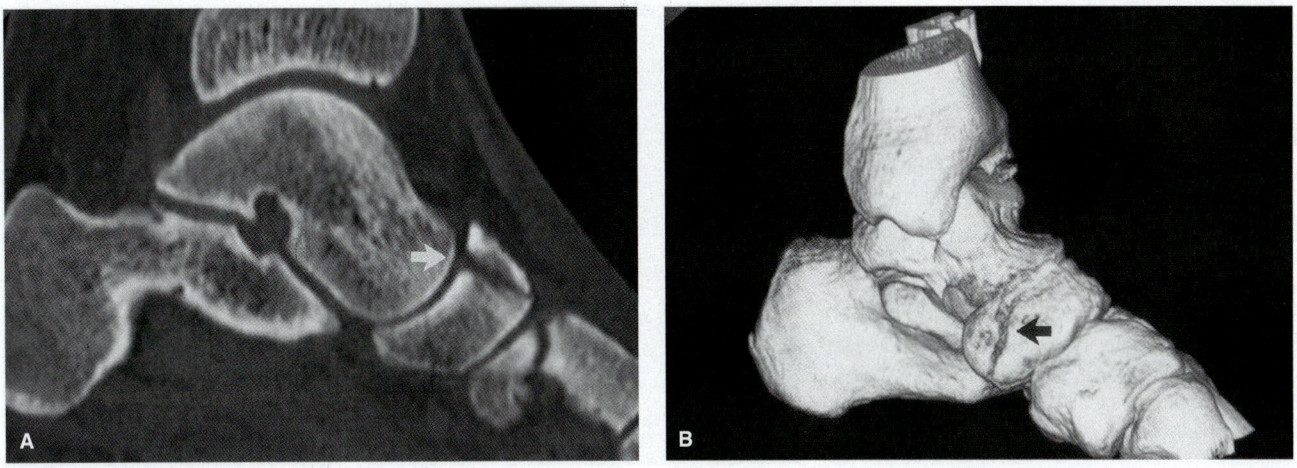

FIGURE 3.7 CT of the navicular fracture. Sagittal CT reformatted image **(A)** and 3D CT reconstruction **(B)** show a fracture of the navicular bone (*arrows*). (From Greenspan A. Lower limbs III: ankle and foot. In: *Orthopedic Imaging: A Practical Approach*. 5th ed. Philadelphia, PA: Lippincott Williams & Wilkins; 2011:356.)

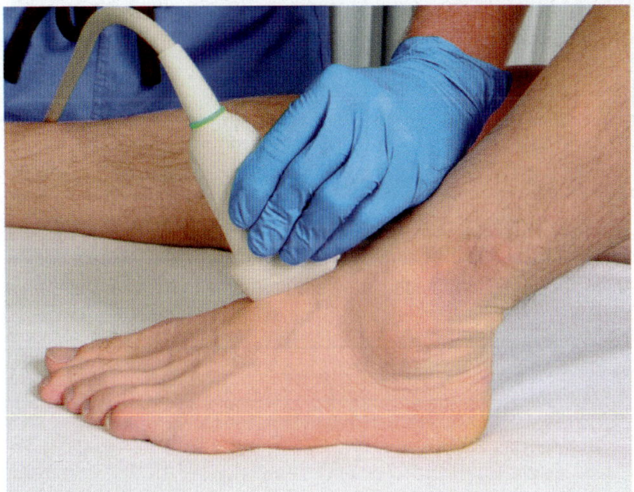

FIGURE 3.8 Correct longitudinal position for ultrasound transducer for ultrasound evaluation of the talonavicular joint.

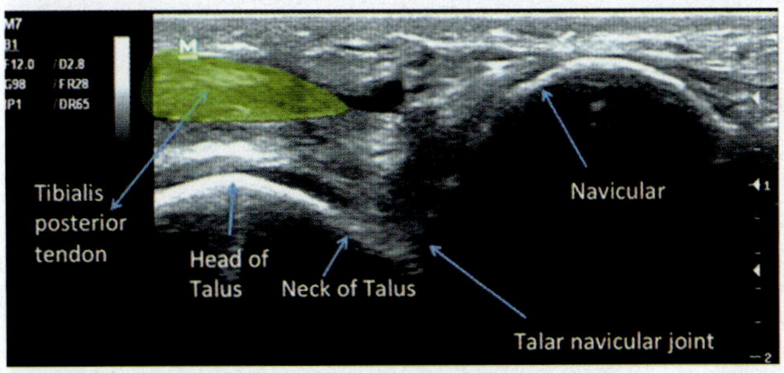

FIGURE 3.9 Longitudinal ultrasound image of the talonavicular joint demonstrating characteristic V shape of the joint.

joint (Fig. 3.9). After the joint space is identified, the joint is evaluated for the presence of arthritis, synovitis, effusion, crystal deposition, and abnormal masses including ganglion cysts (Figs. 3.10 to 3.16). Color Doppler is used to identify the overlying blood vessels (Fig. 3.17).

CLINICAL PEARLS

Bursitis, ligamentous strains and sprains, fractures, tendinopathy, osteoarthritis, synovitis, avascular necrosis, and impingement syndromes may coexist with talonavicular joint disease and may contribute to the patient's pain symptoms. The use of multiple imaging modalities may help clarify the diagnosis and identify occult pathology (Figs. 3.18 to 3.20).

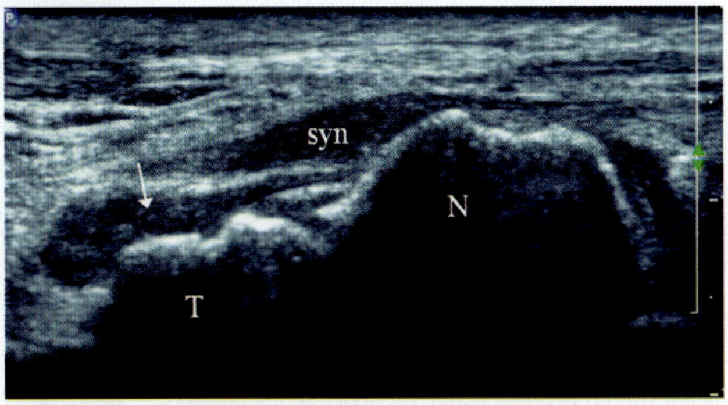

FIGURE 3.10 Psoriatic arthritis. Longitudinal ultrasound scan of dorsal aspect of talonavicular joint shows synovial hypertrophy (syn) and thickening of the proximal insertion of the dorsal talonavicular ligament due to enthesitis (*arrow*). T, talus; N, navicular. (From Lee R, Griffith J. Foot and ankle. In: Beggs I, ed. *Musculoskeletal Ultrasound*. Philadelphia, PA: Lippincott Williams & Wilkins; 2014:229.)

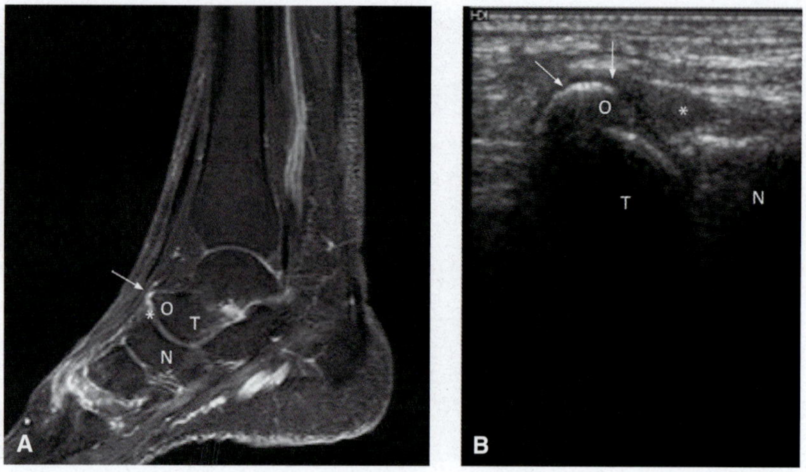

FIGURE 3.11 Sagittal T1-weighted fat saturated after intravenous gadolinium injection MRI **(A)** and ultrasound (anterior longitudinal paramidline plane; **(B)** showing synovitis of the talonavicular joint. Synovitis is highlighted by *arrows* on the MRI image and the *asterisk* on the ultrasound image. T, talus; N, navicular; O, osteophyte. (From Wakefield RJ, Freeston JE, O'Connor P, et al. The optimal assessment of the rheumatoid arthritis hindfoot: a comparative study of clinical examination, ultrasound and high field MRI. *Ann Rheum Dis* 2008;67(12):1678–1682.)

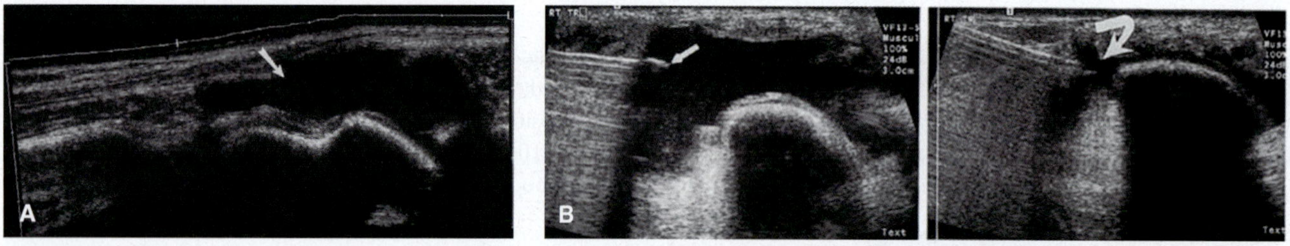

FIGURE 3.12 **A:** Longitudinal extended field-of-view image demonstrating a large multilobulated dorsal ganglion in the midfoot originating from the talonavicular joint capsule (*arrow*). **B:** Short-axis views demonstrating the needle tip within the ganglion cyst (*arrow* at left) and the appearance of the decompressed cyst after aspiration (*arrow* at right). (From Sofka CM, Adler RS. Ultrasound-guided interventions in the foot and ankle. *Semin Musculoskelet Radiol* 2002;6(2):163–168.)

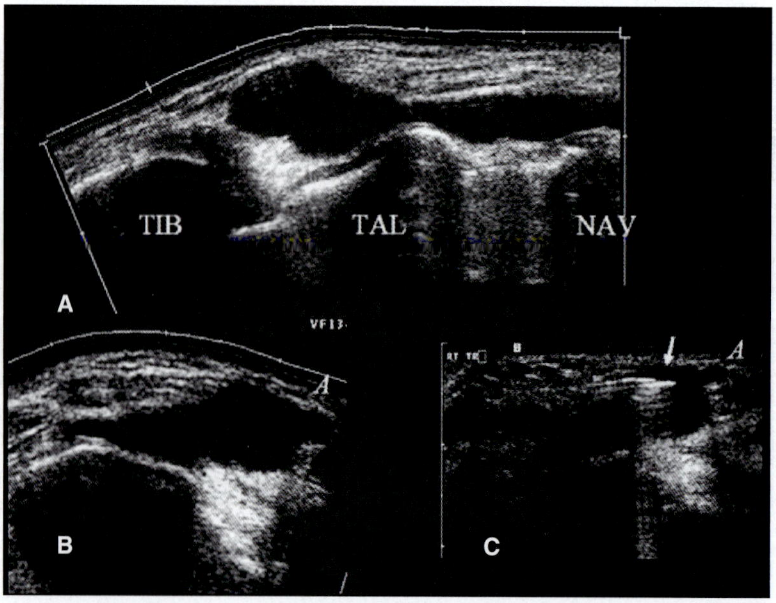

FIGURE 3.13 Three images of the dorsum of the midfoot demonstrating a large ganglion cyst arising from the talonavicular joint capsule. Longitudinal **(A)** and transverse **(B)** extended field-of-view images demonstrate the relationship of the cyst to the bones of the midfoot: tibia (TIB), talus (TAL), and navicular (NAV). **C:** Short-axis view demonstrating a needle (*arrow*) entering the cyst for therapeutic aspiration and injection. A, artery. (From Adler R, Sofka CM, Positano RG. *Atlas of Foot and Ankle Sonography*. Philadelphia, PA: Lippincott Williams & Wilkins; 2004:34.)

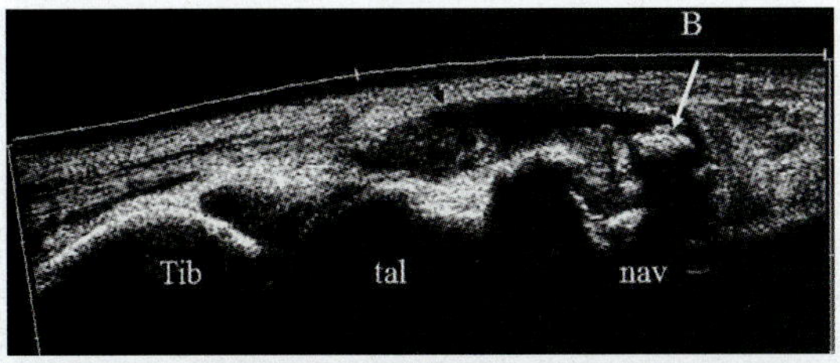

FIGURE 3.14 Longitudinal extended field-of-view image demonstrating a complex synovial cyst (*arrow*) arising from the arthritic talonavicular joint; talus (tal) and navicular (nav) are indicated. Dorsal osteophytosis is seen arising from the navicular as well as an osteochondral body (B) within the cyst. Distension of the tibiotalar joint by an effusion is evident. Tib, tibia. (From Adler R, Sofka CM, Positano RG. *Atlas of Foot and Ankle Sonography*. Philadelphia, PA: Lippincott Williams & Wilkins; 2004:34.)

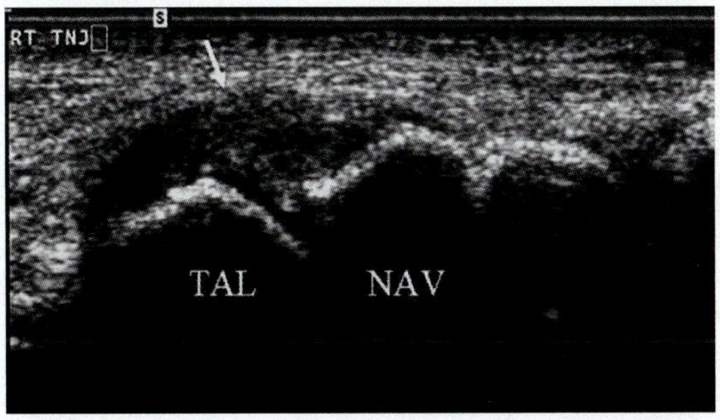

FIGURE 3.15 Longitudinal ultrasound image of the talonavicular joint demonstrating hypoechoic soft tissue arising from the joint space consistent with a distended joint capsule (*arrow*) in a patient with pyrophosphate arthropathy. TAL, talus; NAV, navicular. (From Adler R, Sofka CM, Positano RG. *Atlas of Foot and Ankle Sonography*. Philadelphia, PA: Lippincott Williams & Wilkins; 2004:39.)

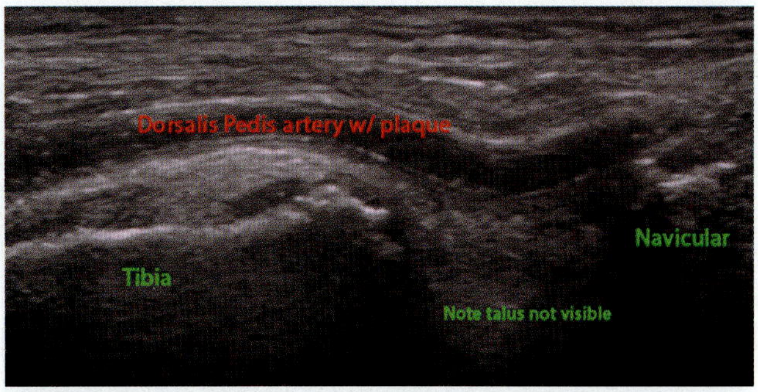

FIGURE 3.16 Longitudinal ultrasound image of the anterior ankle demonstrating avascular necrosis involving the talonavicular joint. Note the plaque in the dorsalis pedis artery.

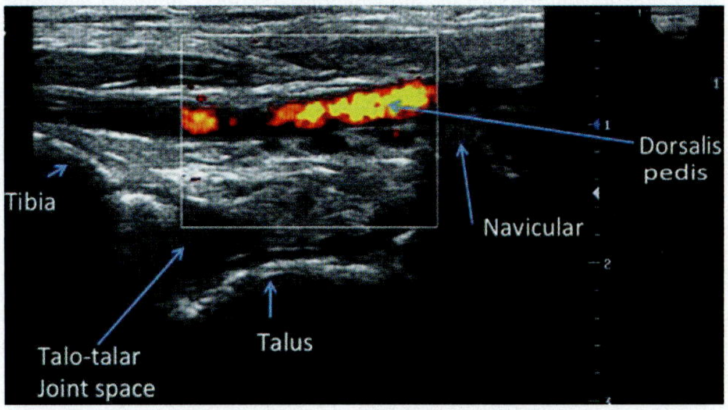

FIGURE 3.17 Longitudinal color Doppler image demonstrating the dorsalis pedis artery overlying the tibiotalar joint.

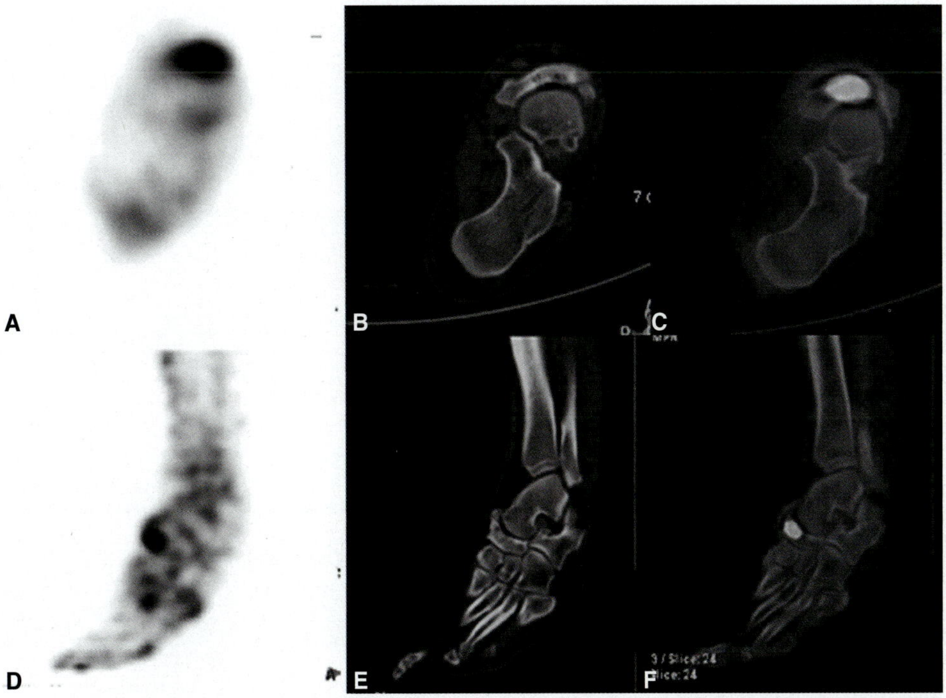

FIGURE 3.18 A 48-year-old man with dorsal foot pain. Axial **(A)** and sagittal **(D)** SPECT, axial **(B)** and sagittal **(E)** CT, and axial **(C)** and sagittal **(F)** fused SPECT/CT images depicting intense uptake in the navicular bone. There are extensive degenerative changes as manifested by joint space loss (with associated vacuum phenomenon), bone sclerosis, and subchondral cyst formation. In addition, there is an accessory navicular bone. SPECT/CT confirms that the underlying cause for the patient's symptoms is secondary osteoarthritis of the navicular bone rather than the accessory ossicle, as there is no uptake associated with the latter. (From Nathan M, Mohan H, Vijayanathan S, et al. The role of 99mTc-diphosphonate bone SPECT/CT in the ankle and foot. *Nucl Med Commun* 2012;33(8):799–807.)

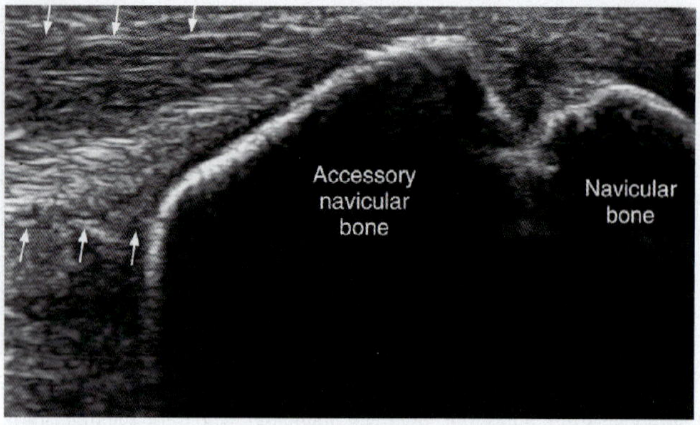

FIGURE 3.19 Longitudinal ultrasound medial aspect of the midfoot showing a quite large accessory navicular bone with attached posterior tibial tendon (*arrows*) fibers. The junction with the main navicular bone is also shown. (From Lee R, Griffith J. Foot and ankle. In: Beggs I, ed. *Musculoskeletal Ultrasound*. Philadelphia, PA: Lippincott Williams & Wilkins; 2014:162.)

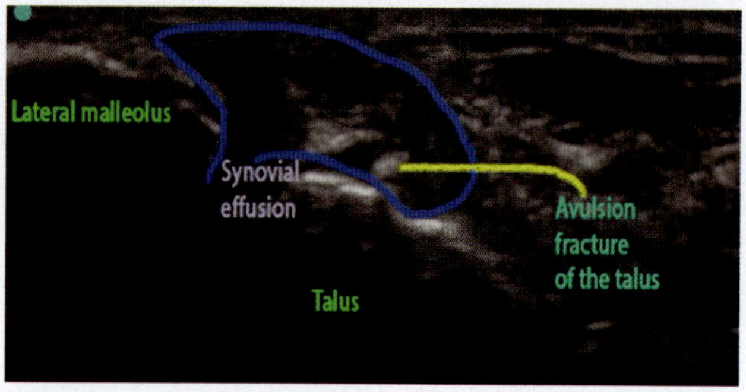

FIGURE 3.20 Longitudinal ultrasound image demonstrating an avulsion fracture of the talus in a patient who suffered a severe inversion injury to the anterior talofibular ligament.

Suggested Readings

De Zordo T, Romagnoli C. Ultrasound-guided procedures: soft tissue masses, joints, tendons, and muscles. *Ultrasound Clin* 2012;7(4):537–550.

Waldman SD. Functional anatomy of the ankle and foot. In: *Pain Review*. Philadelphia, PA: Saunders; 2009:155–156.

Waldman SD. Intra-articular injection of the subtalar joint. In: *Atlas of Pain Management Injection Techniques*. 3rd ed. Philadelphia, PA: Saunders; 2012:413–415.

Waldman SD, Campbell RSD. Anatomy: special imaging considerations of the ankle and foot. In: *Imaging of Pain*. Philadelphia, PA: Saunders; 2011:417–419.

Ward ST, Williams PL, Purkayastha S. Intra-articular corticosteroid injections in the foot and ankle: a prospective 1-year follow-up investigation. *J Foot Ankle Surg* 2008;47(2):138–144.

CHAPTER 4

Abnormalities of the Talofibular Ligament

ANATOMIC CONSIDERATIONS

The ankle is a hinge-type articulation between the distal tibia, the two malleoli, and the talus (Fig. 4.1). The articular surface is covered with hyaline cartilage, which is susceptible to arthritis. The joint is surrounded by a dense capsule that helps strengthen the ankle. The joint capsule is lined with a synovial membrane that attaches to the articular cartilage. The ankle joint is innervated by the deep peroneal and tibial nerves.

The major ligaments of the ankle joint include the talofibular, anterior talofibular, calcaneofibular, and posterior talofibular ligaments, which provide the majority of strength to the ankle joint (Fig. 4.2). The talofibular ligament is not as strong as the deltoid ligament and is susceptible to strain. The talofibular ligament runs from the anterior border of the lateral malleolus to the lateral surface of the talus (Fig. 4.3).

CLINICAL CORRELATES

One of the four major ligaments of the ankle joint, the anterior talofibular ligament runs from anterior border of the lateral malleolus to the lateral surface of the talus (Fig. 4.3). Also known as the medial ligament of talocrural joint, the anterior talofibular ligament is susceptible to strain at the joint line or avulsion at its origin or insertion. The anterior talofibular ligament is frequently injured from inversion injuries to the ankle that occur when tripping when wearing high heels, landing hard or running on hard uneven surfaces, and during dancing, soccer, and basketball (Fig. 4.4). The pain of anterior talofibular ligament damage is localized to the lateral ankle and is made worse with inversion of the ankle joint. Point tenderness just below the lateral malleolus is often present on physical examination. Significant swelling and ecchymosis are often evident

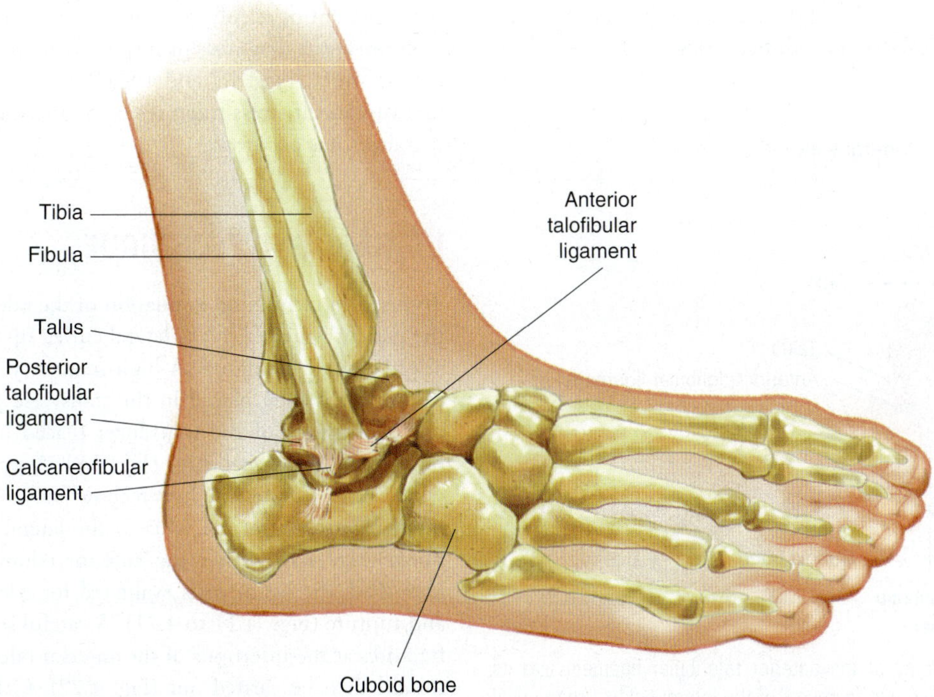

FIGURE 4.1 The articulations of the ankle joint.

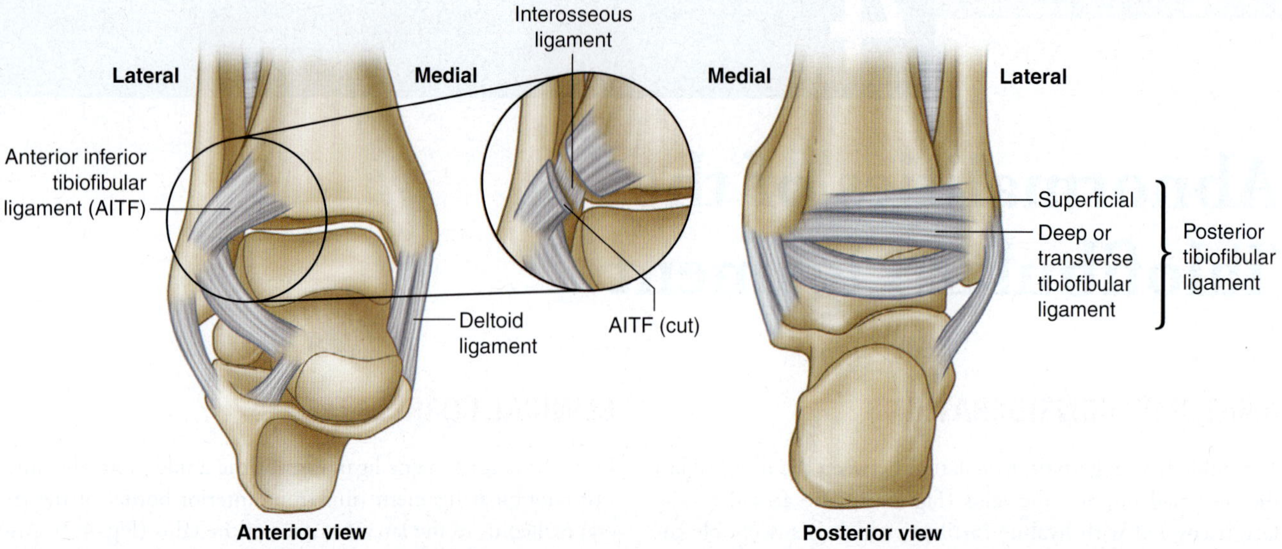

FIGURE 4.2 The major ligaments of the ankle joint include the talofibular, anterior talofibular, calcaneofibular, and posterior talofibular ligaments, which provide the majority of strength to the ankle joint. (From Patel A, Horton G. Anatomy of the foot and ankle. In: Altcheck DW, DiGiovanni CW, Dines JS, et al, eds. *Foot and Ankle Sports Medicine*. Philadelphia, PA: Lippincott Williams & Wilkins; 2013:2.)

after acute injury. Activity, especially involving weight bearing, plantar flexion, and inversion of the ankle will exacerbate the pain. Local heat and decreased activity as well as elevation of the affected ankle may provide a modicum of relief. Sleep disturbance is common in patients suffering from trauma to the anterior talofibular ligament of the ankle. Coexistent fracture, bursitis, tendinitis, arthritis, or internal derangement of the ankle may confuse the clinical picture after trauma to the knee joint making clinical diagnosis difficult (Fig. 4.5).

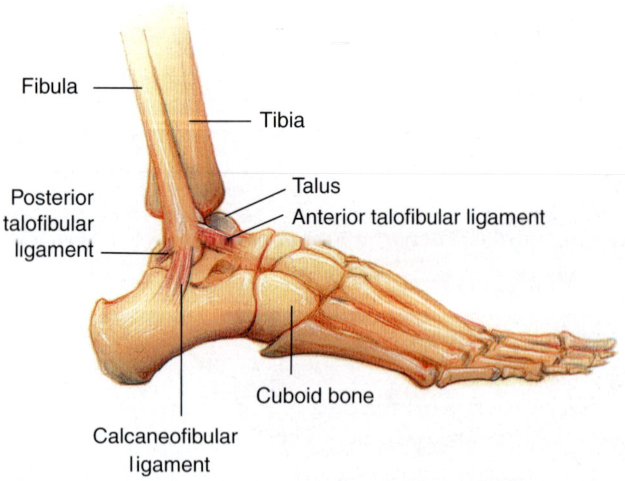

FIGURE 4.3 Anatomy of the anterior talofibular ligament and its relationship with the other ligaments of the lateral ankle. (Anatomical Chart Company, 2013.)

Plain radiographs and/or arthrography are indicated in all patients who present with anterior talofibular ligament pain, especially after ankle trauma (Fig. 4.6). Based on the patient's clinical presentation, additional testing may be indicated, including complete blood cell count, sedimentation rate, and antinuclear antibody testing. MRI or ultrasound imaging of the ankle is indicated if internal derangement or occult mass or tumor is suspected as well as to confirm the diagnosis of suspected anterior talofibular ligament injury (Figs. 4.7 and 4.8). Bone scan may be useful to identify occult stress fractures involving the joint, especially if trauma has occurred.

ULTRASOUND TECHNIQUE

To perform ultrasound evaluation of the talofibular ligament, the patient is placed in the lateral curled up position with the affected ankle facing up. A high-frequency linear ultrasound transducer is then placed in the transverse position with the posterior aspect of the transducer placed just over the bottom of the lateral malleolus (Fig. 4.9). A survey scan is taken which demonstrates the hyperechoic anterior talofibular ligament running from the talus to the lateral malleolus of the fibula (Fig. 4.10). After the anterior talofibular ligament is identified, the ligament is evaluated for edema, strain, tears, and rupture (Figs. 4.11 to 4.21). A careful search for avulsion fractures at the insertions of the anterior talofibular ligaments should then be carried out (Fig. 4.22). Color Doppler may aid in the assessment of the extent of acute ligament injury (Fig. 4.23).

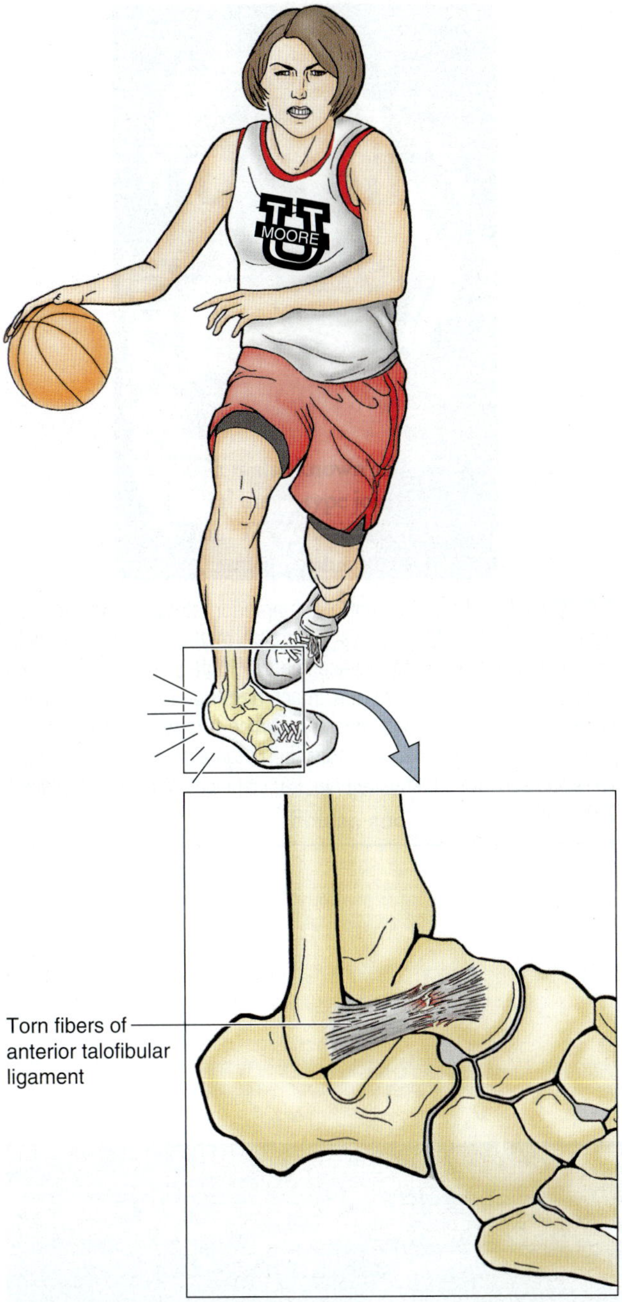

FIGURE 4.4 The anterior talofibular ligament is frequently injured by inversion injuries that occur when tripping when wearing high heels, landing hard on uneven surfaces, and during dancing, soccer, and basketball.

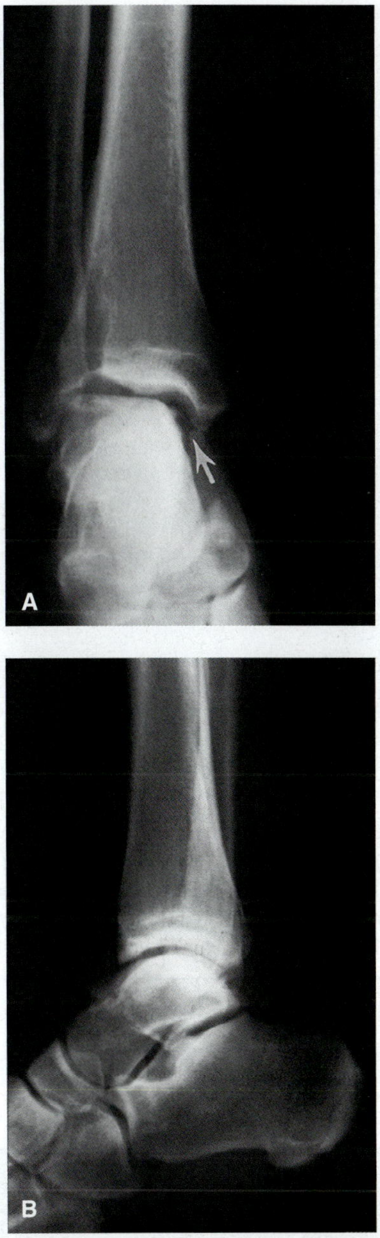

FIGURE 4.5 Anteroposterior **(A)** and lateral **(B)** radiographic views of the ankle in a patient with chronic instability after ankle sprain. There is degenerative arthritis with talar shift, widening of the medial ankle mortise (*arrow*), and intra-articular fragments. (From Berquist TH. Soft tissue trauma and overuse syndromes. In: *Imaging of the Foot and Ankle.* 3rd ed. Philadelphia, PA: Lippincott Williams & Wilkins; 2011:125.)

CLINICAL PEARLS

Bursitis, fractures, tendinopathy, osteoarthritis, synovitis, avascular necrosis, and impingement syndromes may coexist with anterior talofibular ligament pathology and may contribute to the patient's pain symptoms. Ultrasound imaging can also be used to assess the healing of previous damaged ligaments as well as to evaluate the integrity of previous surgical repairs (Figs. 4.24 and 4.25).

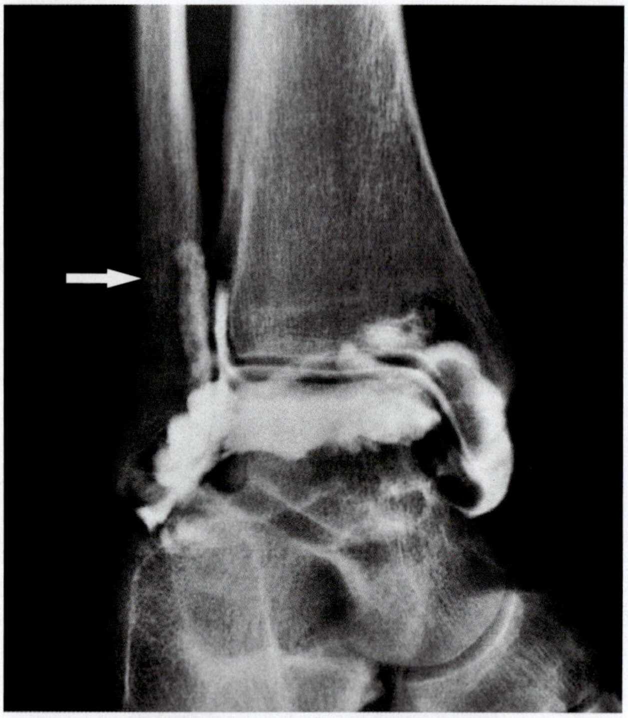

FIGURE 4.6 Tear of the distal anterior tibiofibular ligament. A 29-year-old man injured his ankle during a basketball game. Conventional radiograph and stress examination revealed no abnormalities. On arthrography, however, leak of contrast into the region of the tibiofibular syndesmosis (*arrow*) indicates a tear of the distal anterior tibiofibular ligament. (From Greenspan A. Lower limbs III: ankle and foot. In: *Orthopedic Imaging: A Practical Approach*. 5th ed. Philadelphia, PA: Lippincott Williams & Wilkins; 2011:346.)

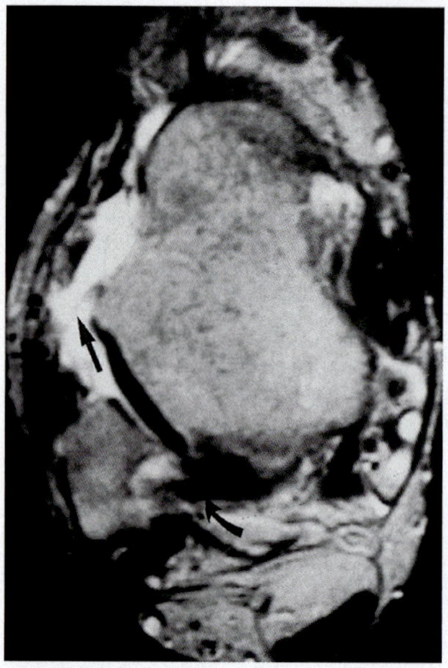

FIGURE 4.7 MRI of the tear of the anterior talofibular ligament. An axial T2-weighted MRI shows disruption of the anterior talofibular ligament resulting in its replacement by high–signal-intensity fluid (*straight arrow*). Note that the intact posterior talofibular ligament shows normal low signal intensity (*curved arrow*). (From Greenspan A. Lower limbs III: ankle and foot. In: *Orthopedic Imaging: A Practical Approach*. 5th ed. Philadelphia, PA: Lippincott Williams & Wilkins; 2011:346.)

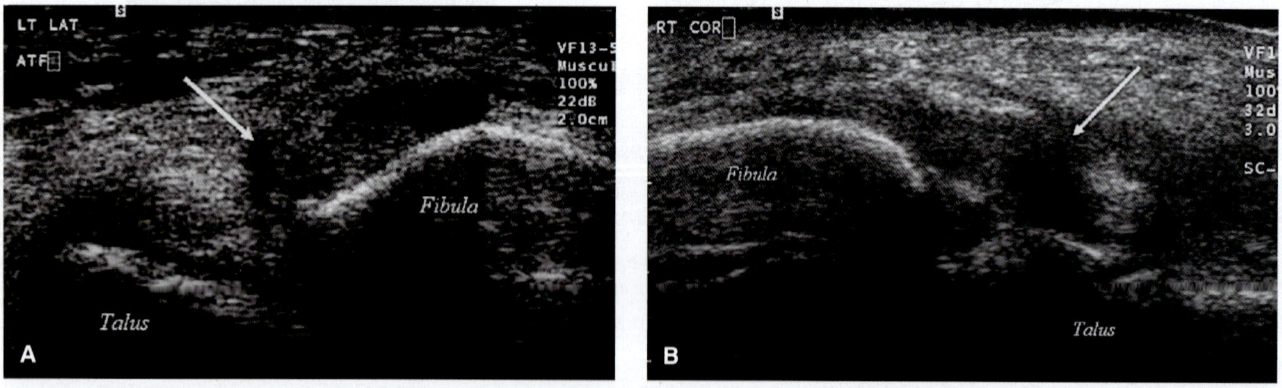

FIGURE 4.8 **A:** Ultrasound image along the lateral aspect of the ankle demonstrates a focal tear of anterior talofibular ligament (*arrow*). Note the discontinuity of the ligament apparent as a discrete hypoechoic defect (*arrow*). **B:** Full-thickness tear (*arrow*) of the ATF in another patient. (From Adler R, Sofka CM, Positano RG. *Atlas of Foot and Ankle Sonography*. Philadelphia, PA: Lippincott Williams & Wilkins; 2004:69.)

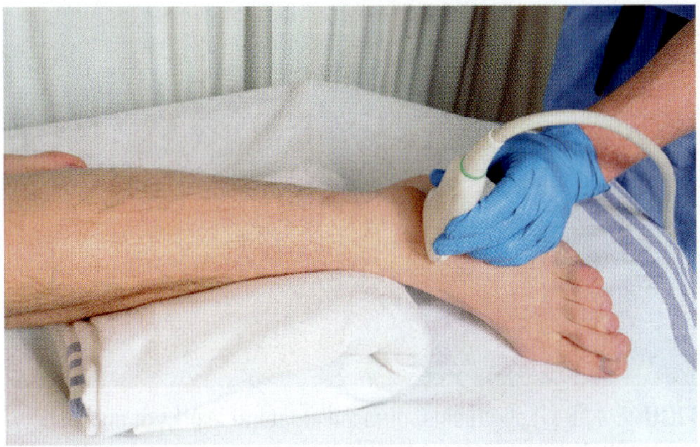

FIGURE 4.9 Correct transverse position for the ultrasound transducer for ultrasound evaluation of the anterior talofibular ligament. Note the posterior aspect of the ultrasound transducer is lying over the bottom of the lateral malleolus.

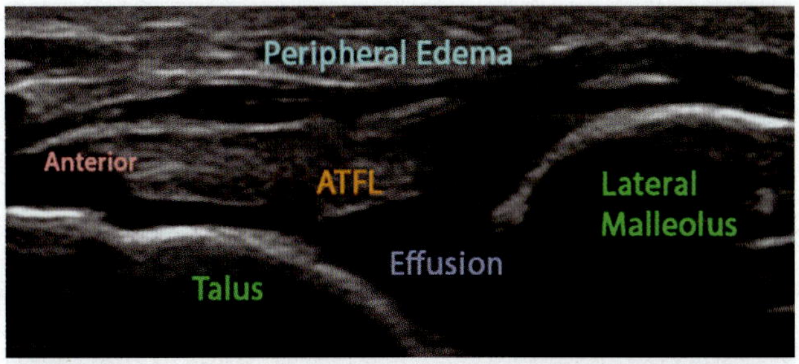

FIGURE 4.12 Ultrasound image of the anterior talofibular ligament (ATFL) in a patient with an acute ankle sprain. Note the peripheral edema and the effusion beneath the ligament.

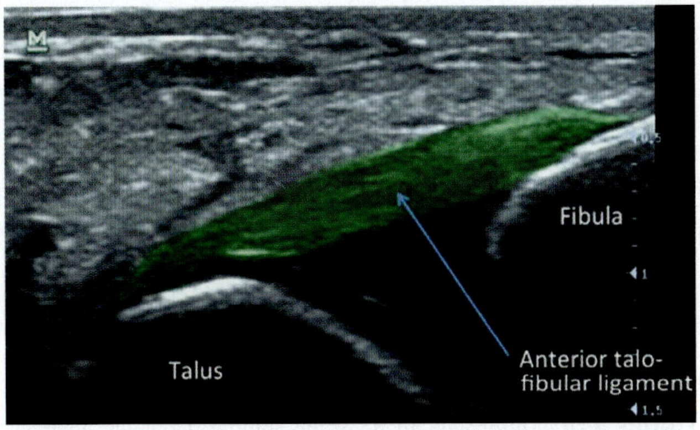

FIGURE 4.10 Transverse ultrasound image demonstrating the anterior talofibular ligament. Anterior is to the left and posterior to the right.

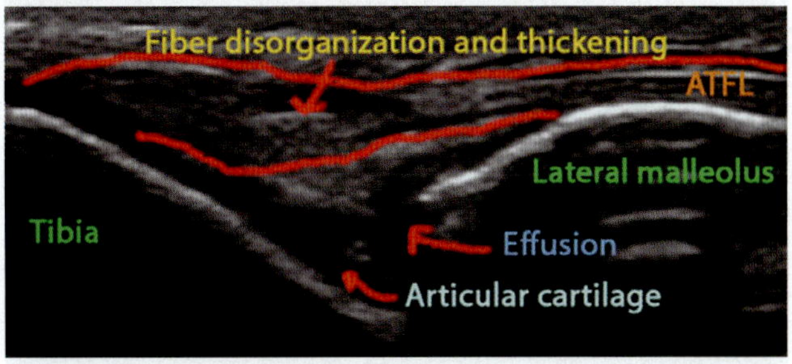

FIGURE 4.13 Sprained anterior talofibular ligament (ATFL) in a 16-year-old male basketball player. The sprained ligament (*arrowheads*) is thickened and heterogeneous.

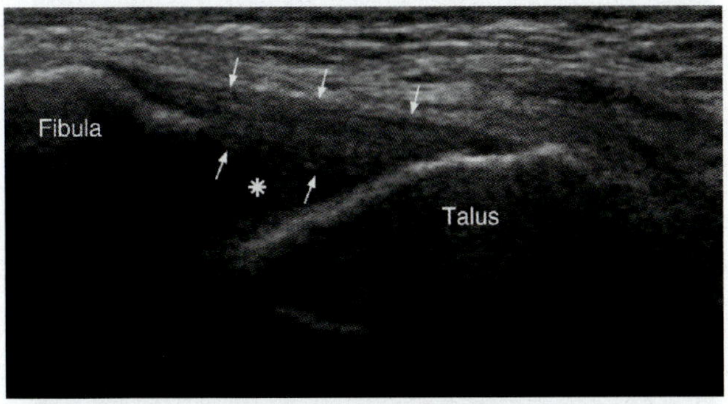

FIGURE 4.11 Transverse ultrasound showing normal anterior talofibular ligament (*arrows*). There is a small amount of fluid in the anterolateral ankle recess (*asterisk*). (From Lee R, Griffith J. Foot and ankle. In: Beggs I, ed. *Musculoskeletal Ultrasound*. Philadelphia, PA: Lippincott Williams & Wilkins; 2014:152.)

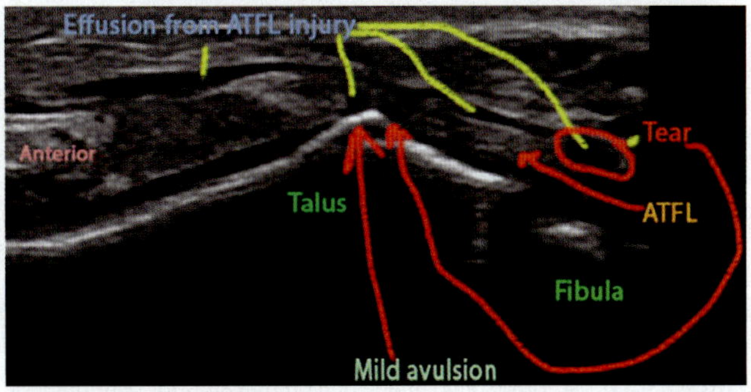

FIGURE 4.14 Transverse ultrasound image of the anterior talofibular ligament (ATFL) demonstrating a small avulsion fracture, ligamentous tearing, and effusion from the acute ankle trauma.

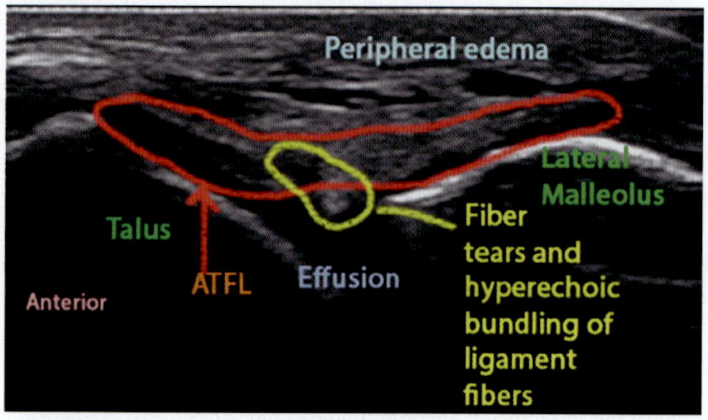

FIGURE 4.15 Ultrasound image of an acutely strained anterior talofibular ligament in a patient who twisted his ankle when stepping off a curb. Note the peripheral edema associated with the acute injury as well as an effusion and tearing and hyperechoic bundling of the ligament.

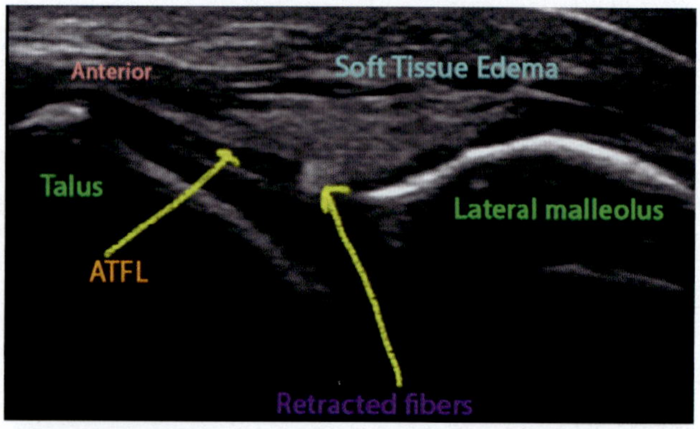

FIGURE 4.16 Ultrasound image of a high-grade tear of the anterior talofibular ligament (ATFL) in a patient with an acute ankle injury. Note the retracted ligament fibers and peripheral edema.

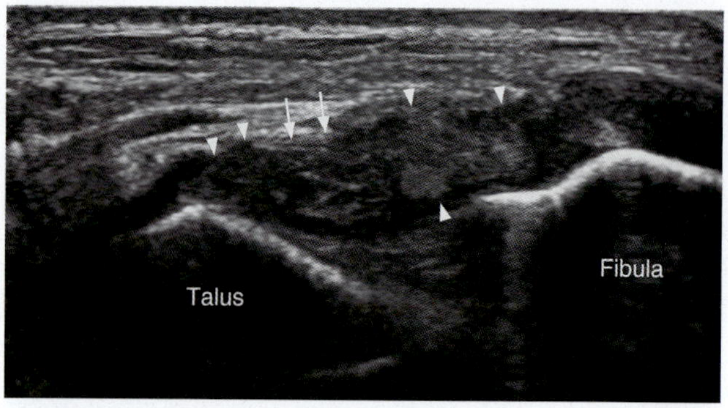

FIGURE 4.18 Longitudinal ultrasound lateral aspect of ankle showing complete tear of anterior talofibular ligament. The ligament (*arrowheads*) is very swollen with a complete tear (*arrows*) close to the talar attachment. (From Lee R, Griffith J. Foot and ankle. In: Beggs I, ed. *Musculoskeletal Ultrasound.* Philadelphia, PA: Lippincott Williams & Wilkins; 2014:167.)

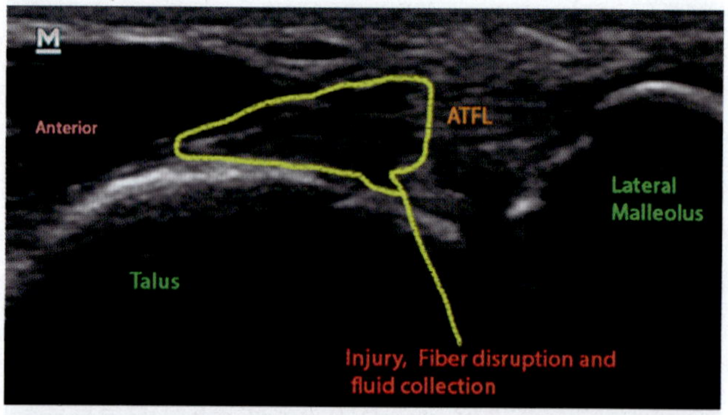

FIGURE 4.19 Ultrasound image of the anterior talofibular ligament in a patient with an acute ankle inversion injury. Note the significant disruption of the ligament fibers and associated edema.

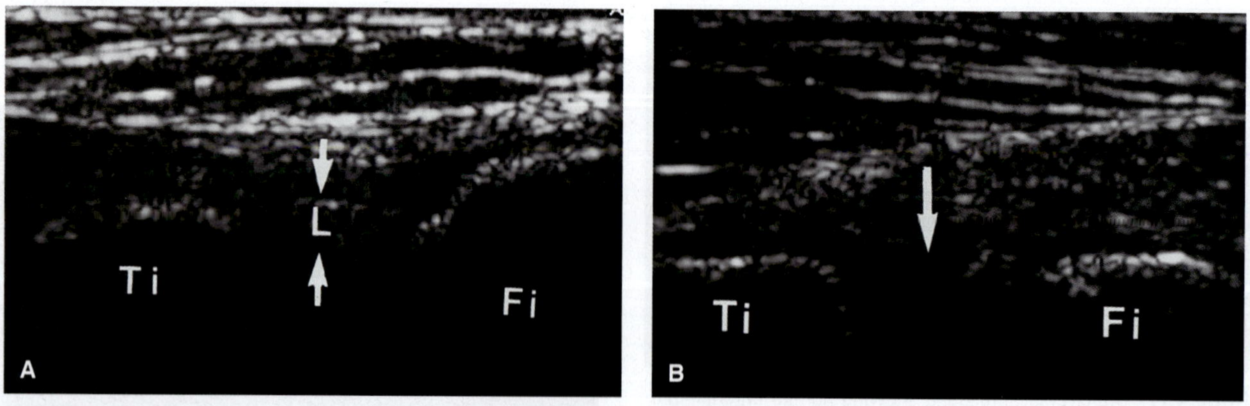

FIGURE 4.17 **A:** Ultrasound image of a normal anterior talofibular ligament. The talus and fibula are labeled. The L indicates the anterior talofibular ligament, which is hyperechoic, and the thickness is labeled. **B:** Ultrasound image of a complete tear of the anterior talofibular ligament. The *arrow* points to the ligament tear, which shows no hyperechoic area. Fi, fibula; Ti, talus. (From Farley FA, Kuhns L, Jacobson JA, et al. Ultrasound examination of ankle injuries in children. *J Pediatr Orthop* 2001;21(5):604–607; Fig. 1AB.)

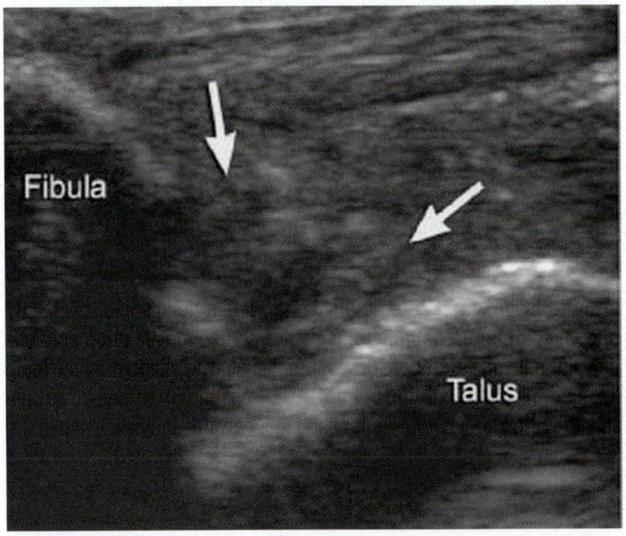

FIGURE 4.20 Full-thickness anterior talofibular ligament tear. Sonogram longitudinal to the anterior talofibular ligament shows abnormal heterogeneous hypoechogenicity in the expected location of the anterior talofibular ligament (*arrows*). No normal fibrillar ligament fibers were identified. (From Jacobson JA. Musculoskeletal ultrasound and MRI: which do I choose? *Semin Musculoskelet Radiol* 2005;9(2):135–149.)

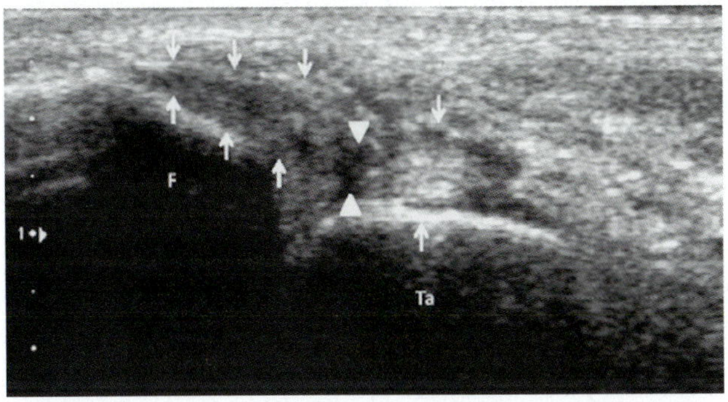

FIGURE 4.21 Rupture of anterior talofibular ligament. Longitudinal 12 MHz US image reveals hypoechoic discontinuity (*triangles*) of the anterior talofibular ligament (*arrows*). F, fibula; Ta, talus. (From Bong DA, Palau-Gonzalez J, Saenz I. Ligaments of the wrist, ankle and foot: sonoanatomy and sonopathology. *Curr Rheum Rev* 2011;7(3):212–230.)

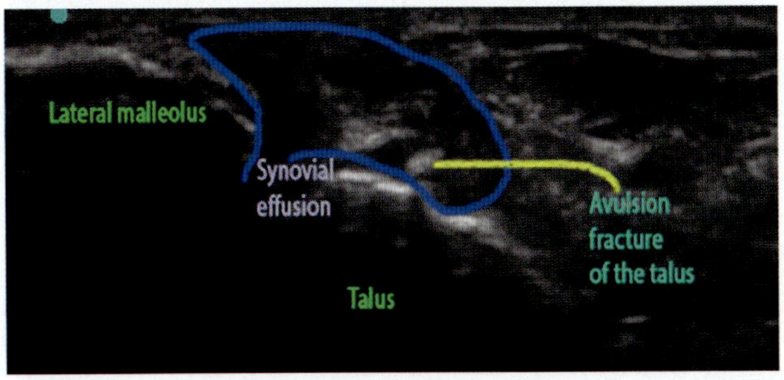

FIGURE 4.22 Longitudinal ultrasound image demonstrating an avulsion fracture of the talus in a patient who suffered a severe inversion injury to the anterior talofibular ligament.

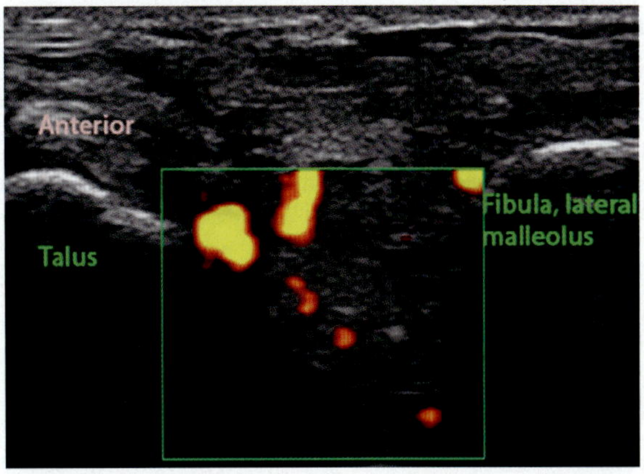

FIGURE 4.23 Color Doppler image of an acute sprain of the anterior talofibular ligament. Note the significant neovascularity.

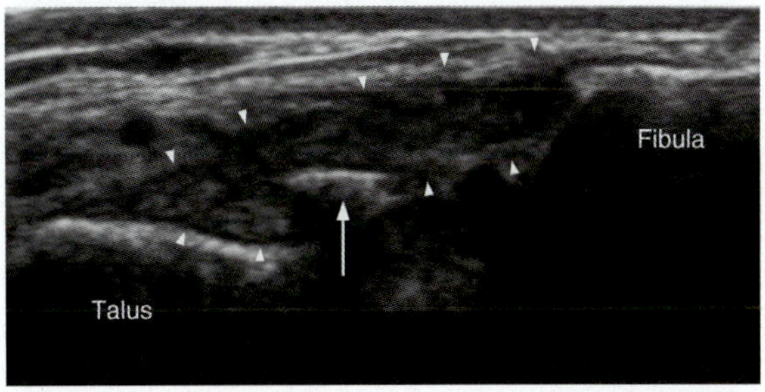

FIGURE 4.24 Longitudinal ultrasound anterolateral aspect of ankle. There is a healing tear of the ATFL with moderate ligament thickening (*arrowheads*) and a small avulsion fracture (*arrow*) most likely from the fibular tip. Overall, ligament continuity is maintained. (From Lee R, Griffith J. Foot and ankle. In: Beggs I, ed. *Musculoskeletal Ultrasound*. Philadelphia, PA: Lippincott Williams & Wilkins; 2014:167.)

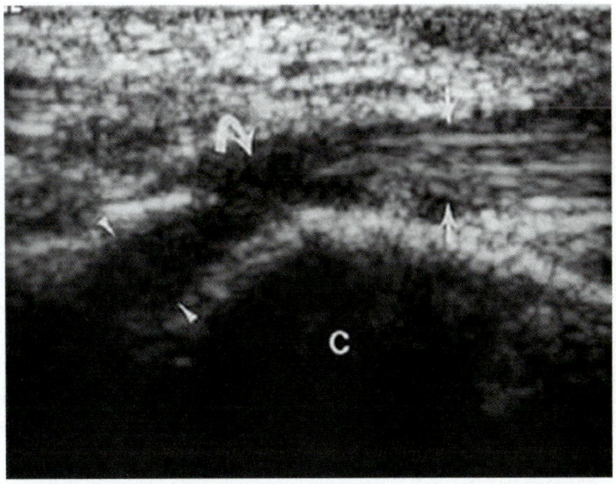

FIGURE 4.25 Anterior talofibular ligament reconstruction using peroneus brevis tendon (Chrisman–Snook procedure). A portion of the peroneus brevis tendon (one-half of the diameter) (*arrows*) is redirected through fibular and calcaneal (C) tunnels and attached at the talus to stabilize the ankle. Note anisotropy (*curved arrow*) of the peroneus brevis tendon at the calcaneal tunnel (*arrowheads*). (From Jacobson JA, Lax MJ. Musculoskeletal sonography of the postoperative orthopedic patient. *Semin Musculoskelet Radiol* 2002;6(1):67–77.)

Suggested Readings

Bonnel F, Toullec E, Mabit C, et al. Chronic ankle instability: biomechanics and pathomechanics of ligaments injury and associated lesions. *Orthop Traumatol Surg Res* 2010;96(4):424–432.

Haller J, Bernt R, Seeger T, et al. MR-imaging of anterior tibiotalar impingement syndrome: agreement, sensitivity and specificity of MR-imaging and indirect MR-arthrography. *Eur J Radiol* 2006;58(3):450–460.

Waldman SD. Anterior talofibular ligament. In: *Pain Review.* Philadelphia, PA: Saunders; 2009:158.

Waldman SD. Functional anatomy of the ankle and foot. In: *Pain Review.* Philadelphia, PA: Saunders; 2009:155–156.

Waldman SD. Intra-articular injection of the anterior talofibular joint. In: *Atlas of Pain Management Injection Techniques.* 3rd ed. Philadelphia, PA: Saunders; 2012:427–430.

Waldman SD, Campbell RSD. Anterior talofibular ligament tear. In: *Imaging of Pain.* Philadelphia, PA: Saunders; 2011:437–438.

CHAPTER 5

Abnormalities of the Deltoid Ligament

ANATOMIC CONSIDERATIONS

The ankle is a hinge-type articulation between the distal tibia, the two malleoli, and the talus (Fig. 5.1). The articular surface is covered with hyaline cartilage, which is susceptible to arthritis. The joint is surrounded by a dense capsule that helps strengthen the ankle. The joint capsule is lined with a synovial membrane that attaches to the articular cartilage. The ankle joint is innervated by the deep peroneal and tibial nerves.

The major ligaments of the ankle joint include the deltoid, anterior talofibular, calcaneofibular, and posterior talofibular ligaments, which provide the majority of strength to the ankle joint (Fig. 5.2). The deltoid ligament is exceptionally strong and is not so subject to strain as the anterior talofibular ligament. The triangular-shaped deltoid ligament is made up of a number of smaller separate ligaments including the anterior tibiotalar ligament, tibiocalcaneal ligament, posterior tibiotalar ligament, and tibionavicular ligament (Fig. 5.3). These ligaments are arranged in two layers. Both layers attach above to the medial malleolus. A deep layer attaches below to the medial body of the talus, with the superficial fibers attaching to the medial talus, the sustentaculum tali of the calcaneus, and the navicular tuberosity (Fig. 5.4).

CLINICAL CORRELATES

One of the four major ligaments of the ankle joint, the deltoid ligament is a strong, triangular-shaped, bilaminar ligament that runs from the medial malleolus, with the deep layer of the ligament attaching below to the medial body of the talus, and the superficial layer of the ligament attaching to the medial talus, the sustentaculum tali of the calcaneus, and the navicular tuberosity (Fig. 5.3). Also known as the medial ligament of talocrural joint, the deltoid ligament is susceptible to strain at the joint line or avulsion at its origin or insertion. The deltoid ligament is frequently injured from eversion injuries to the ankle that occur when tripping when wearing high heels, landing hard on uneven surfaces, and during dancing, soccer, and American football (Fig. 5.4). The pain of deltoid ligament damage is localized to the medial ankle and is made worse with plantar flexion and eversion of the ankle joint. Significant swelling and ecchymosis

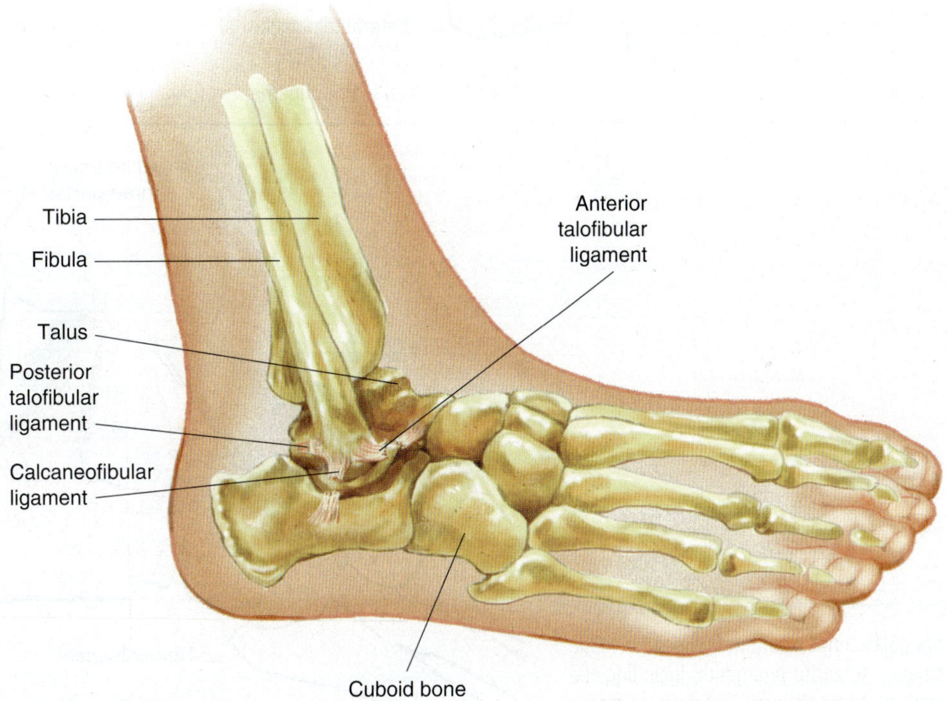

FIGURE 5.1 The articulations of the ankle joint.

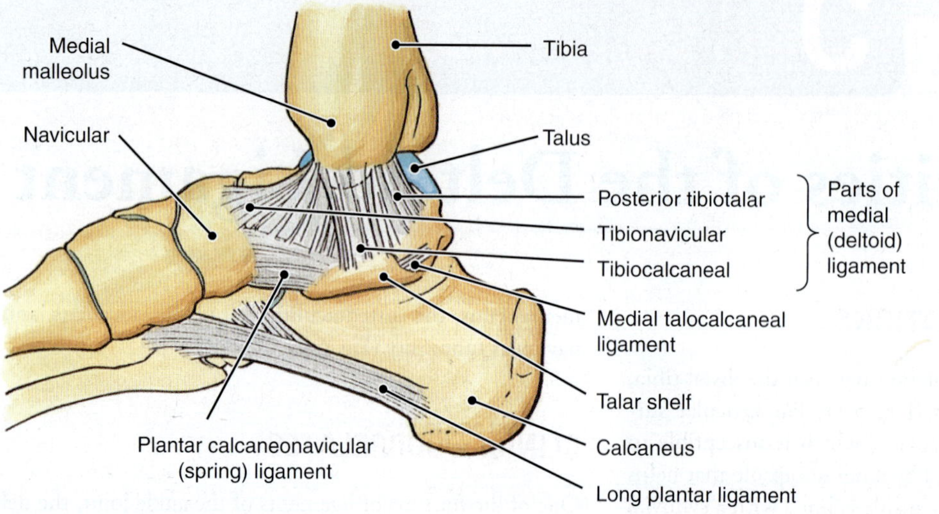

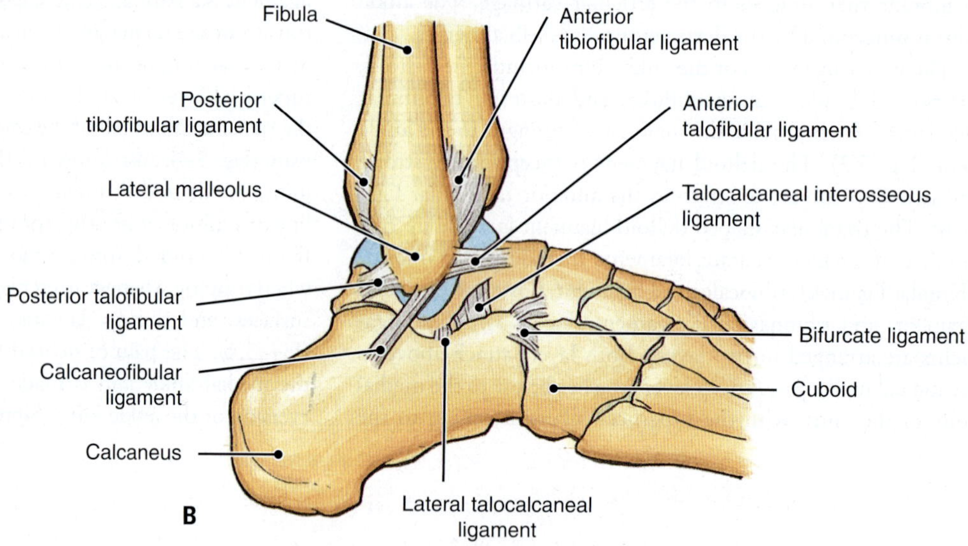

FIGURE 5.2 **A,B:** The anatomy of the deltoid ligament and its relationship with the other ligaments of the medial ankle.

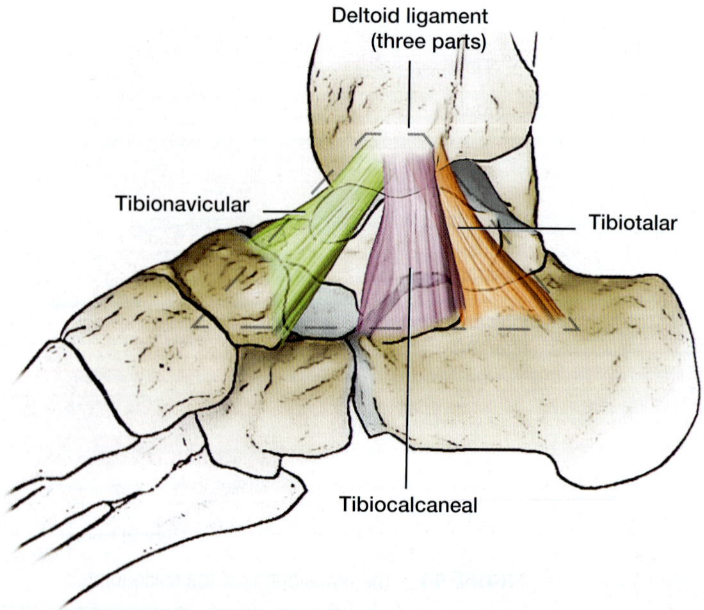

FIGURE 5.3 The triangular-shaped deltoid ligament is made up of a number of smaller separate ligaments, including the anterior tibiotalar ligament, tibiocalcaneal ligament, posterior tibiotalar ligament, and tibionavicular ligament.

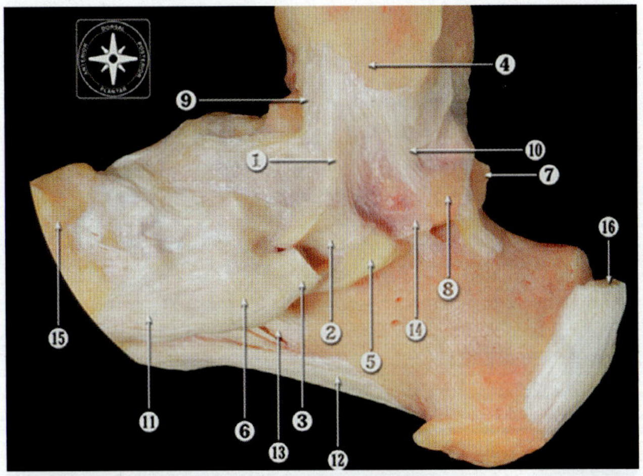

FIGURE 5.4 Medial view of one osteoarticular dissection showing the components of the superficial layer of the deltoid ligament, especially the tibiospring ligament (major component). (1) Tibiospring ligament. (2) Spring ligament (superomedial calcaneonavicular ligament). (3) Posterior tibial tendon (cut). (4) Medial malleolus. (5) Sustentaculum tali. (6) Navicular tuberosity. (7) Lateral process of the talus. (8) Medial process of the talus. (9) Tibionavicular ligament (major component). (10) Superficial tibiotalar ligament or superficial posterior tibiotalar ligament (additional band). (11) Medial cuneonavicular ligament. (12) Long plantar ligament. (13) Plantar calcaneocuboid ligament. (14) Medial talocalcaneal ligament. (15) Medial cuneiform. (16) Calcaneal or Achilles tendon (cut). (From Hintermann B, Golano P. The anatomy and function of the deltoid ligament. *Techn Foot Ankle Surg* 2014;13(2):67–72.)

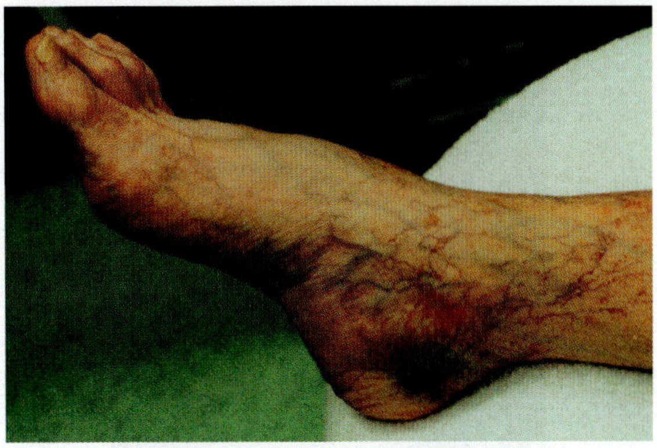

FIGURE 5.6 Swelling and ecchymosis are frequently identified on physical examination following deltoid ligament injury. (From Berg D, Worzala K. *Atlas of Adult Physical Diagnosis*. Philadelphia, PA: Lippincott Williams & Wilkins; 2006.)

are often evident after acute injury (Fig. 5.5). Activity, especially involving weight bearing, plantar flexion, and eversion of the ankle will exacerbate the pain. Local heat and decreased activity as well as elevation of the affected ankle may provide a modicum of relief. Sleep disturbance is common in patients suffering from trauma to the deltoid ligament of the ankle. Coexistent fracture, bursitis, tendinitis, arthritis, or internal derangement of the ankle may confuse the clinical picture after trauma to the knee joint making clinical diagnosis difficult.

Plain radiographs are indicated in all patients who present with deltoid ligament pain, especially after ankle trauma (Fig. 5.6). An external stress rotation mortise view will aid in identification of disruption of the deltoid ligament (Fig. 5.7). Based on the patient's clinical presentation, additional testing may be indicated, including complete blood cell count, sedimentation rate, and antinuclear antibody testing. Magnetic resonance imaging, computerized tomography, and/or ultrasound imaging of the ankle are indicated if internal derangement or occult mass or tumor is suspected as well as to confirm the diagnosis of suspected deltoid ligament injury (Figs. 5.8 to 5.10).

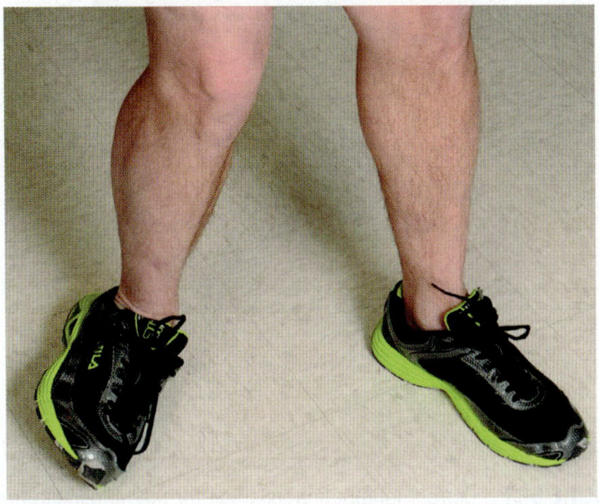

FIGURE 5.5 The deltoid ligament is frequently injured by eversion injuries that occur when tripping when wearing high heels, landing hard on uneven surfaces, and during dancing, soccer, and American football.

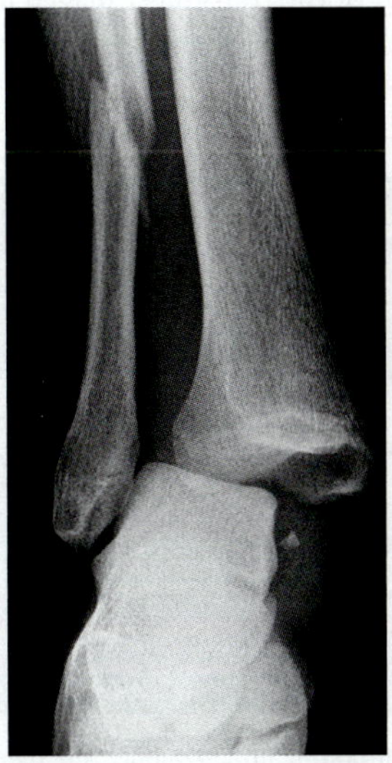

FIGURE 5.7 Radiograph demonstrating a fracture dislocation of the ankle with complete disruption of the deltoid ligament. (From Mulholland MW, Maier RV, Lillemoe KD, et al. *Greenfield's Surgery: Scientific Principles and Practice*. 4th ed. Philadelphia, PA: Lippincott Williams & Wilkins; 2006.)

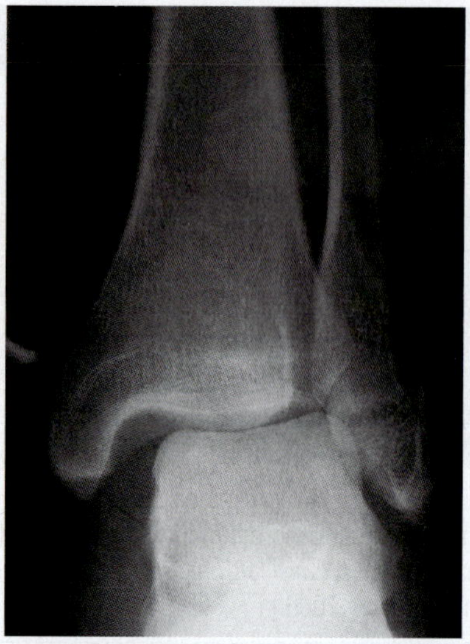

FIGURE 5.8 A positive external rotation stress mortise radiograph. (From DeAngelis NA, Eskander MS, French BG. Does medial tenderness predict deep deltoid ligament incompetence in supination-external rotation type ankle fractures? *J Orthop Trauma* 2007;21(4):244–247.)

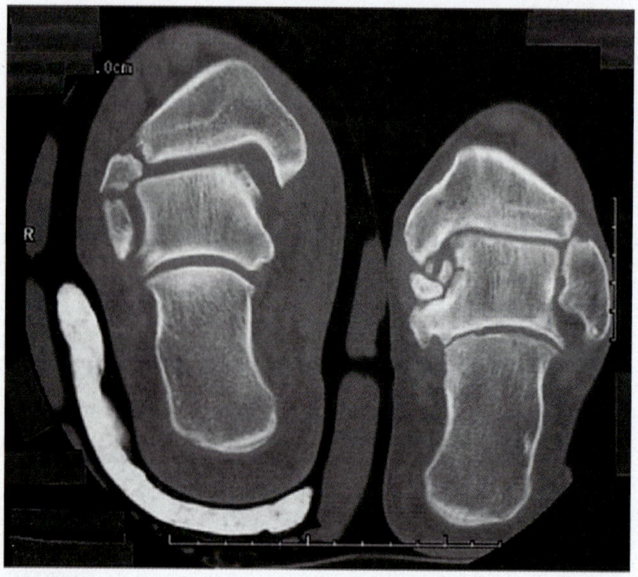

FIGURE 5.10 Coronal CT view of both ankles showing widening of the medial clear space of the right ankle in comparison with the left ankle, which indicates a deltoid ligament disruption. There was an old injury of the talus on the left side. (From DeAngelis NA, Eskander MS, French BG. Does medial tenderness predict deep deltoid ligament incompetence in supination-external rotation type ankle fractures? *J Orthop Trauma* 2007;21(4):244–247.)

Bone scan may be useful to identify occult stress fractures involving the joint, especially if trauma has occurred.

ULTRASOUND TECHNIQUE

To perform ultrasound evaluation of the deltoid ligament, patient is then placed in the supine position with the lower extremity externally rotated. A high-frequency linear ultrasound transducer is placed in the longitudinal position with the superior aspect of the transducer placed just over the center of the medial malleolus and rotated toward the Achilles tendon (Fig. 5.11). A survey scan is taken which demonstrates the triangular-shaped deltoid ligament nestled between the medial malleolus and talus (Fig. 5.12). After the deltoid ligament is identified, the ligament is evaluated for fluid accumulation, strain, tears, and rupture (Figs. 5.13 and 5.14). Color Doppler may aid in identification of neovascularization of the deltoid ligament following injury (Fig. 5.15).

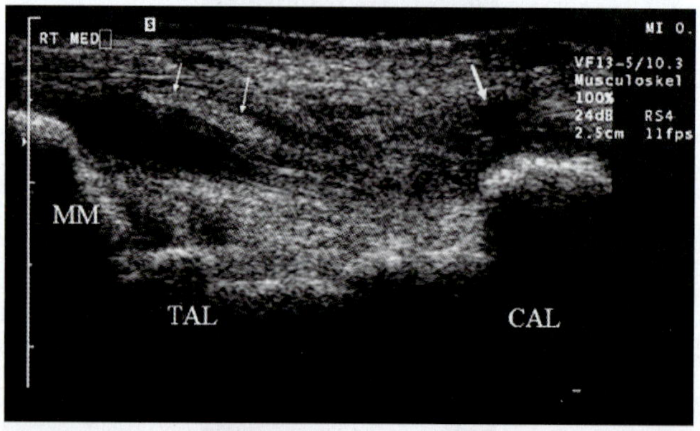

FIGURE 5.9 Longitudinal image along the medial joint line demonstrates tears of the superficial (talocalcaneal) and tibionavicular fibers of the deltoid ligament (*arrows*). CAL, calcaneus; MM, medial malleolus; TAL, talus. (From Adler R, Sofka CM, Positano RG. *Atlas of Foot and Ankle Sonography*. Philadelphia, PA: Lippincott Williams & Wilkins; 2004:71.)

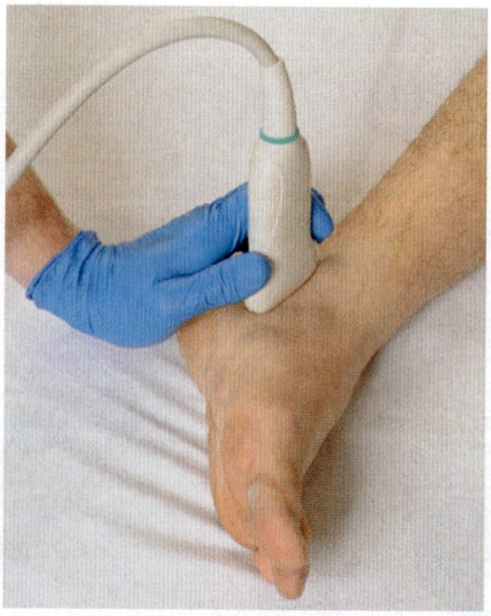

FIGURE 5.11 Correct longitudinal position for the ultrasound transducer for ultrasound evaluation of the deltoid ligament. Note the superior aspect of the ultrasound transducer is slightly rotated toward the Achilles tendon.

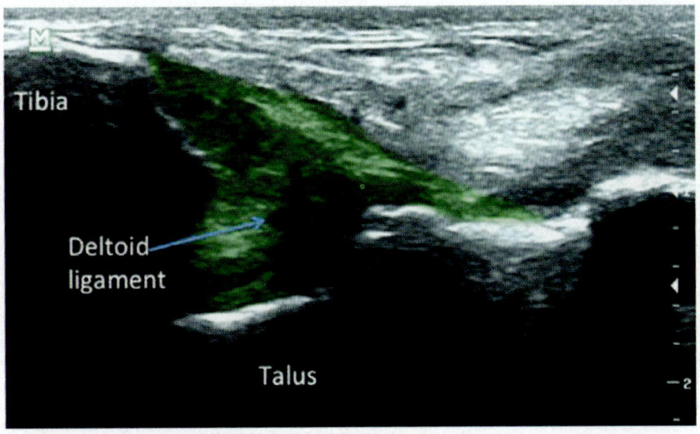

FIGURE 5.12 Longitudinal ultrasound image demonstrating the triangular-shaped deltoid ligament.

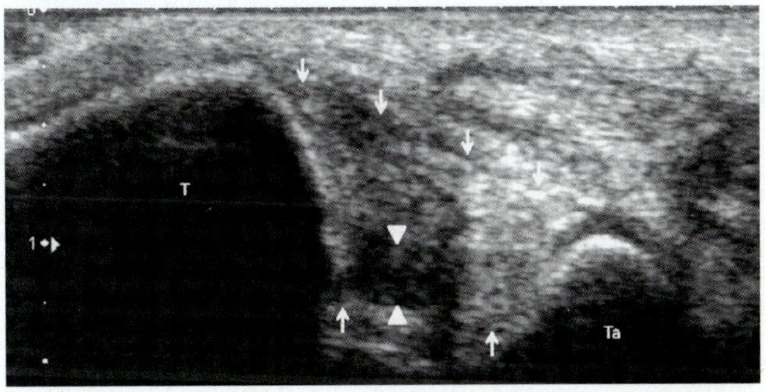

FIGURE 5.13 Longitudinal ultrasound image demonstrating a hypoechoic discontinuity (*arrowheads*) of the deep posterior tibiotalar component of the deltoid ligament (*arrows*). T, tibia; Ta, talus. (From Bong DA, Palau-Gonzalez J, Saenz I. Ligaments of the wrist, ankle, and foot: sonoanatomy and sonopathology. *Curr Rheum Rev* 2011;7(3): 212–230.)

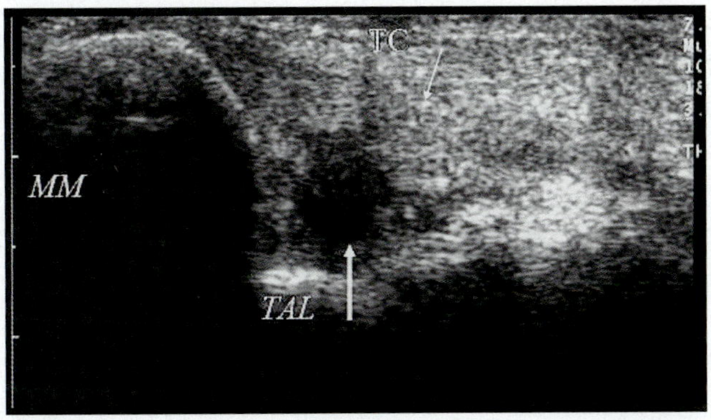

FIGURE 5.14 Longitudinal image along the medial ankle demonstrates a tear of the deep fibers of the deltoid ligament (*thick arrow*). The more superficial talocalcaneal (TC) fibers (*thin arrow*) remain in continuity. MM, medial malleolus; TAL, talus. (From Adler R, Sofka CM, Positano RG. *Atlas of Foot and Ankle Sonography*. Philadelphia, PA: Lippincott Williams & Wilkins; 2004:70.)

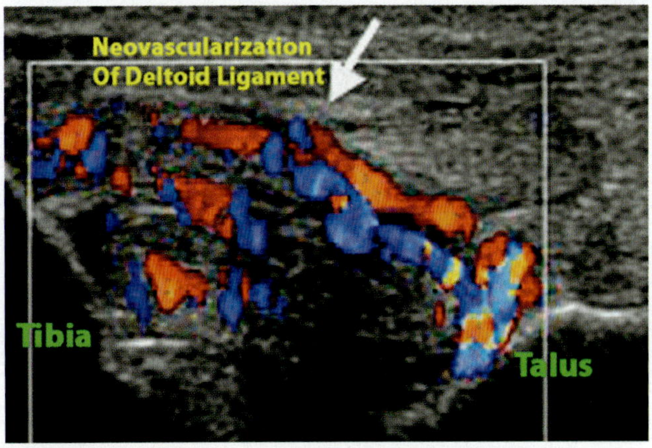

FIGURE 5.15 Color Doppler may aid in identification of neovascularization of the deltoid ligament following injury.

CLINICAL PEARLS

Bursitis, fractures, tendinopathy, osteoarthritis, synovitis, avascular necrosis, and impingement syndromes may coexist with deltoid ligament pathology and may contribute to the patient's pain symptoms. The use of multiple imaging modalities may help clarify the diagnosis and identify occult pathology (Fig. 5.16).

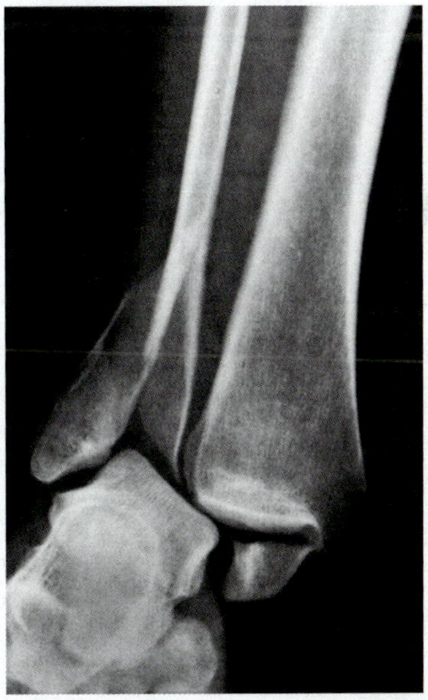

FIGURE 5.16 Weber type B fracture. A 24-year-old woman injured her right ankle in a skiing accident. Anteroposterior radiograph of the ankle demonstrates a spiral fracture of the fibula beginning at the level of the tibiofibular syndesmosis with consequent tear of the inferoposterior portion of the syndesmotic complex; the interosseous membrane is intact. The site of the fracture of the medial malleolus suggests that the deltoid ligament may be intact. According to the Weber classification, this is a type B fracture. (From Greenspan A. Lower limb III: ankle and foot. In: *Orthopedic Imaging: A Practical Approach*. 5th ed. Philadelphia, PA: Lippincott Williams & Wilkins; 2011:342.)

Suggested Readings

Beals TC, Crim J, Nickisch F. Deltoid ligament injuries in athletes: techniques of repair and reconstruction. *Oper Techn Sports Med* 2010;18(1):11–17.

Boss AP, Hintermann B. Anatomical study of the medial ankle ligament complex. *Foot Ankle Int* 2002;23:547–553.

Hintermann B, Knupp M, Pagenstert GI. Deltoid ligament injuries: diagnosis and management. *Foot Ankle Clin*2006;11(3):625–637.

Waldman SD. The deltoid ligament. In: *Pain Review.* Philadelphia, PA: Saunders,; 2009:157.

Waldman SD. Functional anatomy of the ankle and foot. In: *Pain Review.* Philadelphia, PA: Saunders; 2009:155–156.

Waldman SD. Intra-articular injection of the deltoid ligament. In: *Atlas of Pain Management Injection Techniques.* 3rd ed. Philadelphia, PA: Saunders; 2012:419–421.

Waldman SD, Campbell RSD. Deltoid ligament tear. In: *Imaging of Pain.* Philadelphia, PA: Saunders; 2011:439–441.

CHAPTER 6

Abnormalities of the Calcaneofibular Ligament

ANATOMIC CONSIDERATIONS

The ankle is a hinge-type articulation between the distal tibia, the two malleoli, and the talus (Fig. 6.1). The articular surface is covered with hyaline cartilage, which is susceptible to arthritis. The joint is surrounded by a dense capsule that helps strengthen the ankle. The joint capsule is lined with a synovial membrane that attaches to the articular cartilage. The ankle joint is innervated by the deep peroneal and tibial nerves.

The major ligaments of the ankle joint include the talofibular, anterior talofibular, calcaneofibular, and posterior talofibular ligaments, which provide the majority of strength to the ankle joint (Fig. 6.2). The calcaneofibular ligament is not as strong as the deltoid ligament and is susceptible to strain. The calcaneofibular ligament runs from the anterior border of the lateral malleolus to the lateral surface of the calcaneus (Figs. 6.3 and 6.4).

CLINICAL CORRELATES

The calcaneofibular ligament runs from the anterior border of the lateral malleolus to the lateral surface of the calcaneus (Fig. 6.3). Also known as the fibulocalcaneal ligament, the calcaneofibular ligament is susceptible to strain at the joint line or avulsion at its origin or insertion. The calcaneofibular ligament is frequently injured from inversion injuries to the ankle that occur when tripping when wearing high heels, stepping off a high curb, landing hard or running on hard uneven surfaces, and during dancing, soccer, and basketball. The pain of calcaneofibular ligament damage is localized anterior and inferior to the lateral malleolus and is made worse with inversion of the ankle joint. Point tenderness just below and behind the lateral malleolus is often present on physical examination. Significant swelling and ecchymosis are often evident after acute injury. Activity, especially involving weight bearing, plantar flexion,

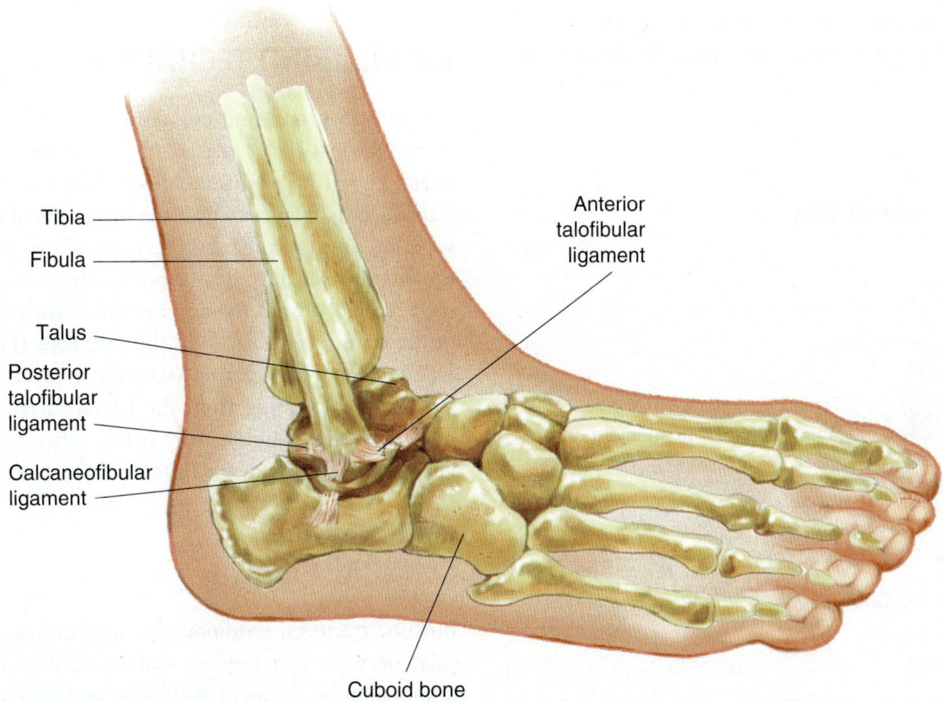

FIGURE 6.1 The articulations of the ankle joint.

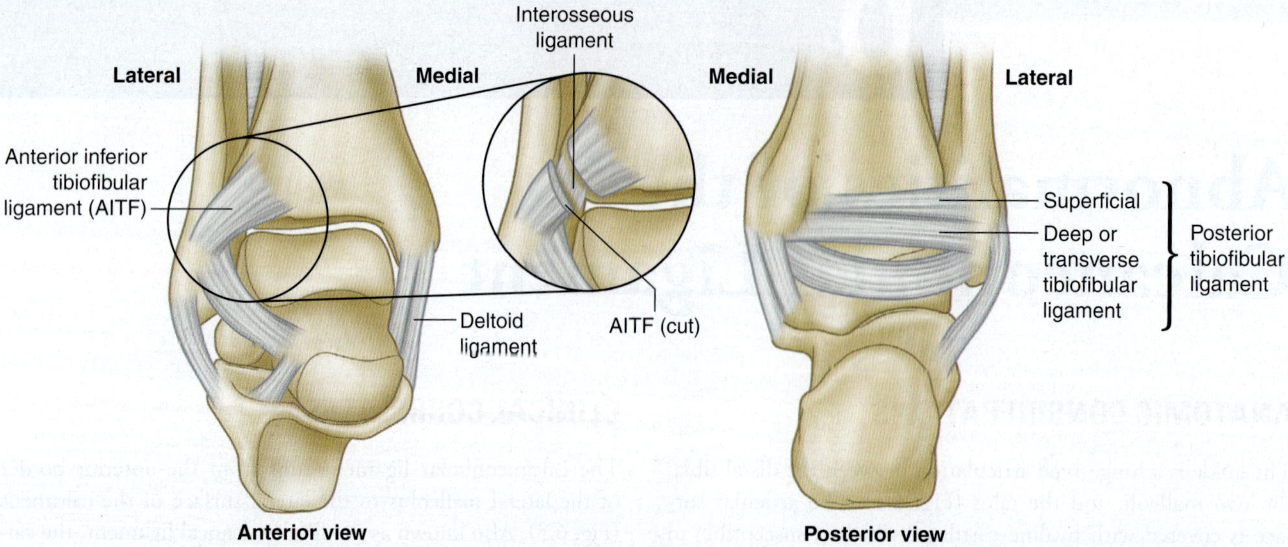

FIGURE 6.2 The major ligaments of the ankle joint include the talofibular, anterior talofibular, calcaneofibular, and posterior talofibular ligaments, which provide the majority of strength to the ankle joint. (From Patel A, Horton G. Anatomy of the foot and ankle. In: Altcheck DW, DiGiovanni CW, Dines JS, et al., eds. *Foot and Ankle Sports Medicine.* Philadelphia, PA: Lippincott Williams & Wilkins; 2013:2.)

and inversion of the ankle will exacerbate the pain. Local heat and decreased activity as well as elevation of the affected ankle may provide a modicum of relief. Sleep disturbance is common in patients suffering from trauma to the calcaneofibular ligament of the ankle. Coexistent fracture, bursitis, tendinitis, arthritis, or internal derangement of the ankle may confuse the clinical picture after trauma to the knee joint making clinical diagnosis difficult.

Plain radiographs and/or arthrography are indicated in all patients who present with calcaneofibular ligament pain, especially after ankle trauma (Figs. 6.5 and 6.6). Based on the patient's clinical presentation, additional testing may be indicated, including complete blood cell count, sedimentation rate, and antinuclear antibody testing. Magnetic resonance imaging, arthrography, and/or ultrasound imaging of the ankle are indicated if internal derangement or occult mass or tumor is suspected as well as to confirm the diagnosis of suspected calcaneofibular ligament injury (Fig. 6.7). Bone scan may be useful to identify occult stress fractures involving the calcaneus, especially if trauma has occurred (Fig. 6.8).

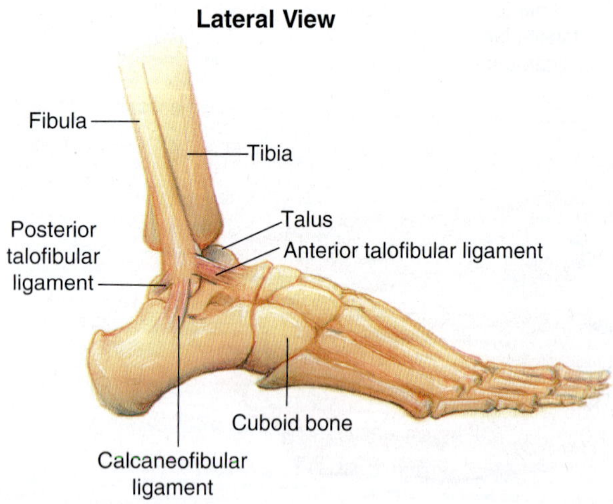

FIGURE 6.3 The anatomy of the calcaneofibular ligament and its relationship with the other ligaments of the lateral ankle.

ULTRASOUND TECHNIQUE

To perform ultrasound evaluation of the calcaneofibular ligament, the patient is placed in the supine position with the lateral curled up position. A high-frequency linear ultrasound transducer is then placed in the longitudinal position with the superior aspect of the transducer placed just over the bottom of the lateral malleolus. The superior aspect of the transducer is then rotated toward the anterior ankle with the inferior aspect of the transducer pointed at the calcaneus (Fig. 6.9). A survey scan is taken which demonstrates the hyperechoic calcaneofibular ligament running from the lateral calcaneus to the lateral malleolus of the fibula (Fig. 6.10). After the calcaneofibular ligament is identified, the ligament is evaluated (Fig. 6.11).

CLINICAL PEARLS

Bursitis, fractures, tendinopathy, osteoarthritis, synovitis, avascular necrosis, and impingement syndromes may coexist with calcaneofibular ligament pathology and may contribute to the patient's pain symptoms. Because of vasculopathy in diabetic patients, calcaneal insufficiency fractures are common (Fig. 6.12).

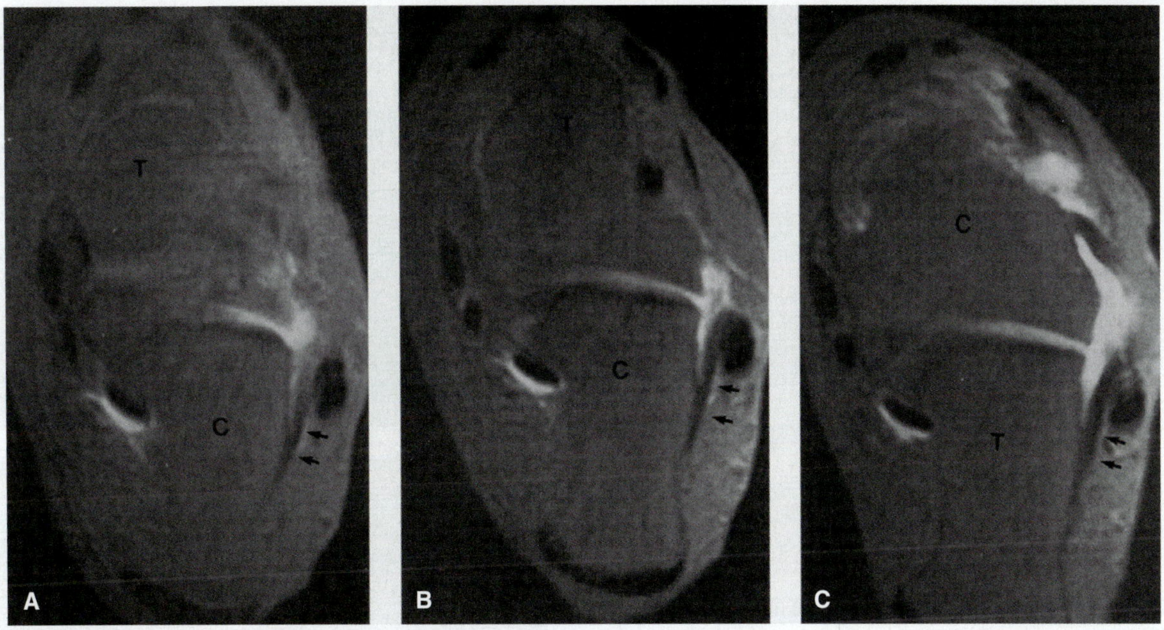

FIGURE 6.4 Axial T1-weighted images of the ankle at the level of calcaneofibular (CF) ligament with intra-articular gadolinium contrast agent. Three different approaches to optimally visualize CF ligament are demonstrated. **A:** This axial image is obtained with the ankle in neutral position. Although no special positioning or modification of the axial plane has been used, the CF ligament (*arrows*) is well seen with gadolinium contrast agent outlining the capsular side of the ligament. C, calcaneus; T, talus. **B:** This axial image is taken with the ankle in plantar flexion in which the ligament assumes a more horizontal course. The CF ligament (*arrows*) is well demonstrated deep to the peroneus tendons. The presence of the intra-articular gadolinium agent leads to displacement of the CF ligament away from the calcaneal cortex of low signal intensity and enhances its visualization. **C:** This is an oblique axial image of the ankle in neutral position. The obliquity of the axial slice has been determined by the axis of the body of the calcaneus, which parallels the long axis of the CF ligament. Here, the CF ligament (*arrows*) is seen well with the help of both the intra-articular contrast agent and the oblique axial plane programmed along the length of the CF ligament. (From Lee SH, Jacobson J, Trudell D, et al. Ligaments of the ankle: normal anatomy with MR arthrography. *J Comp Assist Tomogr* 1998;22(5):807–813.)

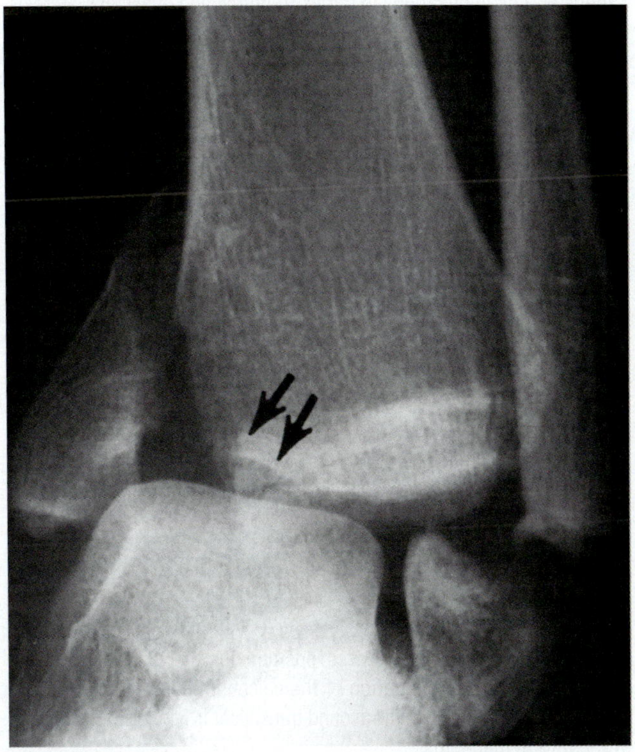

FIGURE 6.5 A 45-year-old woman sustained an inversion injury of her ankle. An anteroposterior radiograph illustrates a classic supination–adduction injury pattern. The medial malleolus fracture is vertical, and the fibula fracture is very distal and transverse. There is an impacted fragment in the medial aspect of the remaining tibial plafond (*arrows*). (From Bucholz RW, Heckman JD. *Rockwood & Green's Fractures in Adults.* 5th ed. Philadelphia, PA: Lippincott Williams & Wilkins; 2001.)

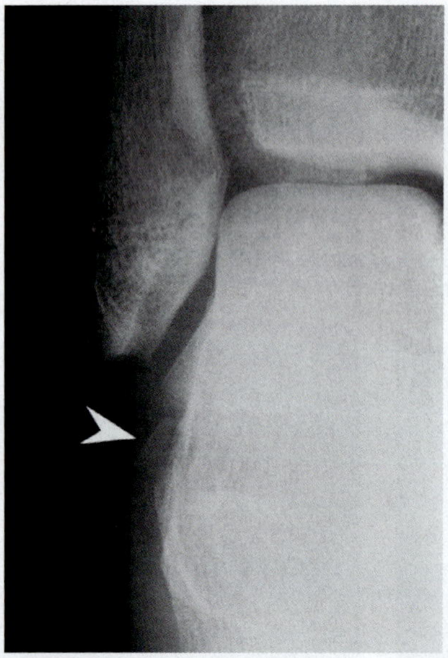

FIGURE 6.6 Anteroposterior radiographs of the right ankle taken at the first examination showed a small bone fragment beneath the lateral malleolus suggestive of an avulsion injury of the calcaneofibular ligament (*arrowhead*). (From Sugimoto K, Kasanami R, Iwai M, et al. Achilles tendon rupture associated with injury of the calcaneofibular ligament. *J Orthop Trauma* 2003;17(7):534–535.)

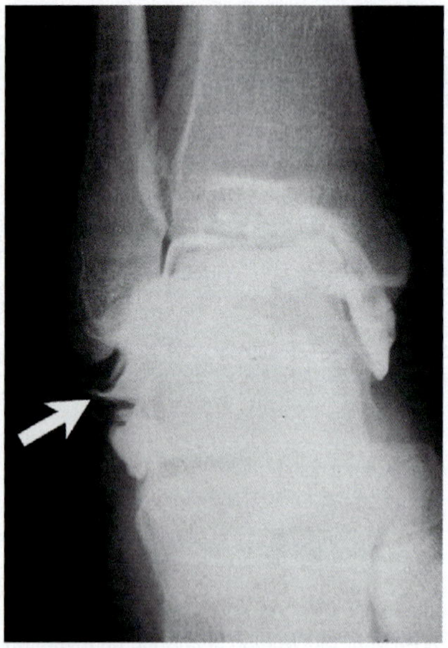

FIGURE 6.7 A 28-year-old man sustained an inversion sprain on uneven ground. The AP view of the subtalar arthrography showed a lateral recess (*arrow*). Combined injuries of the anterior talofibular ligament and calcaneofibular ligament were seen during surgery. (From Sugimoto K, Takakura Y, Samoto N, et al. Subtalar arthrography in recurrent instability of the ankle. *Clin Orthop Relat Res* 2002;394: 169–176.)

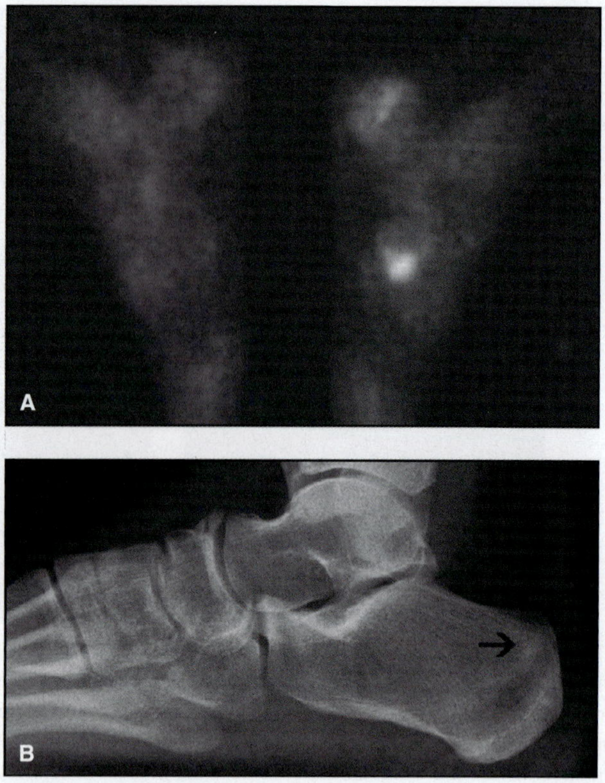

FIGURE 6.8 **A:** Bone scan showing superior posterior calcaneal focal linear uptake with less intensity than expected for an acute stress fracture, likely representing a healing stress fracture. Incidental increased uptake in the ipsilateral midfoot likely represents an additional stress fracture within the midfoot not definitely seen on the previous radiograph. **B:** Lateral ankle radiograph reveals a linear sclerotic band along the posterior superior calcaneus (*arrow*), consistent with fatigue stress fracture. (From Flores R, Bui-Mansfield LT. Vascular anatomy of the calcaneus and its implications in stress fractures and avascular necrosis. *Contemp Diagn Radiol* 2013;36(5):1–6.)

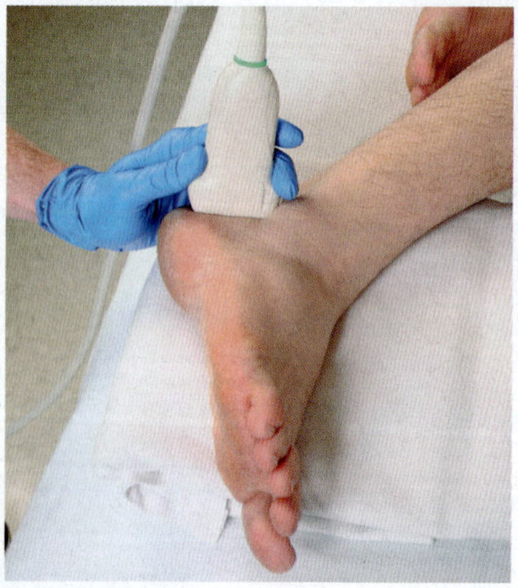

FIGURE 6.9 Correct transverse position for the ultrasound transducer for ultrasound evaluation of the calcaneofibular ligament. Note the posterior aspect of the ultrasound transducer is lying over the bottom of the lateral malleolus.

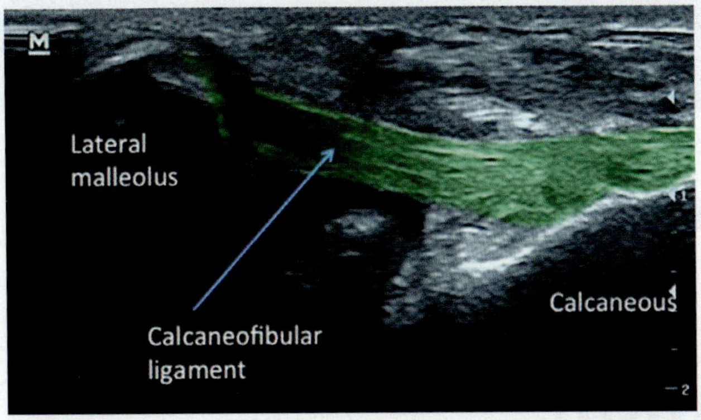

FIGURE 6.10 Longitudinal ultrasound image demonstrating the calcaneofibular ligament.

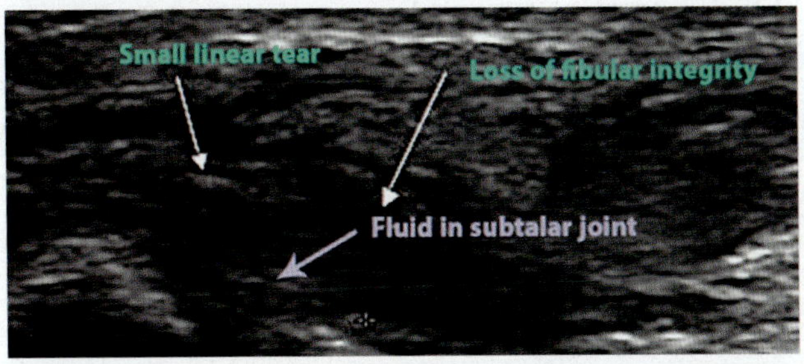

FIGURE 6.11 Longitudinal ultrasound image demonstrating loss of fibular integrity of the calcaneofibular ligament as evidenced by hypoechoic linear tearing and thickening of the ligament. Note fluid in the subtalar joint.

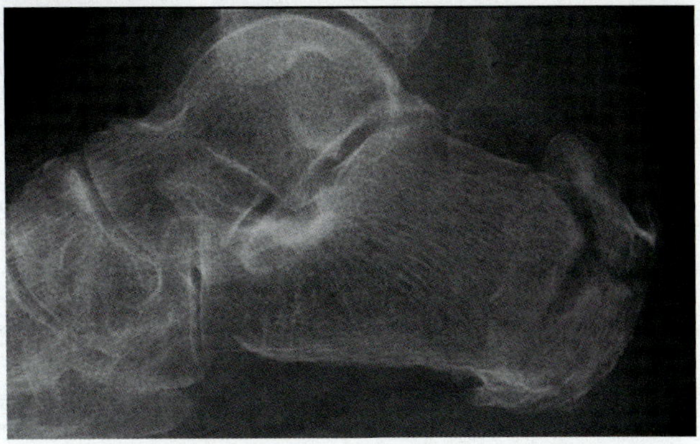

FIGURE 6.12 Lateral ankle radiograph reveals a calcaneal insufficiency avulsion fracture in a diabetic patient with heel pain. Note the associated vascular calcifications. (From Flores R, Bui-Mansfield LT. Vascular anatomy of the calcaneus and its implications in stress fractures and avascular necrosis. *Contemp Diagn Radiol* 2013;36(5):1–6; Fig. 5.)

Suggested Readings

Bonnel F, Toullec E, Mabit C, et al. Chronic ankle instability: biomechanics and pathomechanics of ligaments injury and associated lesions. *Orthop Traumatol Surg Res* 2010;96(4):424–432.

Haller J, Bernt R, Seeger T, et al. MR-imaging of anterior tibiotalar impingement syndrome: agreement, sensitivity and specificity of MR-imaging and indirect MR-arthrography. *Eur J Radiol* 2006;58(3):450–460.

Waldman SD. Calcaneofibular ligament. In: *Pain Review.* Philadelphia, PA: Saunders; 2009:158.

Waldman SD. Functional anatomy of the ankle and foot. In: *Pain Review.* Philadelphia, PA: Saunders; 2009:155–156.

Waldman SD. Injection of the calcaneofibular ligament. In: *Atlas of Pain Management Injection Techniques.* 3rd ed. Philadelphia, PA: Saunders; 2012:427–430.

Waldman SD, Campbell RSD. Calcaneofibular ligament tear. In: *Imaging of Pain.* Philadelphia, PA: Saunders; 2011:437–438.

CHAPTER 7

Posterior Tibialis Tendinitis and Other Abnormalities of the Posterior Tibialis Tendon

ANATOMIC CONSIDERATIONS

The posterior tibialis muscle plantarflexes the foot at the ankle and inverts the foot at the subtalar and transverse tarsal joints. The muscle finds its origin from the posterior tibia and fibula (Fig. 7.1). The tendon of the muscle passes behind the medial malleolus, running beneath the flexor retinaculum, and into the sole of the foot where it inserts on the navicular bone (Fig. 7.2). The posterior tibialis tendon is susceptible to the development of tendinitis as it curves around the medial malleolus (Fig. 7.3).

CLINICAL CORRELATES

Posterior tibialis tendinitis is a clinical syndrome characterized by sharp, constant, and severe inner ankle pain. This painful condition is often seen as a result of acute eversion injuries to the ankle although it is also seen with overuse or misuse of the ankle in foot, as seen in long distance running with improper shoes. Recently, there have been a number of reports of posterior tibialis tendinitis in Irish dancers as a result of the "leap over move" that is a common part of their dance routine.

Patients suffering from posterior tibialis tendinitis often splint the inflamed posterior tibialis tendon by adopting an antalgic gait to avoid using the affected tendon. This dysfunctional gait may cause a secondary bursitis and tendinitis around the foot and ankle, which may both confuse the clinical picture and further increase the patient's pain and disability. Pain on palpation of the posterior tibialis tendon as it passes behind the medial malleolus is a consistent finding in patients with posterior tibialis tendinitis as is exacerbation of pain with active resisted inversion and passive eversion of the ankle (Fig. 7.4). The inner aspect of the ankle may feel hot and appear swollen, which may be misdiagnosed as superficial thrombophlebitis or cellulitis. Patients suffering from posterior tibialis tendinitis will also often complain that it feels like their shoes are rubbing the inside of their ankles raw, although on examination the skin appears normal. A creaking or grating sensation may be palpated when passively inverting and everting the ankle. Untreated, posterior tibialis tendinitis will result in increasing pain and functional disability calcium deposition around the tendon occurring, making subsequent treatment more difficult. Continued trauma to the inflamed tendon ultimately may result in tendon rupture (Fig. 7.5). Rupture of the posterior tibialis tendon will result if disruption of the normal architecture of the foot resulting in the loss of the arch of the foot and development of the pes planus deformity (Fig. 7.6).

Plain radiographs are indicated in all patients who present with medial ankle pain. Based on the patient's clinical presentation, additional testing may be indicated, including complete blood cell count, sedimentation rate, and antinuclear antibody testing. MRI or ultrasound imaging of the ankle is indicated if posterior tibialis tendinitis, rupture, or joint instability is suggested (Figs. 7.7 to 7.11). Radionuclide bone scanning is useful to identify stress fractures of the tibia not seen on plain radiographs.

ULTRASOUND TECHNIQUE

Ultrasound-guided evaluation of the posterior tibialis tendinitis is carried out by placing the patient in the supine position with the arms resting comfortably along the patient's chest and the affected lower extremity externally rotated. A total of 4 mL of local anesthetic and 80 mg of depot steroid are drawn up in a 12-mL sterile syringe. The medial malleolus is then identified by palpation. A linear high-frequency ultrasound transducer is placed in a longitudinal plane, with the middle of the ultrasound transducer lying over the posterior border of the medial malleolus (Fig. 7.12). This will put the ultrasound transducer parallel to the posterior tibialis tendon as it passes behind the medial malleolus. An ultrasound survey scan is taken. The posterior tibialis tendon can be seen lying just behind the medial malleolus as a fibular linear structure (Figs. 7.13 and 7.14). When the posterior tibialis tendon is identified on ultrasound imaging, the tendon is evaluated for fluid, extrinsic compression, tendinosis, tendinitis, tears, and rupture (Figs. 7.15 to 7.31). Ultrasound imaging is also useful in assessing the effect of implantable hardware on surrounding structures.

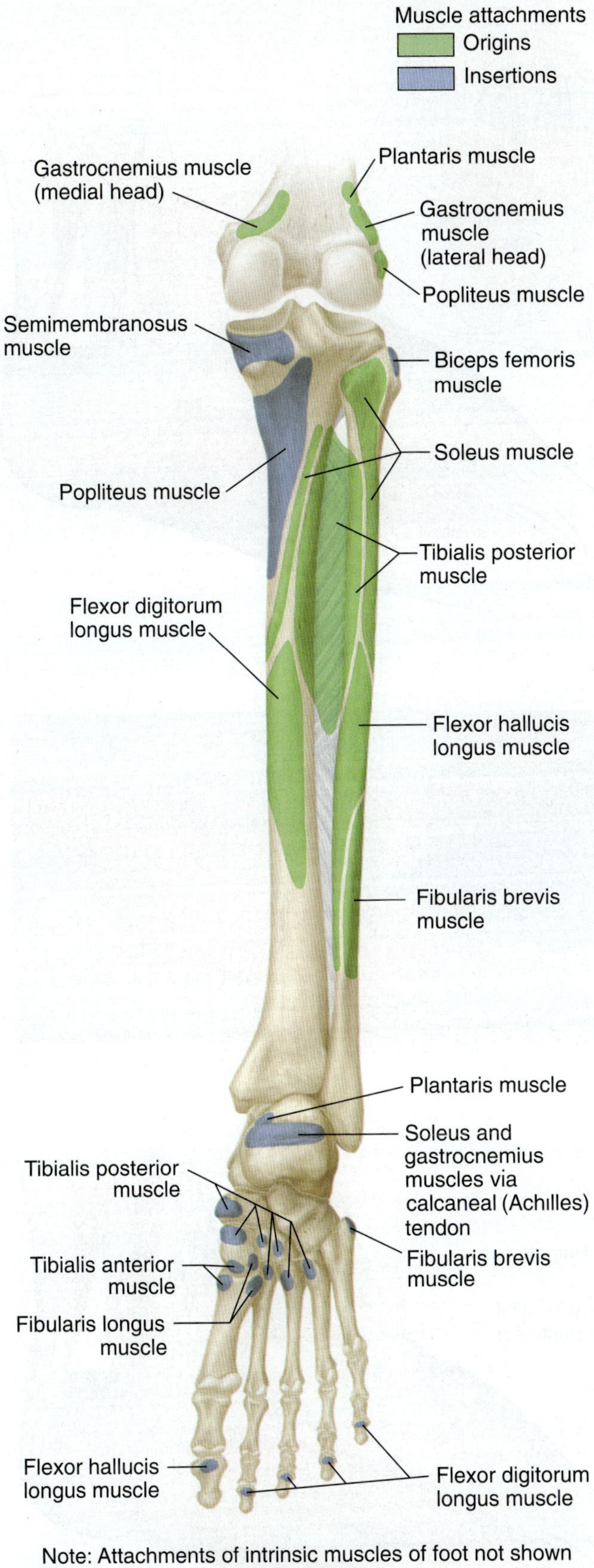

FIGURE 7.1 The posterior tibialis muscle finds its origin at the posterior tibia and fibula. (From Tank PW, Gest TR. The lower limb. In: *Lippincott Williams & Wilkins Atlas of Anatomy*. Philadelphia, PA: Lippincott Williams & Wilkins; 2009:116.)

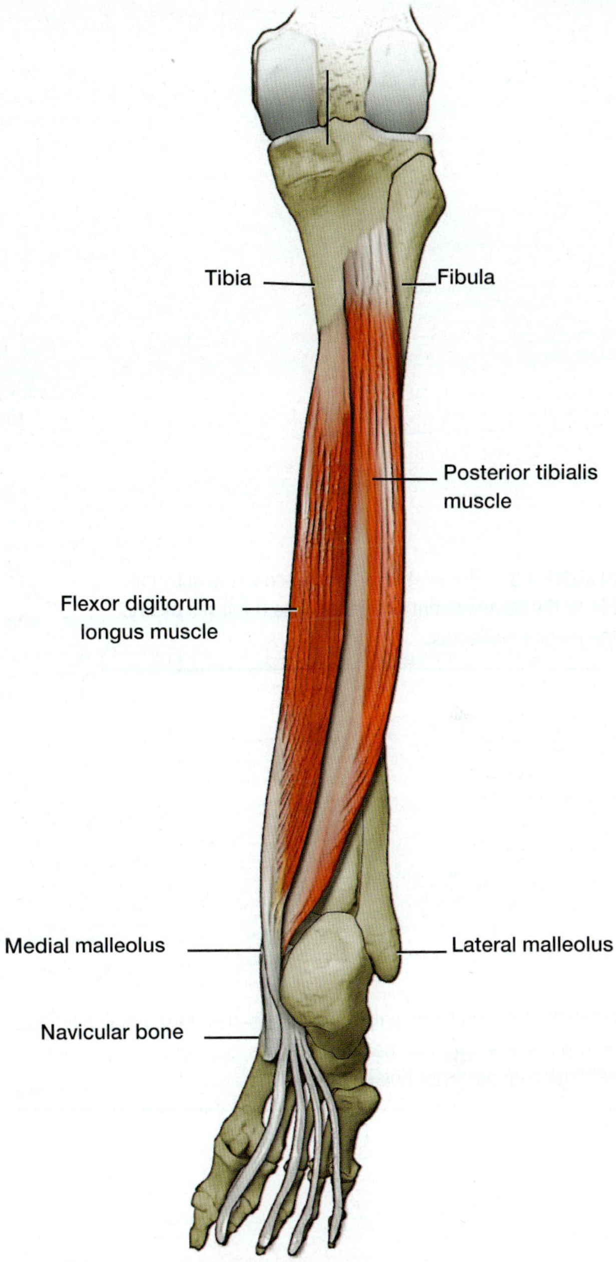

FIGURE 7.2 Anatomy of the posterior tibialis muscle.

CLINICAL PEARLS

Bursitis and arthritis of the ankle and foot may coexist with posterior tibialis tendinitis and may contribute to the patient's pain symptoms. It is important to timely diagnose posterior tibialis tendonitis and to identify the activity and/or pathology responsible for its evolution and then initiate prompt treatment to avoid tendon rupture.

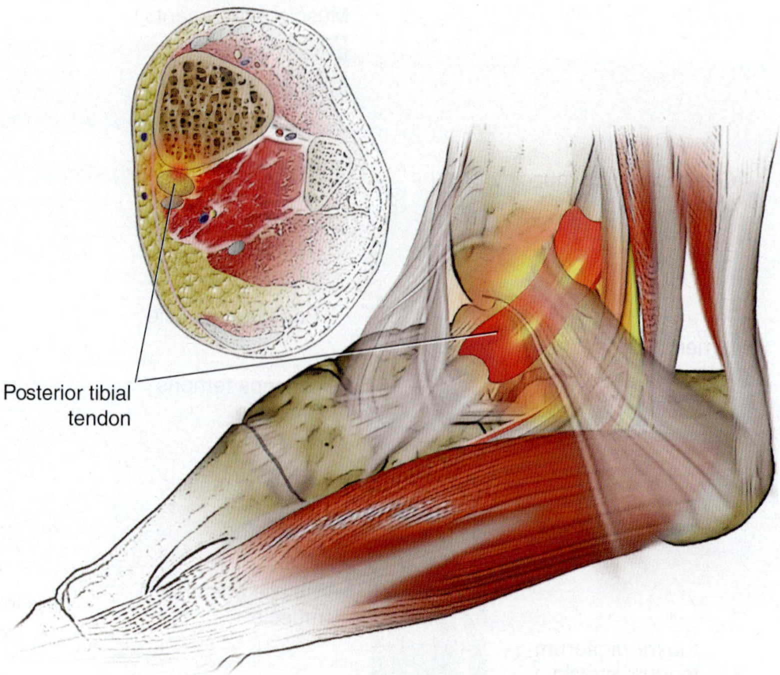

FIGURE 7.3 The posterior tibialis tendon is susceptible to the development of tendinitis as it passes behind the medial malleolus.

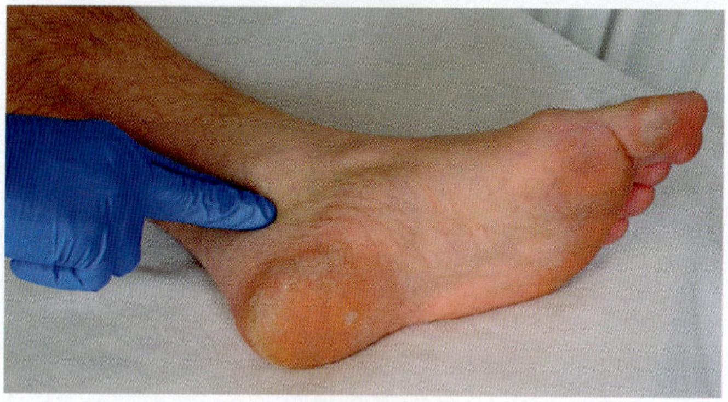

FIGURE 7.4 Pain on palpation of the posterior tibialis tendon as it passes behind the medial malleolus is a consistent finding in patients with posterior tibialis tendinitis.

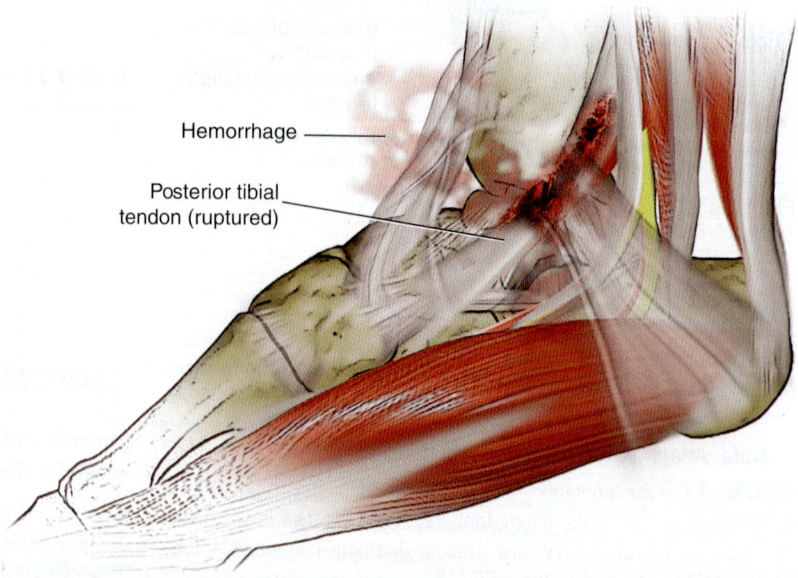

FIGURE 7.5 Failure to aggressively treat posterior tibialis tendinitis may result in rupture of the tendon.

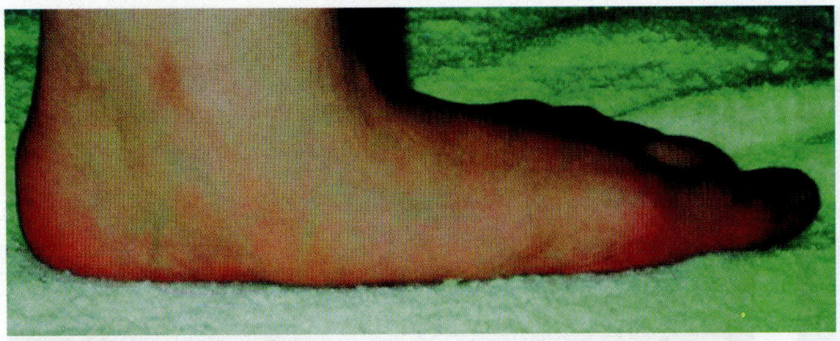

FIGURE 7.6 Rupture of the posterior tibialis tendon will result if disruption of the normal architecture of the foot resulting in the loss of the arch of the foot and development of the pes planus deformity.

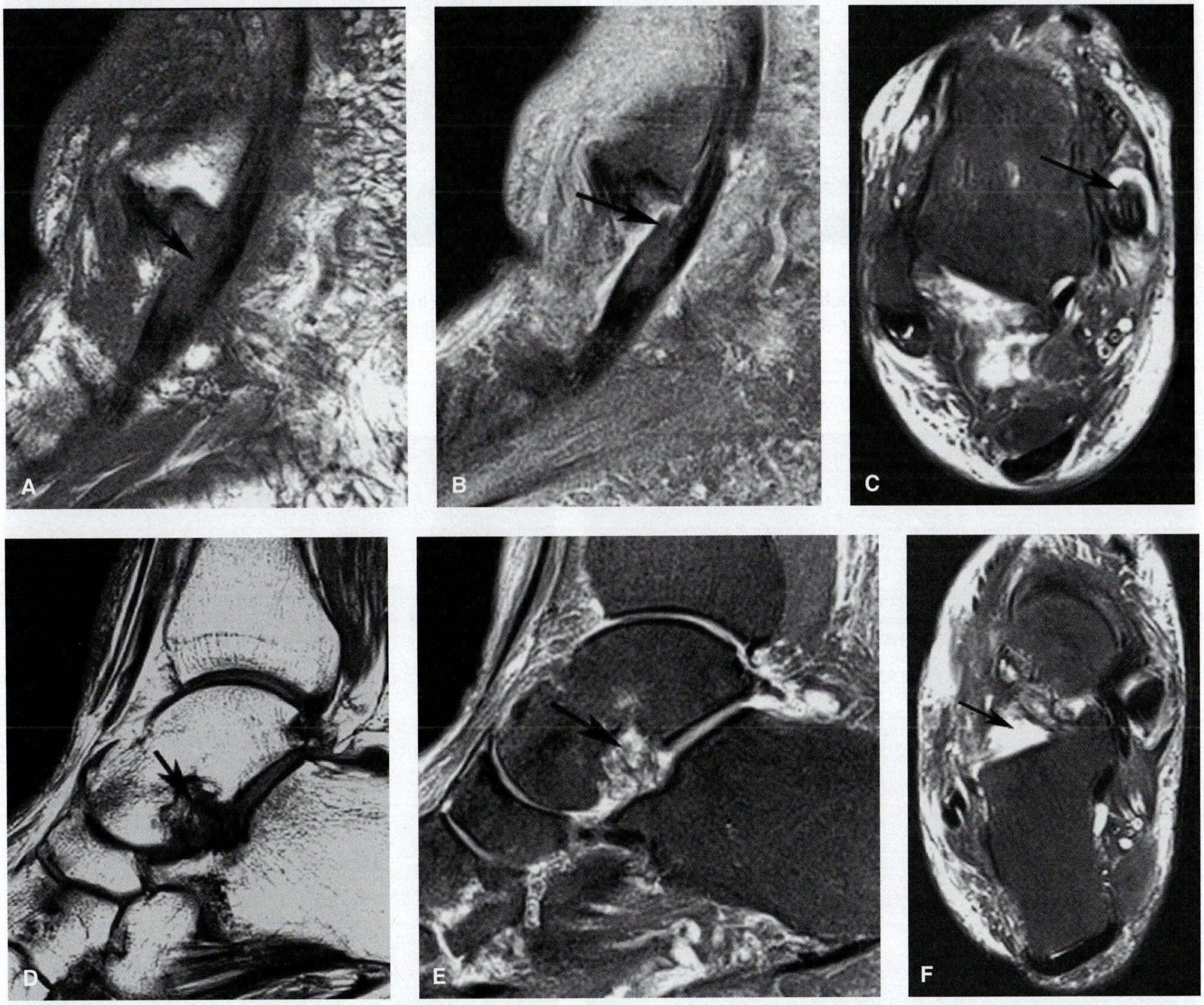

FIGURE 7.7 Partial (type II) tear of the posterior tibial tendon with associated sinus tarsi syndrome. Sagittal T1- **(A)** and T2- **(B)** weighted and axial T2-weighted **(C)** images through the posterior tibial tendon demonstrate a tear at the malleolar tip (*arrow*) with thickening of the tendon and fluid in the tendon sheath. Sagittal T1- **(D)** and sagittal **(E)** and axial **(F)** T2-weighted images demonstrate abnormal signal intensity in the tarsal canal and sinus (*arrow*) due to associated sinus tarsi syndrome. (From Berquist TH. Soft tissue trauma and overuse syndromes. In: *Imaging of the Foot and Ankle.* 3rd ed. Philadelphia, PA: Lippincott Williams & Wilkins; 2011:114–204.)

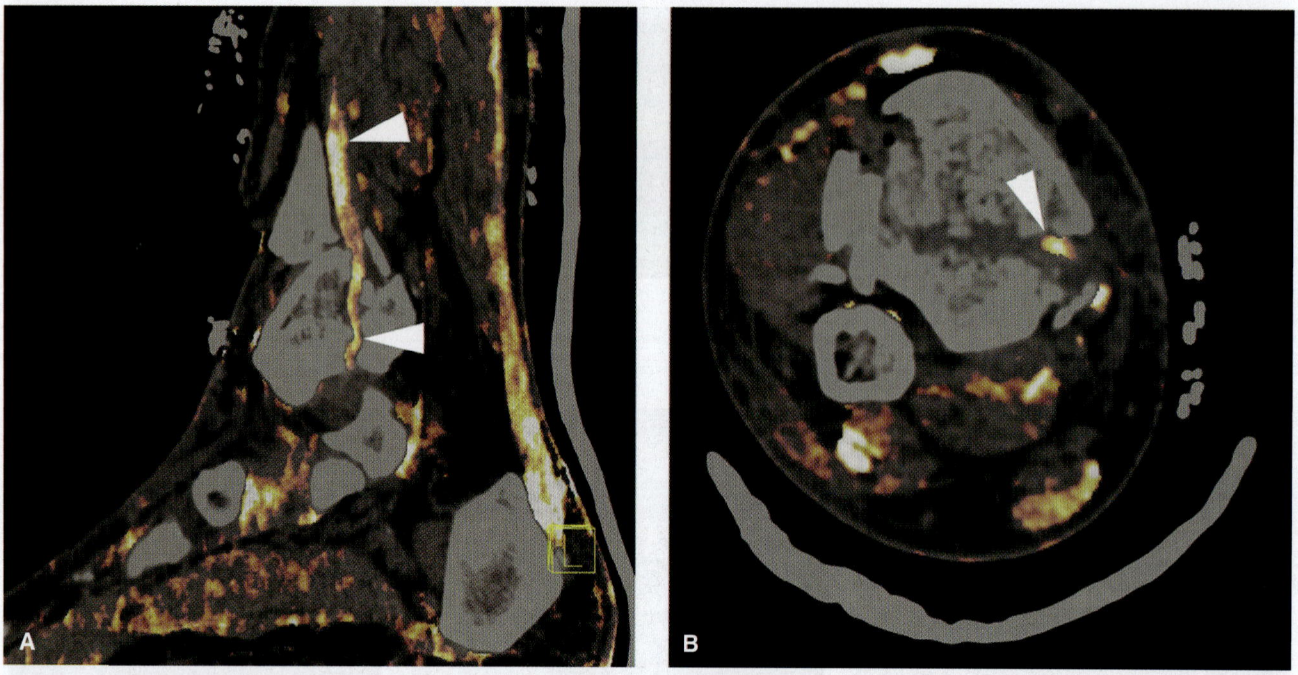

FIGURE 7.8 **A:** Sagittal DECT image of the comminuted distal tibia with the tibialis posterior tendon trapped between the fragments (*arrowheads*). **B:** Axial DECT image of the comminuted distal tibia with the tibialis posterior tendon trapped between the fragments (*arrowhead*). (From Mallinson P, Antoniades G, McLaughlin P, et al. Dual-energy computed tomographic tendon algorithm in acute trauma: initial experiences. *J Comp Assist Tomogr* 2014;38(3):348–351.)

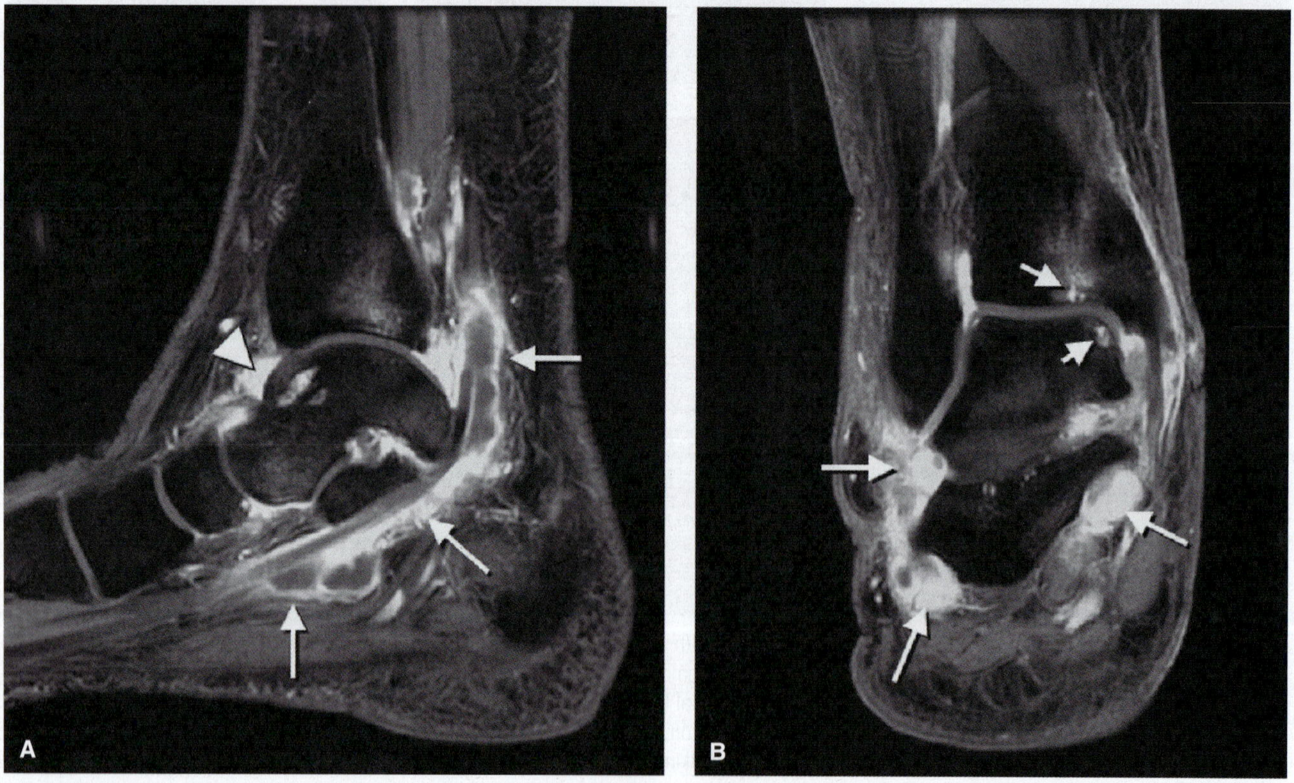

FIGURE 7.9 Sagittal **(A)** and coronal **(B)** postgadolinium fat-suppressed two-dimensional fast SPGR sequences of the ankle and hindfoot in a 32-year-old patient with enhancing periarticular synovitis (*arrowhead*), complex tenosynovitis (*long arrows*), and periarticular erosions (*short arrows*) caused by rheumatoid arthritis. (From Collins MS, Felmlee JP. 3T magnetic resonance imaging of ankle and hindfoot tendon pathology. *Top Magn Reson Imaging* 2009;20(3):175–188; Fig. 3AB.)

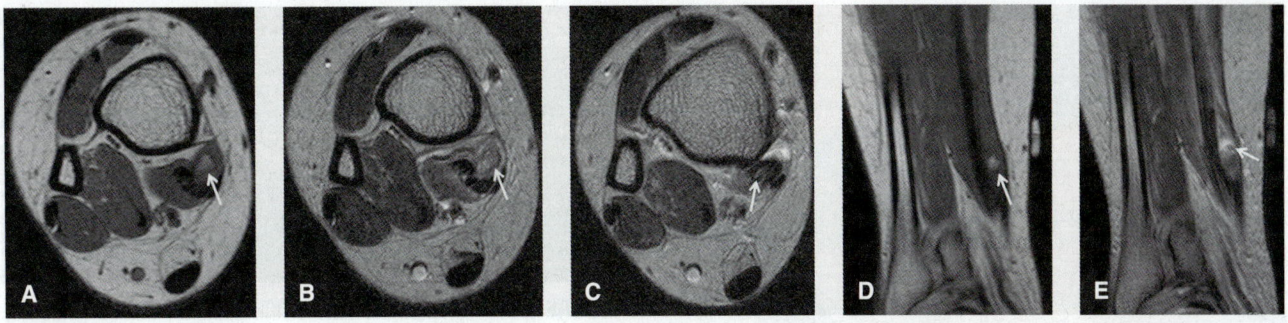

FIGURE 7.10 T1- **(A)** and T2- **(B)** weighted axial magnetic resonance imaging (MRI) scan showing bony mass (*arrow*) displacing the tibialis posterior (TP) tendon. **C:** T2-weighted axial MRI scan at the level of the distal conjoined TP tendon showing the osteochondroma and TP tendon (*arrow*), in which signal changes are noted, suggesting the tendon tear. **D:** T1-weighted coronal MRI scan showing tip of bony mass (*arrow*) protruding within the TP tendon and muscle. **E:** T2-weighted coronal MRI scan clearly showing osteochondroma (*arrow*) with overlying cartilage cap abutting the TP tendon. (From Kim YC, Ahn JH, Lee JW. Osteochondroma of the distal tibia complicated by a tibialis posterior tendon tear. *J Foot Ankle Surg* 2012;51(5):660–663.)

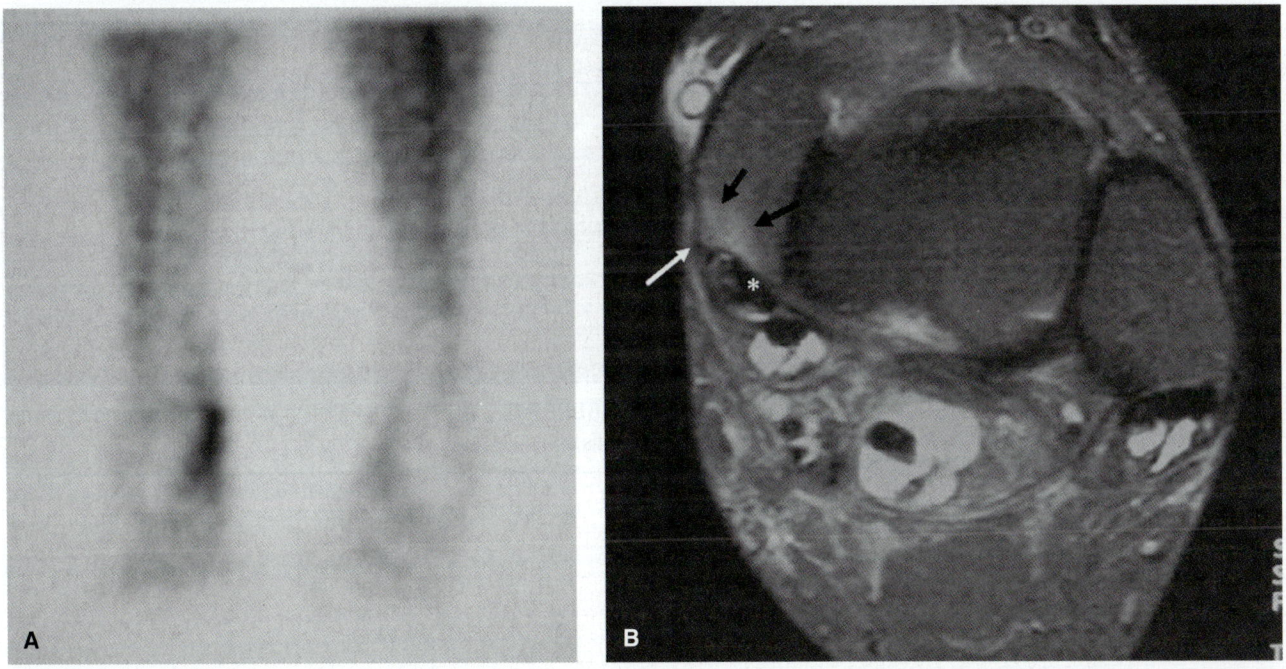

FIGURE 7.11 Anterior view of blood pool phase of NMS bone scan **(A)** and axial fat-suppressed T2-weighted image **(B)** in a patient with symptomatic tenosynovitis and attrition-type tear of the tibialis posterior tendon. Increased vascularity is seen on blood pool image along the medial aspect of the ankle in the course of the tibialis posterior tendon, and the MRI shows attrition of the normal size of the tibialis posterior tendon (*asterisk*) with torn tendon debris adjacent to it. Reactive bone marrow edema in the adjacent tibia (*black arrows*), a posteromedial tibial spur (*white arrow*), and extensive reactive edema in the soft tissues of the posteromedial ankle are present. Fluid in flexor digitorum longus and flexor hallucis longus tendon sheaths also noted. (From Peduto AJ, Read JW. Imaging of ankle tendinopathy and tears. *Top Magn Reson Imaging* 2010;21(1):25–36.)

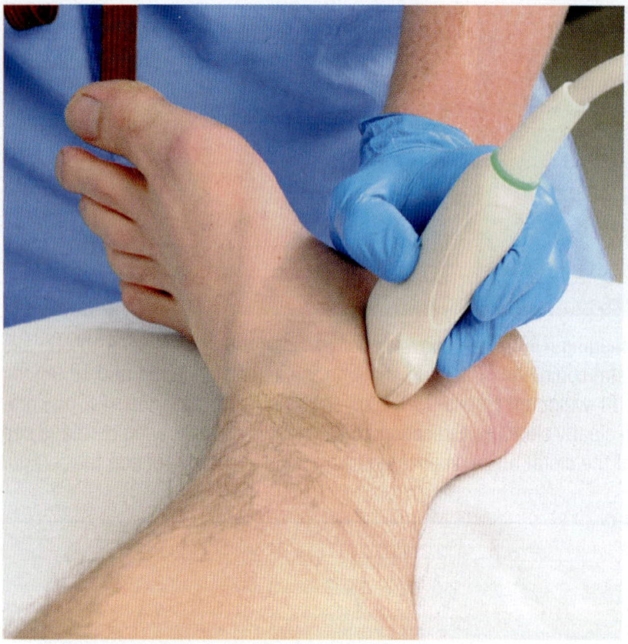

FIGURE 7.12 Proper longitudinal ultrasound transducer placement for ultrasound evaluation of the posterior tibialis tendon.

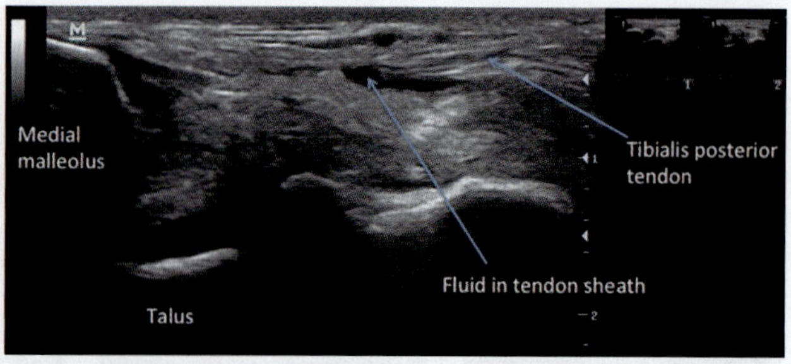

FIGURE 7.14 Longitudinal view of the posterior tibialis tendon as it passes behind the medial malleolus demonstrating fluid within the tendon sheath.

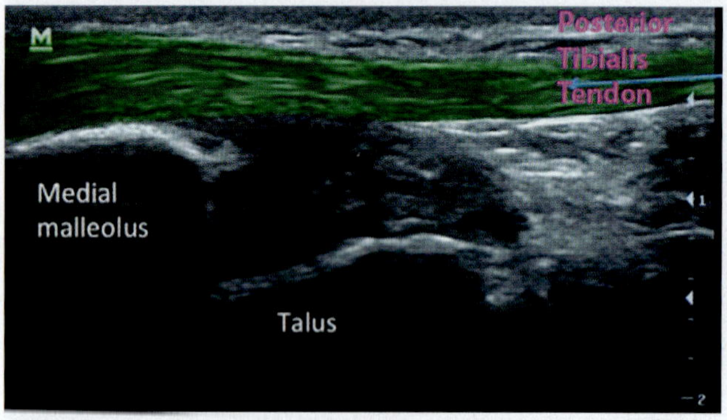

FIGURE 7.13 Longitudinal view of the posterior tibialis tendon as it passes behind the medial malleolus.

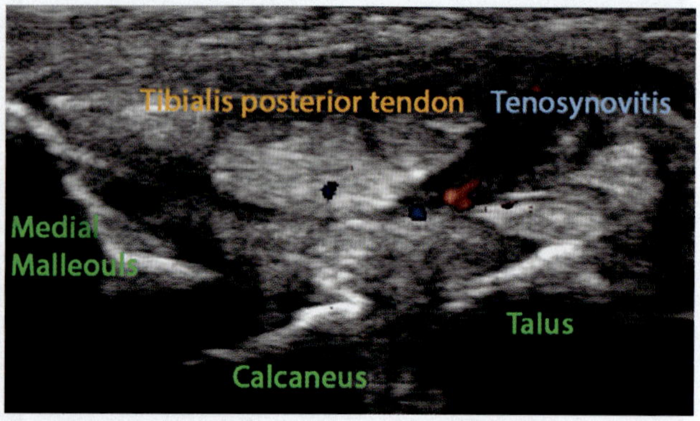

FIGURE 7.15 Transverse ultrasound image demonstrating tenosynovitis of the tibialis posterior tendon.

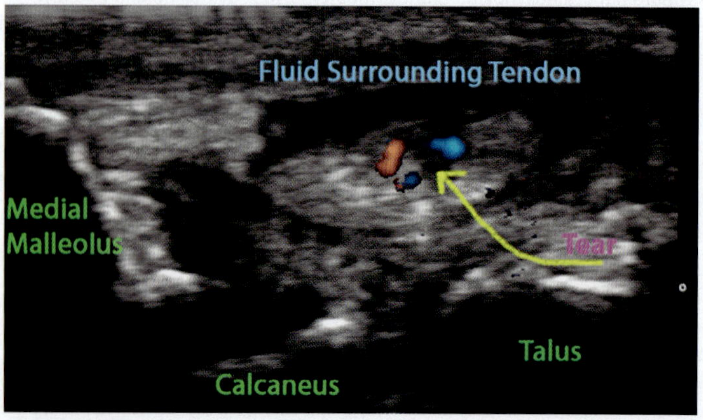

FIGURE 7.16 Transverse color Doppler image demonstrating an acute tear of the tibialis posterior tendon. Note fluid surrounding the tendon.

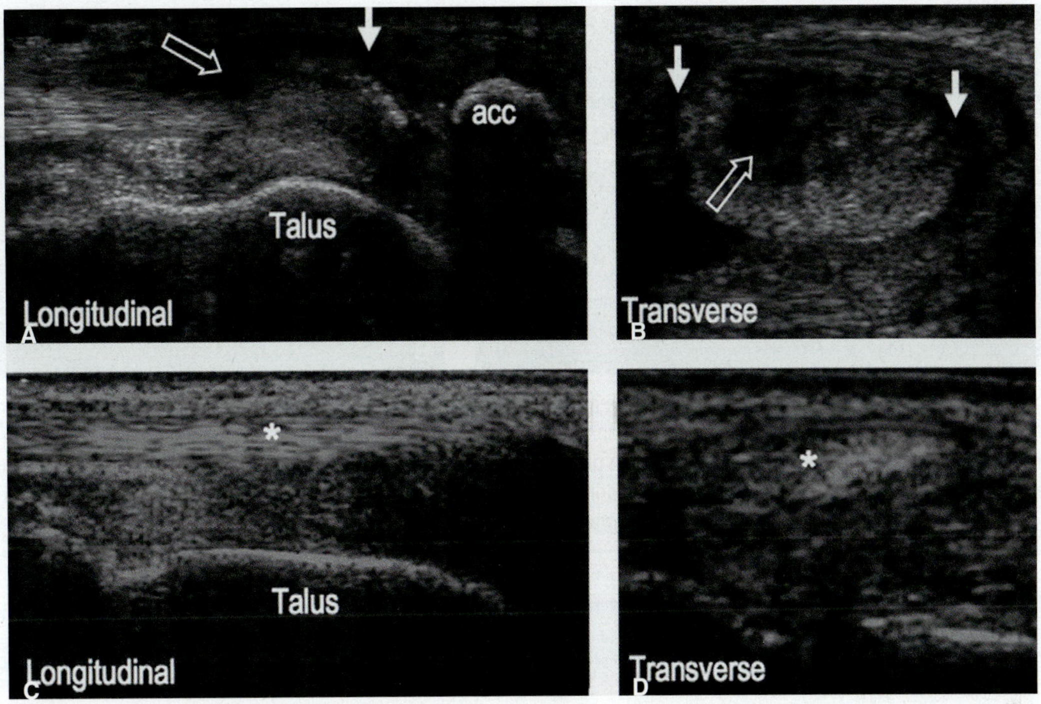

FIGURE 7.17 Tibialis posterior tendinosis. **A:** Longitudinal ultrasound image of the distal tibialis posterior tendon with a degenerative tear (*open arrow*) just proximal to the accessory navicular (acc). *Arrow*, tenosynovial fluid. **B:** Transverse ultrasound image showing a markedly thickened tendon with hypoechoic cleft (*open arrow*) within the substance of the tendon, consistent with a partial longitudinal tear. A small amount of tenosynovial fluid is seen within the tendon sheath (*arrows*). **C,D:** Normal longitudinal and transverse ultrasound image of the distal tibialis posterior tendon (*asterisk*). (From Chew K, Stevens KJ, Wang TG, et al. Introduction to diagnostic musculoskeletal ultrasound: part 2: examination of the lower limb. *Am J Phys Med Rehab* 2008;87(3):238–248.)

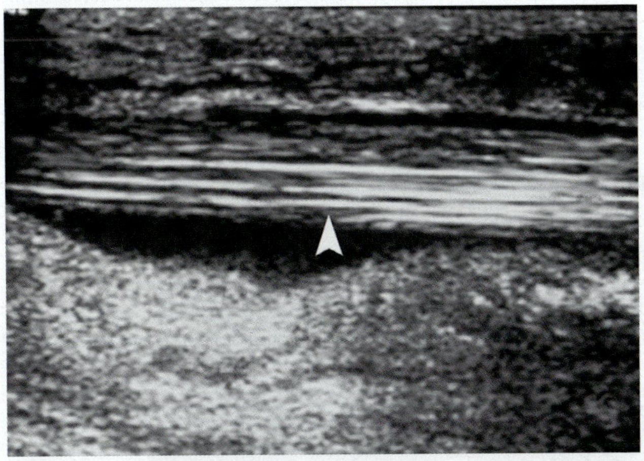

FIGURE 7.18 Longitudinal ultrasound image of the posterior tibial tendon showing anechoic fluid in the tendon sheath surrounding the relatively normal-appearing tendon (*arrowhead*). Note also the edema in the adjacent soft tissue. (From Ahmed R, Nazarian LN. Overview of musculoskeletal sonography. *Ultrasound Q* 2010;26(1):27–35.)

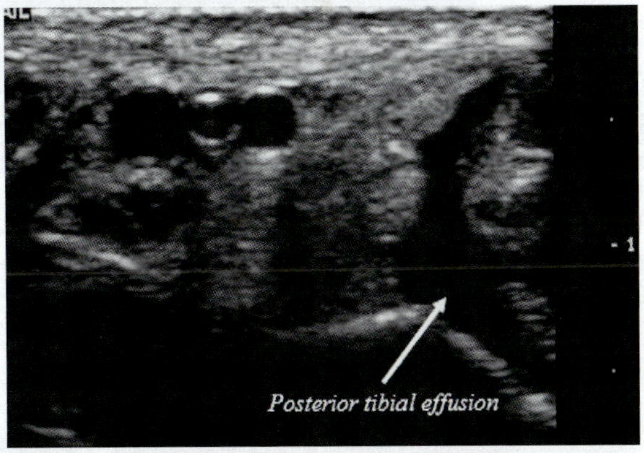

FIGURE 7.19 In this transverse image (anatomic axial plane) obtained over the medial compartment, the posterior tibial tendon and flexor digitorum longus tendons **(right)** are separated by fluid in their common tendon sheath (*arrow*). The neurovascular bundle can be seen to the left of the image. Three rounded hypoechoic structures correspond to the centrally positioned posterior tibial arteries and adjacent vein. An elliptical hypoechoic structure posterior to the vascular structures, containing fine internal structure, corresponds to the posterior tibial nerve. The surrounding echogenic halo corresponds to the investing fibroadipose connective nerve. The surrounding echogenic halo corresponds to the investing fibroadipose connective tissue (or epineurium). The degree to which the nerve appears hypoechoic is variable. (From Adler R, Sofka CM, Positano RG. *Atlas of Foot and Ankle Sonography*. Philadelphia, PA: Lippincott Williams & Wilkins; 2004:48.)

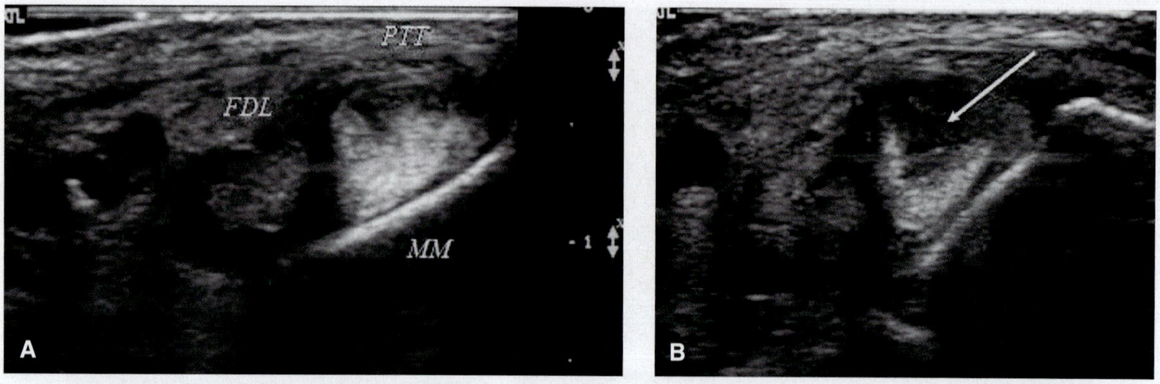

FIGURE 7.20 **A:** Transverse ultrasound image at the tip of the medial malleolus demonstrates tendinosis of the posterior tibial tendon (PTT) and flexor digitorum longus (FDL). MM, medial malleolus. The tendons are enlarged, and there is moderate surrounding fluid. Portions of the neurovascular bundle are evident in the left of the image. **B:** Transverse ultrasound image of the posterior tibial tendon obtained slightly more caudally in the same patient demonstrates moderate tendinosis of the tendon, with a linear hypoechoic split within the periphery of the tendon (*arrow*). (From Adler R, Sofka CM, Positano RG. *Atlas of Foot and Ankle Sonography.* Philadelphia, PA: Lippincott Williams & Wilkins; 2004:56–57.)

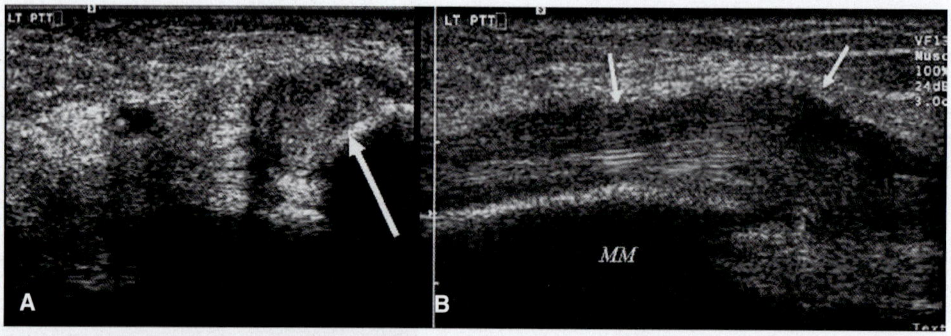

FIGURE 7.21 Tendon abnormalities should be imaged in two planes, as indicated in this case of posterior tibial tendinosis. Although short-axis views are sensitive to subtle tendinosis, the full extent of the tendinopathy, as well as its relationship to other anatomic landmarks, is better appreciated in long axis. **A:** In this case, the short-axis view shows intrasubstance clefts, enlargement, and indistinct margins of the tendon (*arrow*). **B:** The extent of the abnormality (*arrows*) can be better appreciated in the longitudinal image as the tendon passes over the medial malleolus (MM).

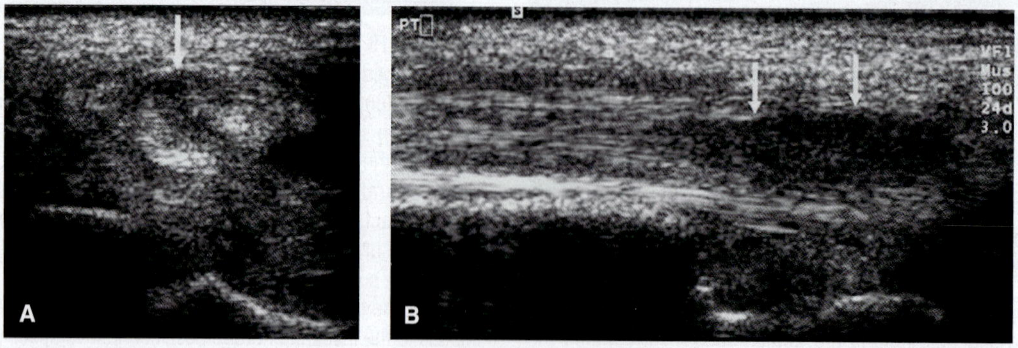

FIGURE 7.22 Transverse **(A)** and longitudinal **(B)** images of the posterior tibial tendon showing a full-thickness longitudinal split tear. This appears as an obliquely oriented hypoechoic defect within the tendon substance (*arrows*). The length of the tear is appreciated on the long-axis view **(B)**. (From Adler R, Sofka CM, Positano RG. *Atlas of Foot and Ankle Sonography.* Philadelphia, PA: Lippincott Williams & Wilkins; 2004:58.)

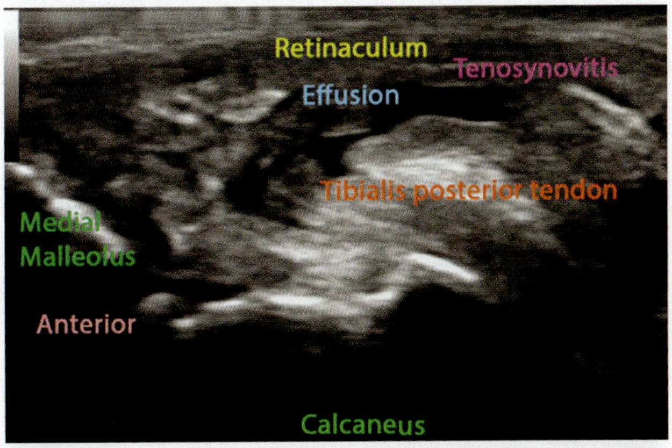

FIGURE 7.23 Ultrasound image demonstrating acute tenosynovitis of the tibialis posterior tendon in a patient who was running on sand.

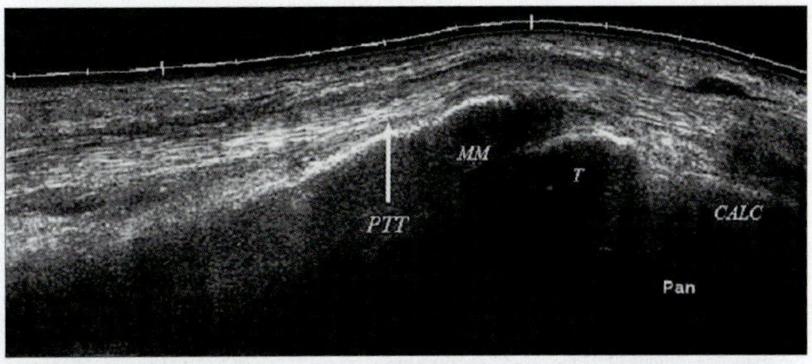

FIGURE 7.25 Extended field of view imaging allows depiction of the full extent of abnormality. This longitudinal extended field of view image along the medial aspect of the ankle in a patient with posterior tibial tendinosis (PTT) demonstrates the extent of the abnormal tendon segment, the relationship between the tendon and the adjacent osseous structures: medial malleolus (MM), talus (T), and calcaneus (CALC). Note the focal distention of the distal tendon sheath **(right)**. (From Adler R, Sofka CM, Positano RG. *Atlas of Foot and Ankle Sonography*. Philadelphia, PA: Lippincott Williams & Wilkins; 2004:60.)

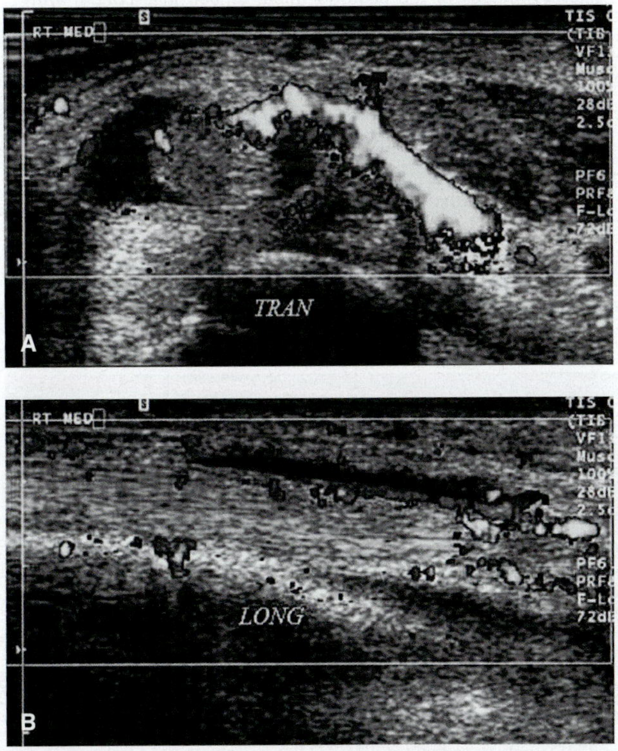

FIGURE 7.24 Transverse **(A)** and longitudinal **(B)** ultrasound images of the posterior tibial tendon demonstrating fluid surrounding the tendon, consistent with a tendon sheath effusion. Of note, the application of power Doppler demonstrates increased vascularity, consistent with posterior tibial tenosynovitis. (From Adler R, Sofka CM, Positano RG. *Atlas of Foot and Ankle Sonography*. Philadelphia, PA: Lippincott Williams & Wilkins; 2004:59.)

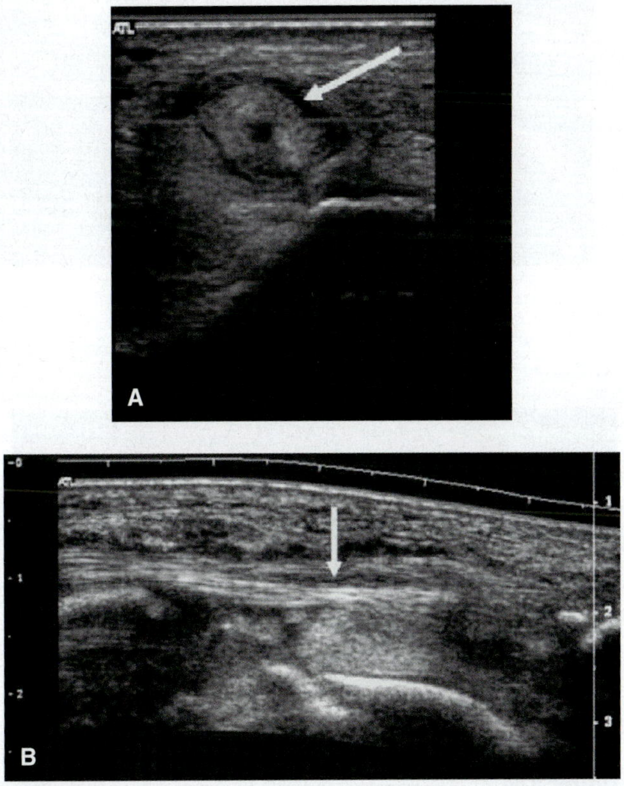

FIGURE 7.26 Short-axis **(A)** and extended field of view longitudinal **(B)** images of the posterior tibial tendon demonstrating tendinosis with a central split within the substance of the tendon. There is nodal thickening of the tendon sheath over the entire visualized segment of the tendon. (From Adler R, Sofka CM, Positano RG. *Atlas of Foot and Ankle Sonography*. Philadelphia, PA: Lippincott Williams & Wilkins; 2004:60.)

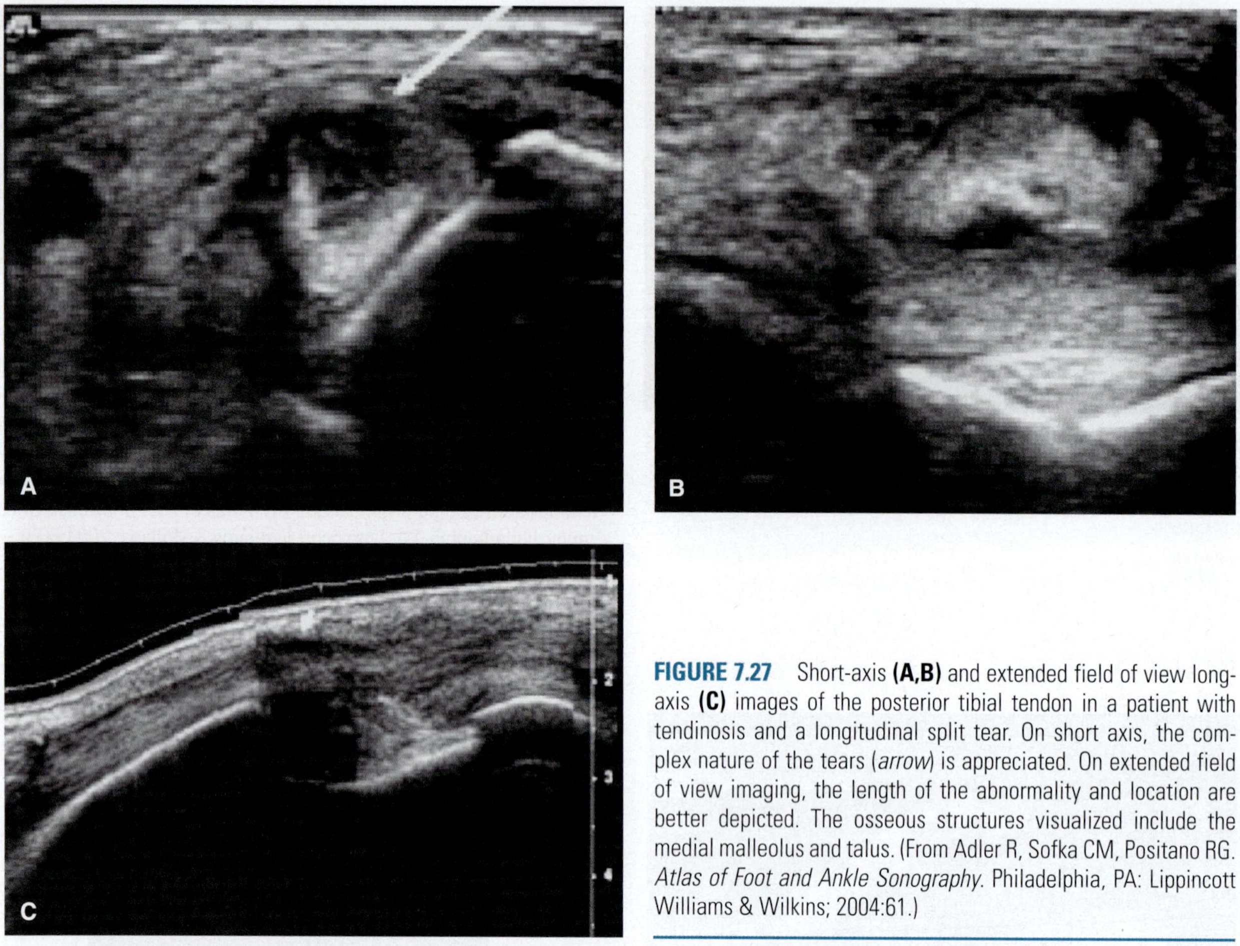

FIGURE 7.27 Short-axis **(A,B)** and extended field of view long-axis **(C)** images of the posterior tibial tendon in a patient with tendinosis and a longitudinal split tear. On short axis, the complex nature of the tears (*arrow*) is appreciated. On extended field of view imaging, the length of the abnormality and location are better depicted. The osseous structures visualized include the medial malleolus and talus. (From Adler R, Sofka CM, Positano RG. *Atlas of Foot and Ankle Sonography*. Philadelphia, PA: Lippincott Williams & Wilkins; 2004:61.)

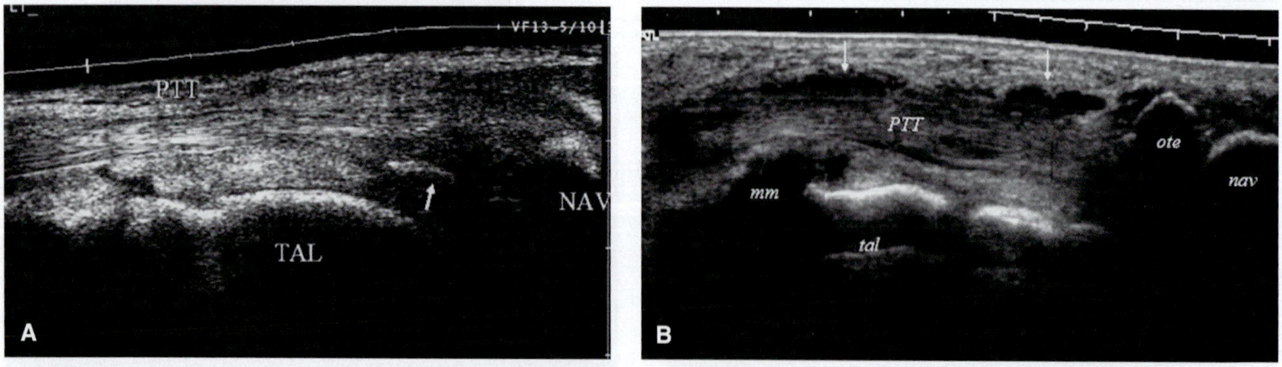

FIGURE 7.28 Longitudinal extended field of view ultrasound images of the distal posterior tibial tendon (PTT) demonstrate the tendon insertion onto the tarsal navicular. It is not uncommon for an intratendinous ossicle to be present at the insertion site of the posterior tibial tendon. These demonstrate significant variability. It is important to recognize these are normal variants. **A:** A thin ossicle is evident along the deep surface of the tendon (*arrow*) just proximal to its insertion (nav). The talus (tal) is labeled. **B:** A much larger ossicle (os tibiale externum [ote]) is present. Large ossicles may show varying degrees of fibrous or bony union with the adjacent navicular bone (nav), resulting in localized pain. There is moderate degeneration of the distal aspect of the posterior tibial tendon (PTT) with loculated fluid in the tendon sheath (*arrows*). mm, medial malleolus. (From Adler R, Sofka CM, Positano RG. *Atlas of Foot and Ankle Sonography*. Philadelphia, PA: Lippincott Williams & Wilkins; 2004:63.)

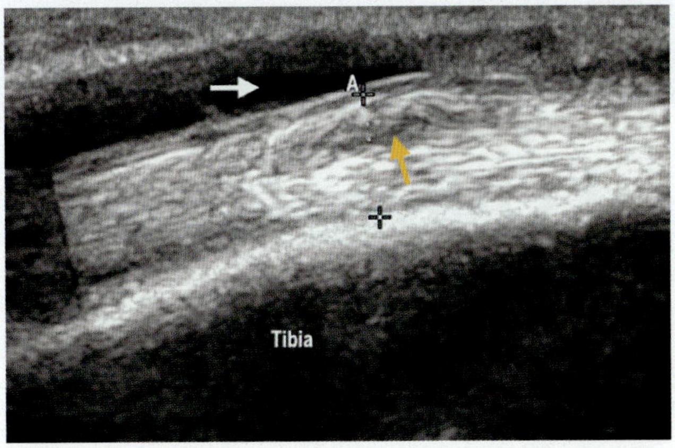

FIGURE 7.29 Longitudinal ultrasound image of the left involved tibialis posterior tendon, taken 2 cm proximal to the tip of the medial malleolus, demonstrated gross tendon enlargement (6.8-mm distance between the cursors) and a hypoechoic focus within the tendon (*yellow arrow*) representing advanced focal degeneration or partial tear. There is also some increased thickening of the paratenon with some surrounding fluid suggestive of inflammation (*white arrow*). (From Neville C, Meyers K, Hojnowski L. Ultrasound assessment of the tibialis posterior tendon. *J Orthopaed Sports Phys Ther* 2010;40(10):667.)

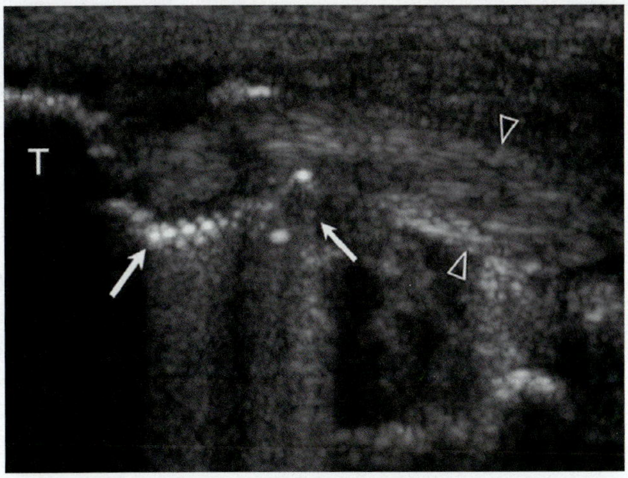

FIGURE 7.31 Screw impingement of posterior tibial tendon. Ultrasound image longitudinal to the posterior tibial tendon (*arrowheads*) shows impingement from screw (*arrows*). Left side of the image is proximal relative to tendon. T, tibia. (From Femino JE, Jacobson JA, Craig CL, et al. Dynamic ultrasound of the foot and ankle: adult and pediatric applications. *Techn Foot Ankle Surg* 2007;6(1):50–61.)

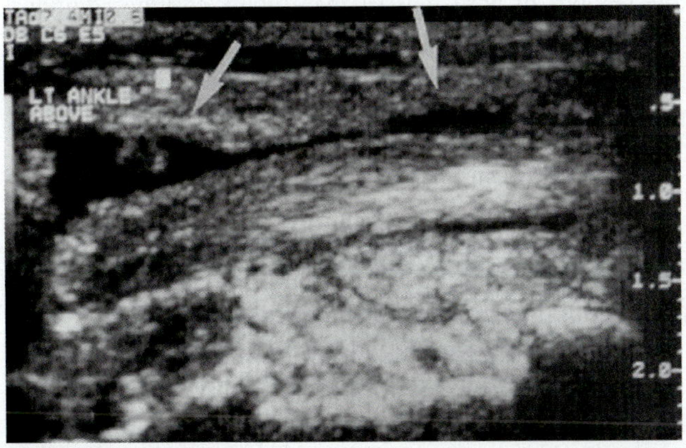

FIGURE 7.30 Longitudinal ultrasound image of the tibialis posterior tendon. Note the fusiform swelling (*arrows*) at the site of the tear, with disruption of the parallelism and increased hypoechoic regions. Also noted is the increased hypoechoic fluid and debris within the sheath. (From Rockett MS, Waitches G, Sudakoff G, et al. Use of ultrasonography versus magnetic resonance imaging for tendon abnormalities around the ankle. *Foot Ankle Intl* 1998;19(9):604–612.)

Suggested Readings

Bowring B, Chockalingam N. Conservative treatment of tibialis posterior tendon dysfunction–a review. *Foot (Edinb)* 2010;20(1):18–26.

Edwards MR, Jack C, Singh SK. Tibialis posterior dysfunction. *Curr Orthop* 2008; 22(3):185–192.

Shibuya N, Ramanujam CL, Garcia GM. Association of tibialis posterior tendon pathology with other radiographic findings in the foot. *J Foot Ankle Surg* 2008;47(6):546–553.

Waldman SD. Injection technique for posterior tibialis tendinitis. In: *Atlas of Pain Management Injection Techniques.* 3rd ed. Philadelphia, PA: Saunders; 2012: 662–663.

Waldman SD. Posterior tibialis tendinitis. In: *Pain Review.* Philadelphia, PA: Saunders; 2009:325.

Waldman SD, Campbell RSD. Posterior tibialis tendinitis. In: *Atlas of Uncommon Pain Syndromes.* 2nd ed. Philadelphia, PA: Saunders; 2009:300–304.

Waldman SD, Campbell RSD. Posterior tibialis tendon rupture. In: *Imaging of Pain.* Philadelphia, PA: Saunders; 2011:435–436.

CHAPTER 8

Peroneal Tendinitis and Other Abnormalities of the Peroneus Longus and Brevis Tendons

ANATOMIC CONSIDERATIONS

The peroneus longus and brevis muscles lie within the lateral peroneal compartment and function to help stabilize the ankle as well as plantarflex the foot at the ankle and evert the foot at the subtalar and transverse tarsal joints (Fig. 8.1). The peroneus longus muscle (which is also known as the fibularis longus muscle) finds its origin on the head and upper body of the fibula as well as the intermuscular septum and inserts via a strong tendon on the plantar side of the cuneiform bone and the first metatarsal (Fig. 8.2). The distal tendon of the peroneus longus muscle passes behind the lateral malleolus, lying within a groove along with the distal tendon of the peroneus brevis muscle (Fig. 8.3). The distal tendon of the peroneus longus muscle then passes beneath the superior fibular retinaculum extending obliquely across the lateral aspect of the calcaneus below the peroneal tubercle (which is also known as the trochlear process of the calcaneus) and inferior to the distal tendon of the peroneus brevis muscle. Crossing the lateral aspect of the cuneiform bone, the tendon then passes beneath peroneus brevis tendon and the cuneiform within a groove to pass obliquely across the sole of the foot to insert into the lateral aspect of the first metatarsal and the lateral side of the medial cuneiform bone (Figs. 8.4 and 8.5). It is at the two points where the tendon changes direction that it is most susceptible to the development of tendinitis.

The peroneus brevis muscle (which is also known as the fibularis brevis muscle) finds its origin more distally on the fibula and inserts at the tuberosity of the fifth metatarsal (Fig. 8.2). The muscle then passes inferiorly in front of and along with the peroneus longus muscle, with the distal tendon of the peroneus brevis muscle passing behind the lateral malleolus to run above the peroneal tubercle on the lateral side of the calcaneus to insert into the lateral side of the base of the fifth metatarsal bone (Figs. 8.3 to 8.5). Both peroneal muscles are supplied by the peroneal nerve.

CLINICAL CORRELATES

Peroneal tendinitis is a clinical syndrome characterized by sharp, constant, and severe ankle pain that is localized behind and just distal to the lateral malleolus. This painful condition is often seen as a result of acute inversion injuries to the ankle although it is also seen with overuse or misuse of the ankle and foot, as seen with repeated jumping and side-to-side movements required when playing soccer, basketball, and football. The problem is also seen in long distance running with improper shoes or from running on soft or uneven surfaces. The pain of peroneal tendinitis will be exacerbated with loading of the foot, especially with toe walking. With injury to the superior peroneal retinaculum, the tendons of both muscles may sublux creating additional ankle instability and a snapping sensation. With rupture of the tendons, pain and decreased strength is noted, especially with lateral cutting movements and push off portion of walking. If the acute insult to the tendons does not heal, the pain and functional disability can become chronic, with the pain waxing and waning depending on the patient's level of activity.

Patients suffering from peroneal tendinitis will often splint the inflamed peroneal tendon by adopting an antalgic gait to avoid using the affected tendon. This dysfunctional gait may cause a secondary bursitis and tendinitis around the foot and ankle which may serve to confuse the clinical picture and further increase the patient's pain and disability. Pain on palpation of the peroneal tendon as it passes behind the lateral malleolus is a consistent finding in patients with peroneal tendinitis as is exacerbation of pain with active resisted eversion and toe walking (Fig. 8.6). The lateral aspect of the ankle may feel hot and appear swollen, which may be misdiagnosed as superficial thrombophlebitis or cellulitis. Patients suffering from peroneal tendinitis will also often complain that it feels like their shoes are rubbing the outside of their ankles raw, although on examination the skin appears normal. A creaking or grating sensation may be palpated when passively everting and inverting the ankle. Untreated, peroneal tendinitis will result in increasing pain, functional disability and calcium deposition around the tendon, which makes subsequent treatment more difficult. Continued trauma to the inflamed tendon ultimately may result in tendon tears and rupture (Figs. 8.7 to 8.9). Rupture of the peroneal tendon will result if disruption of the normal architecture of the tendon leads to alteration of the patient's gait.

Plain radiographs are indicated in all patients who present with lateral ankle pain and foot pain. In the pres-

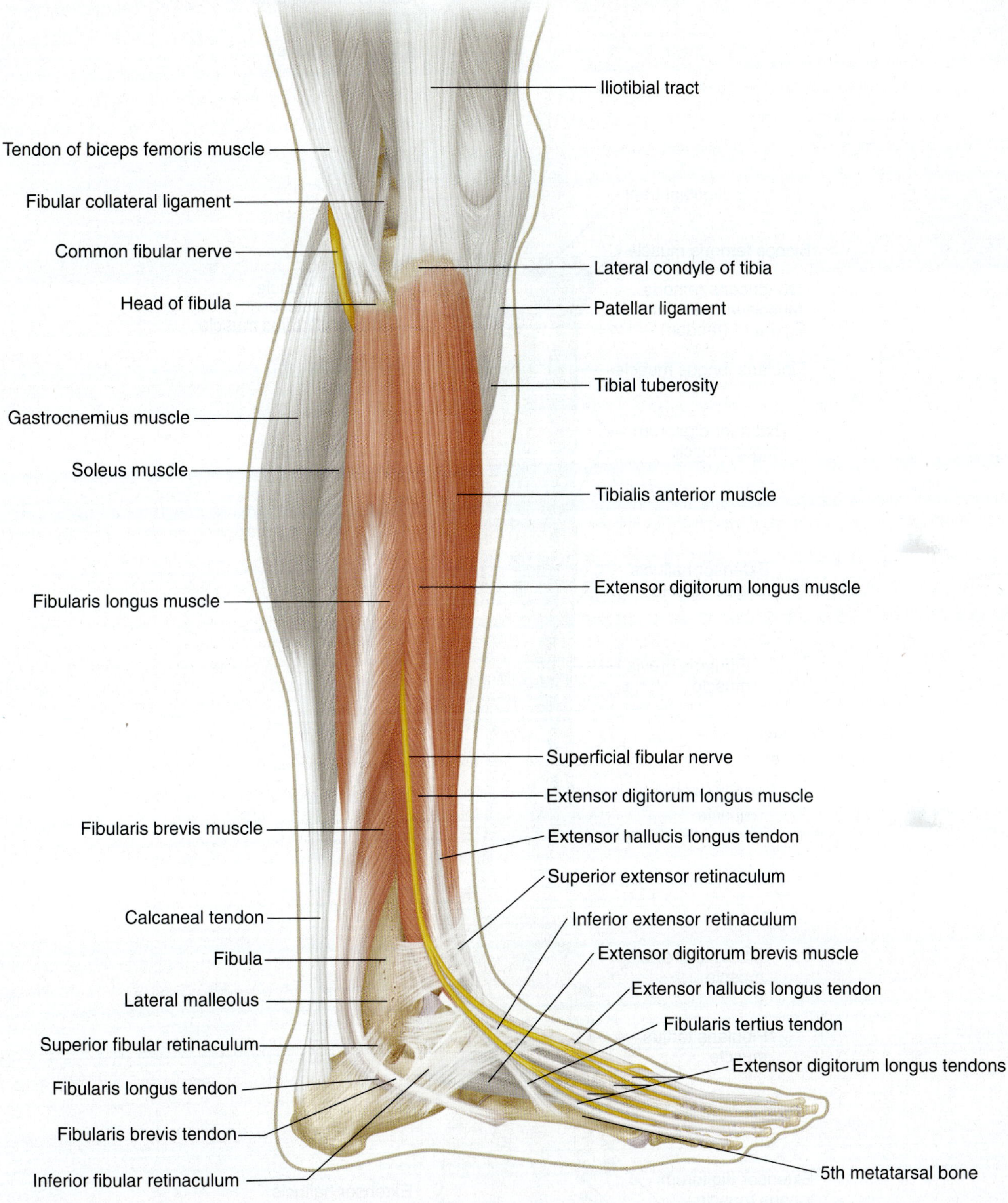

FIGURE 8.1 The anatomy of the peroneus longus and brevis muscles. (From Tank PW, Gest TR. The lower limb. In: *Lippincott Williams & Wilkins Atlas of Anatomy*. Philadelphia, PA: Lippincott Williams & Wilkins; 2009:122.)

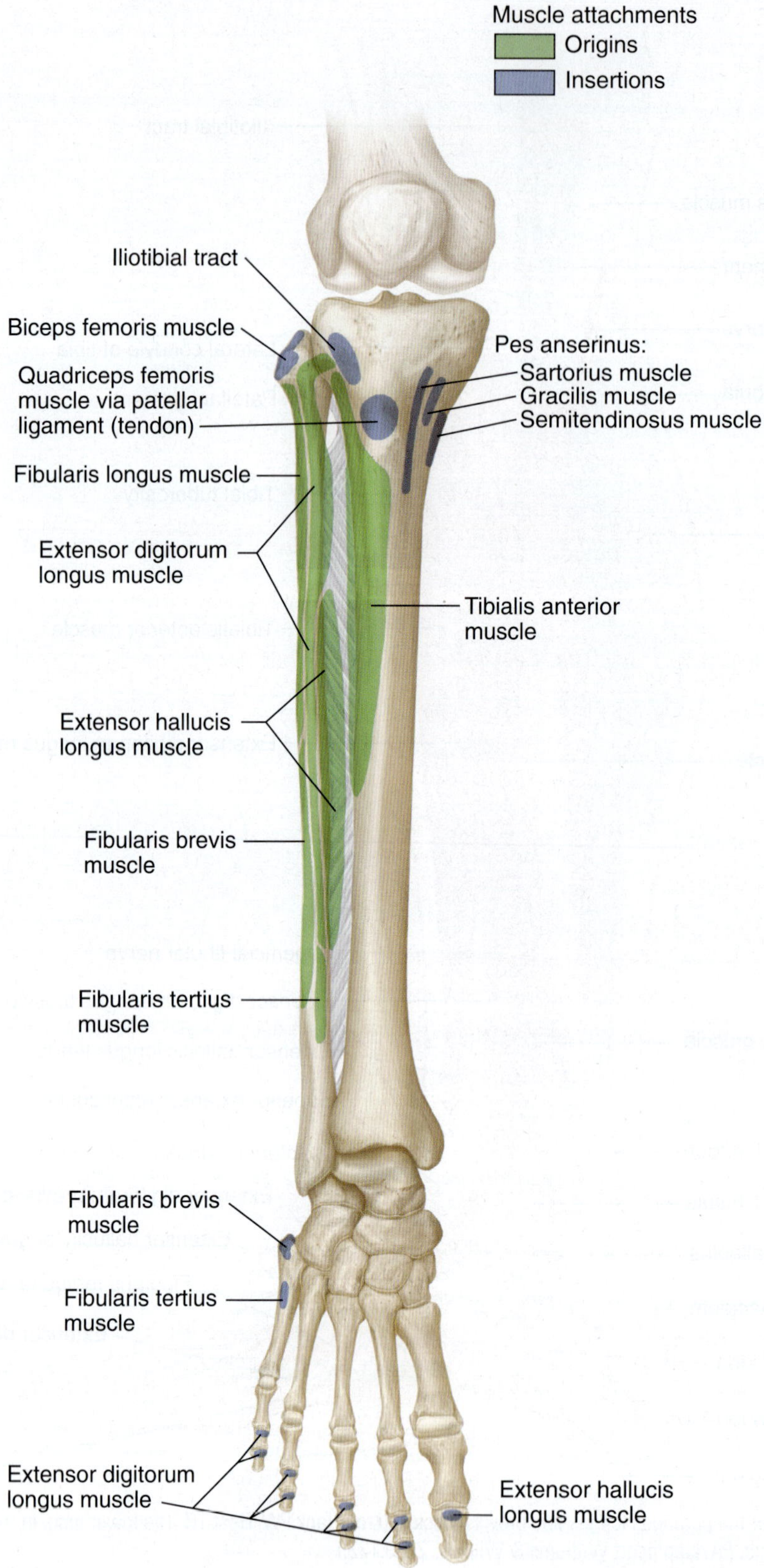

FIGURE 8.2 The peroneus longus muscle (which is also known as the fibularis longus muscle) finds its origin on the head and upper body of the fibula as well as the intermuscular septum and inserts via a strong tendon on the plantar side of the cuneiform bone and the first metatarsal. The peroneus brevis muscle (which is also known as the fibularis brevis muscle) finds its origin more distally on the fibula and inserts at the tuberosity of the fifth metatarsal. (From Tank PW, Gest TR. The lower limb. In: *Lippincott Williams & Wilkins Atlas of Anatomy.* Philadelphia, PA: Lippincott Williams & Wilkins; 2009:116.)

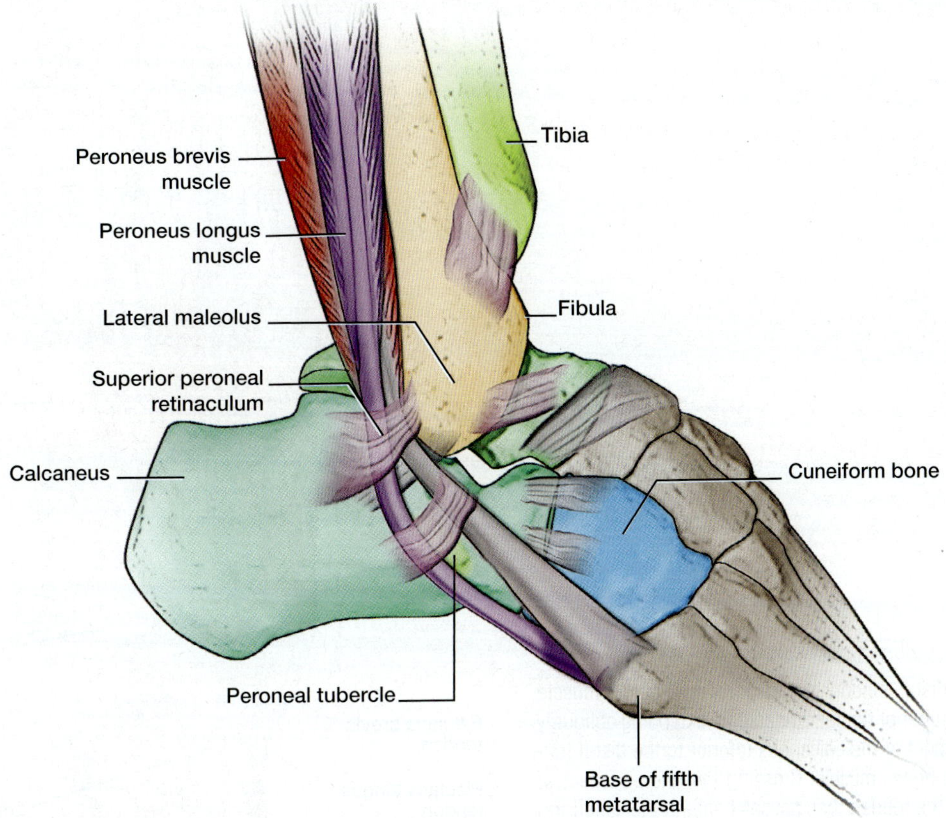

FIGURE 8.3 The peroneus longus and brevis tendons are susceptible to the development of tendinitis as they pass behind the lateral malleolus. The peroneus longus tendon is also suceptible to the development of tendinitis at the point where it turns medially to pass beneath the peroneus brevis tendon.

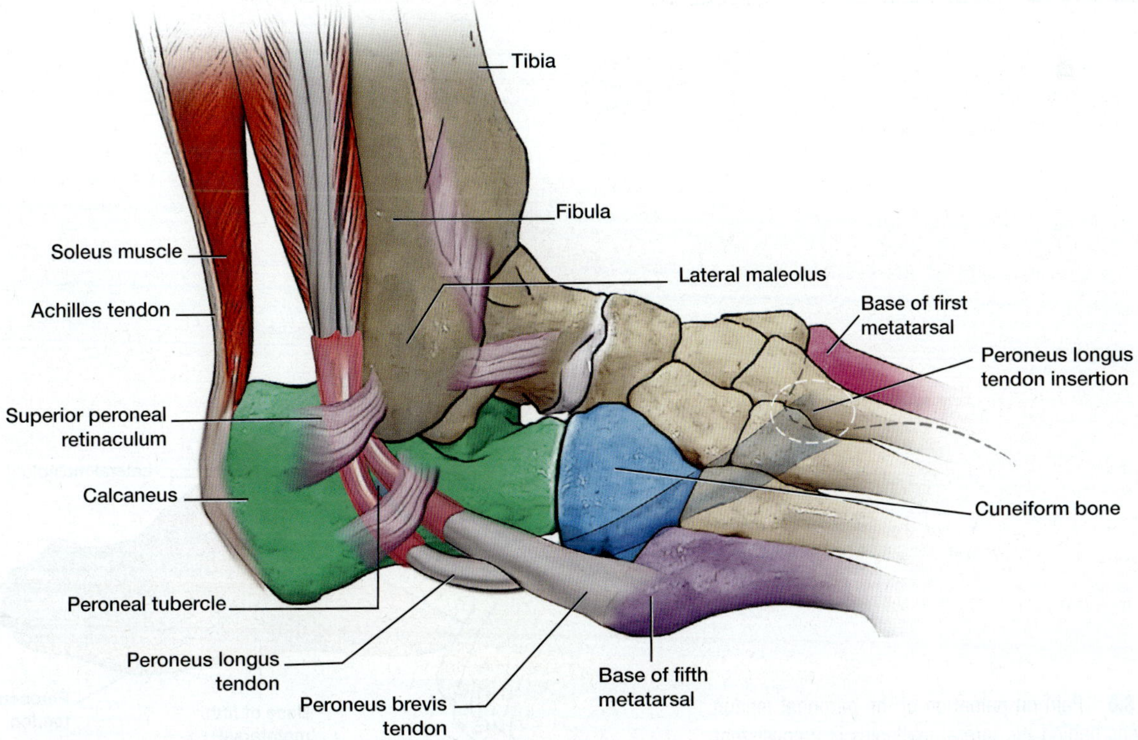

FIGURE 8.4 The peroneus longus and brevis tendons.

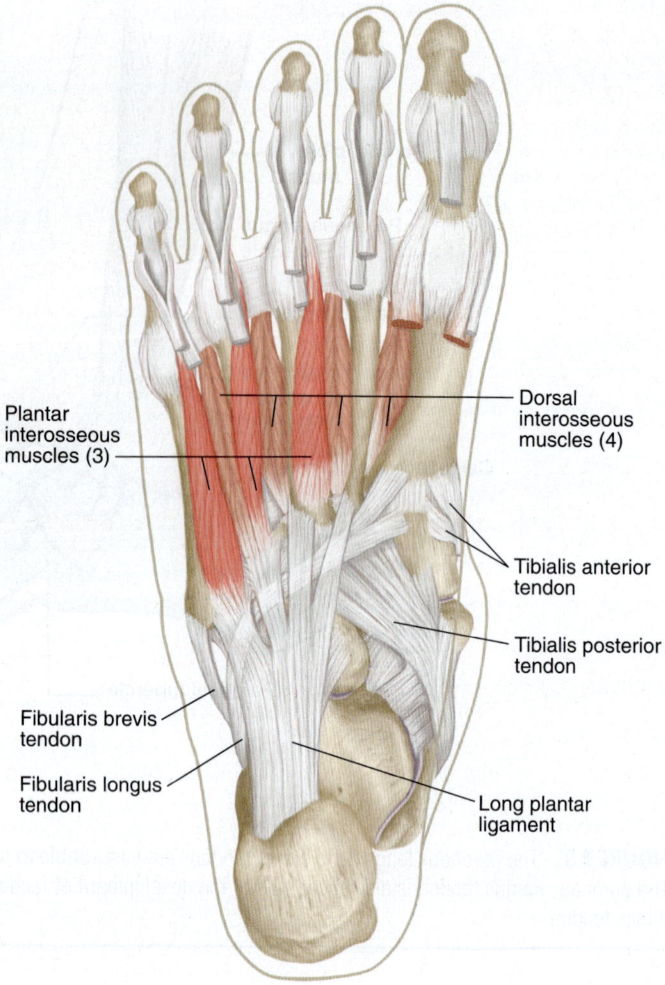

FIGURE 8.5 The distal tendon of the peroneus longus muscle passes beneath the superior fibular retinaculum extending obliquely across the lateral aspect of the calcaneus inferior to the distal tendon of the peroneus brevis muscle. Crossing the lateral aspect of the cuneiform bone, the tendon then passes beneath the cuneiform within a groove to pass obliquely across the sole of the foot to insert into the lateral aspect of the first metatarsal and the lateral side of the medial cuneiform bone. (From Tank PW, Gest TR. The lower limb. In: *Lippincott Williams & Wilkins Atlas of Anatomy*. Philadelphia, PA: Lippincott Williams & Wilkins; 2009:138.)

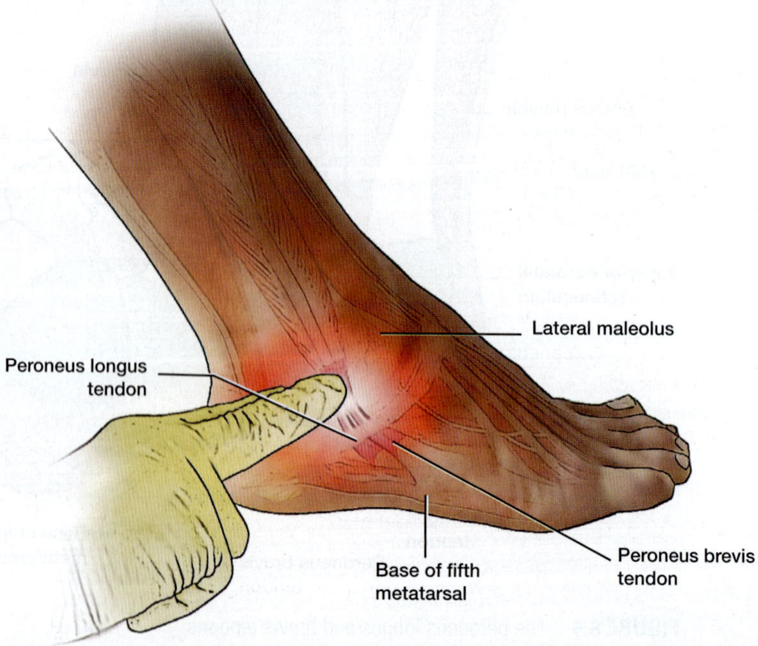

FIGURE 8.6 Pain on palpation of the peroneal tendon as it passes behind the lateral malleolus is a consistent finding in patients with peroneal tendinitis.

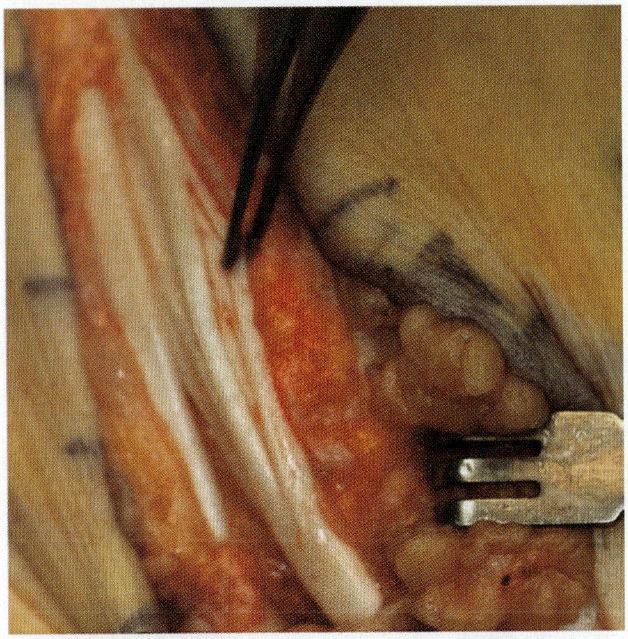

FIGURE 8.7 Longitudinal tear of peroneus brevis. (From Femino JE, Jacobson JA, Craig CL, et al. Dynamic ultrasound of the foot and ankle: Adult and pediatric applications. *Techn Foot Ankle Surg* 2007;6(1): 50–61.)

ence of trauma, a careful search for a Jones fracture of the base of the fifth metatarsal is indicated (Fig. 8.10). Based on the patient's clinical presentation, additional testing may be indicated, including complete blood cell count, sedimentation rate, and antinuclear antibody testing. MRI and/or ultrasound imaging of the ankle is indicated if peroneal tendinitis, rupture, fracture, or joint instability is suggested. Radionuclide bone scanning is useful to identify stress fractures of the bones of the ankle not seen on plain radiographs.

ULTRASOUND TECHNIQUE

Ultrasound evaluation of the peroneus longus and brevis tendons at the ankle can be carried out by placing the patient in the lateral curled up position with the affected leg positioned up on a folded blanket. A linear high frequency ultrasound transducer is placed in a transverse plane approximately just above and behind the lateral malleolus of the ankle and an ultrasound survey scan is taken (Fig. 8.11). The peroneal tendons can be seen lying adjacent to the lateral malleolus (Fig. 8.12). The tendon of the peroneus longus muscle will be seen to course lateral to the tendon of the peroneus brevis muscle. The ultrasound transducer is slowly moved inferiorly and the flattened appearing peroneus brevis tendon can be seen to lie anteromedial to the peroneus longus tendon (Fig. 8.13). Moving inferiorly, the peroneus brevis tendon will move into a position above the peroneus longus tendon. At the inframalleolar region, the tendons diverge as the peroneus brevis tendon passes above the peroneal tubercle of the calcaneus and the peroneus longus tendon passes below the peroneal tubercle of the calcaneus (Fig. 8.14). When the peroneal tendons are identified on ultrasound imaging, the tendons are evaluated for fluid, extrinsic compression, tendinosis, tendinitis, tears, and rupture (Figs. 8.15 to 8.24). Evaluation of the peroneal retinaculum for tears should then be carried out. Ultrasound

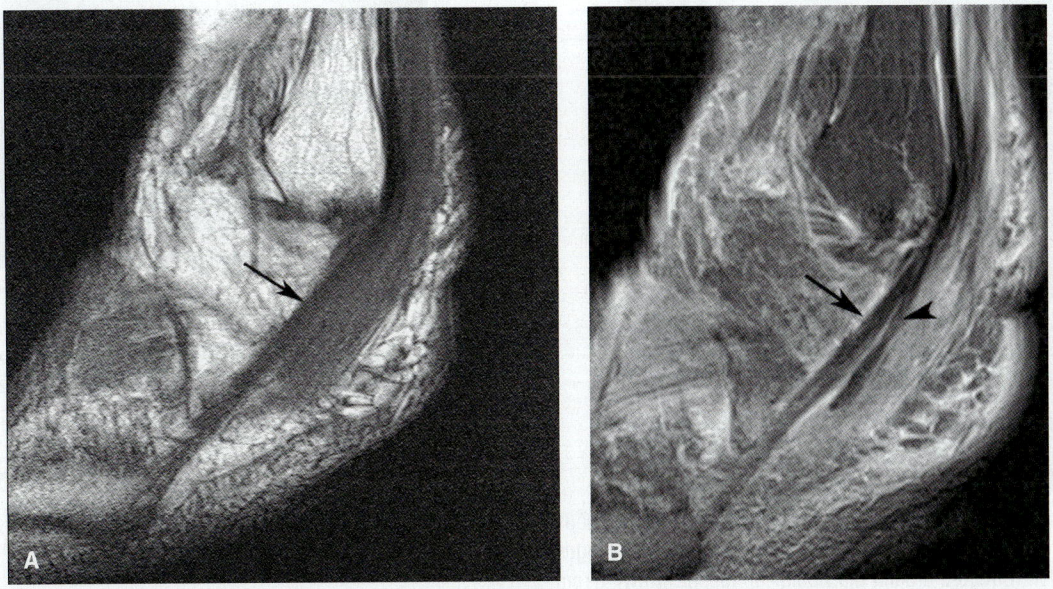

FIGURE 8.8 Acute high-grade peroneus longus tear. Sagittal T1- **(A)** and fast spin echo fat-suppressed T2-weighted **(B)** and an axial proton density weighted (*continued*)

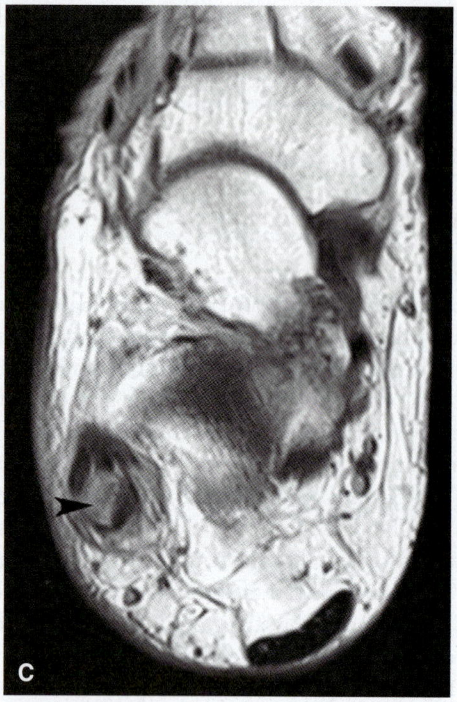

FIGURE 8.8 (*Continued*) **(C)** images demonstrating the peroneus brevis (*arrow* in **A** and **B**) and a thin peroneus longus (*arrowhead* in **B** and **C**) due to a high-grade tear. (From Berquist TH. Foot, ankle, and calf. In: *MRI of the Musculoskeletal System*. 6th ed. Philadelphia, PA: Lippincott Williams & Wilkins; 2013:517.)

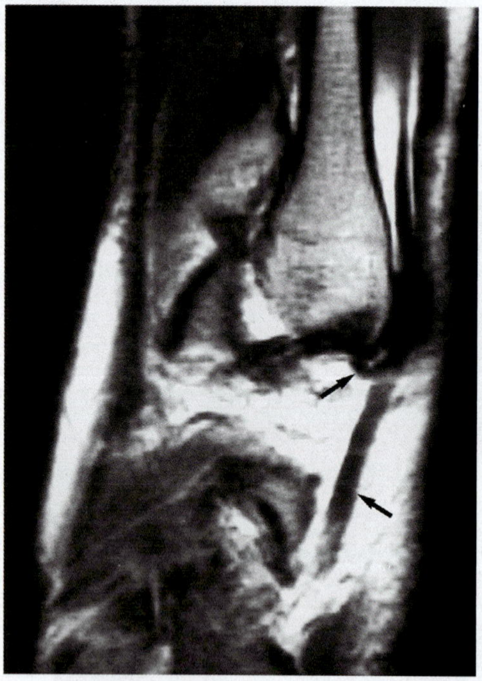

FIGURE 8.9 Sagittal T1-weighted image show a normal peroneus brevis (lower *arrow*) and complete disruption of the peroneus longus with the tendon retracted around the fibular tip (upper *arrow*). (From Berquist TH. Foot, ankle, and calf. In: *MRI of the Musculoskeletal System*. 6th ed. Philadelphia, PA: Lippincott Williams & Wilkins; 2013:516.)

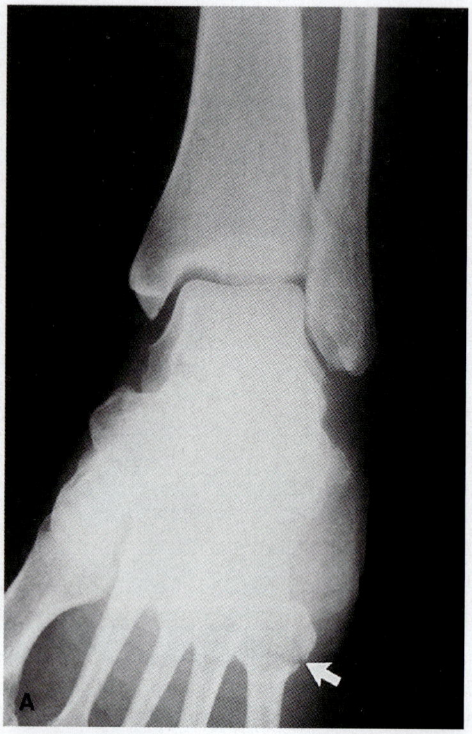

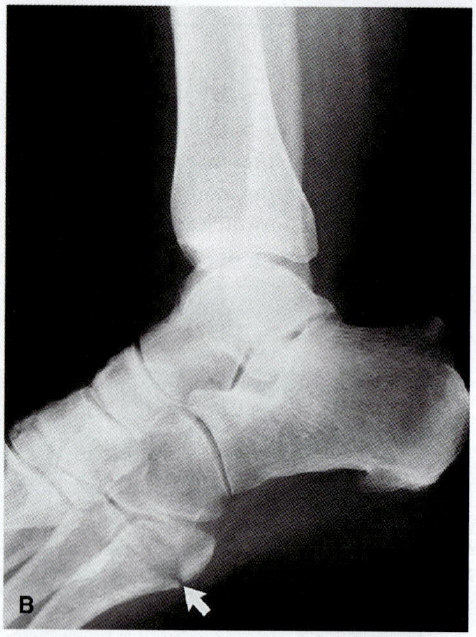

FIGURE 8.10 Jones fracture (dancers fracture): base of the fifth metatarsal. **A:** AP ankle. **B:** Lateral ankle. Note the transverse fracture line at the base of the fifth metatarsal (*arrows*). (From Rowe LJ, Yochum TR, Maola CJ. Trauma. In: *Yochum and Rowes' Essentials of Skeletal Radiology*. 3rd ed. Vol. 1. Philadelphia, PA: Lippincott Williams & Wilkins; 2005.)

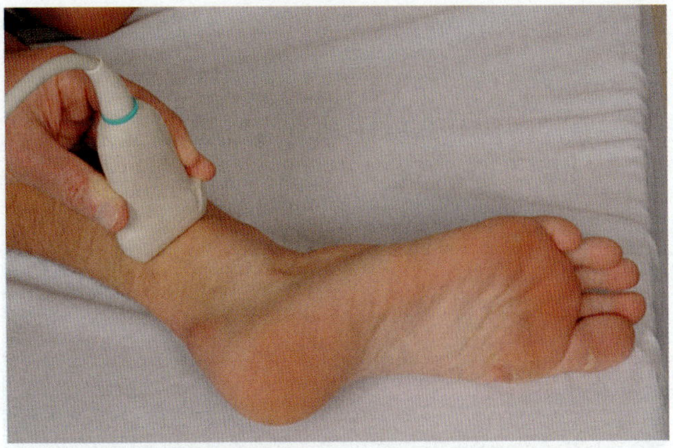

FIGURE 8.11 Proper transverse position of the ultrasound transducer for ultrasound evaluation of the peroneus longus and brevis tendons.

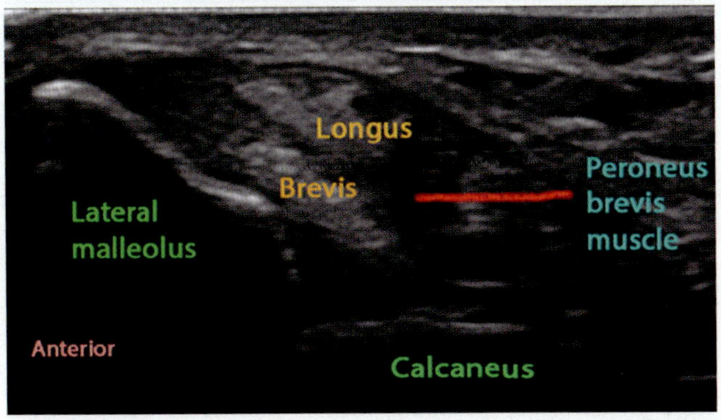

FIGURE 8.12 Transverse ultrasound image of the lateral ankle demonstrating the relationship of the peroneus longus and brevis tendons to the lateral malleolus.

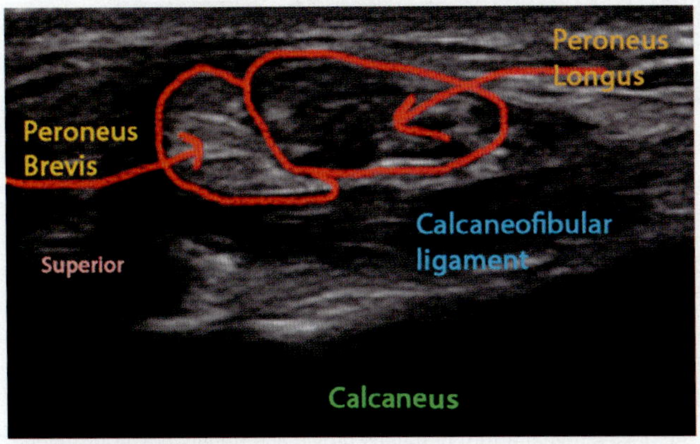

FIGURE 8.13 Transverse ultrasound image at the inferior aspect of lateral malleolus demonstrating the relative positions of the peroneus longus and brevis tendons.

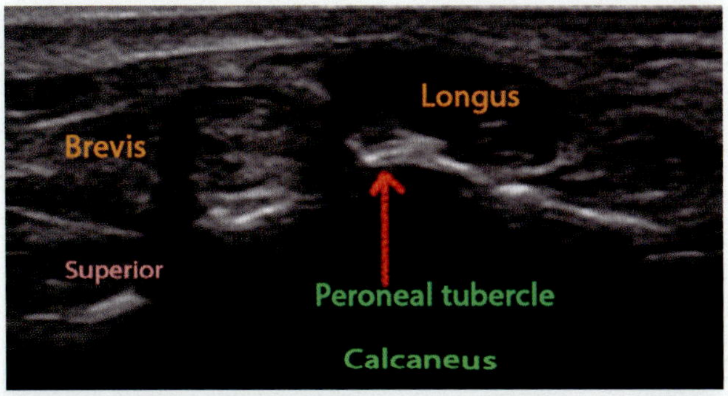

FIGURE 8.14 Transverse ultrasound image demonstrating the separation of the peroneus longus and brevis tendons by the peroneal tubercle of the calcaneus to the lateral malleolus.

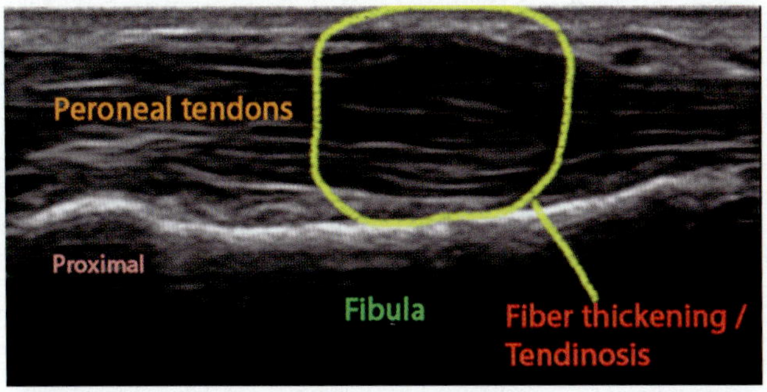

FIGURE 8.15 Peroneal tendinosis. Longitudinal ultrasound image demonstrating thickening of the fibers of the peroneal tendons and loss of normal fibular architecture consistent with tendinosis.

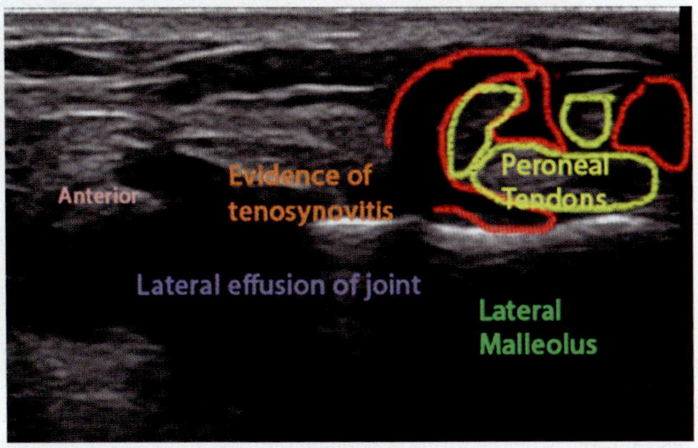

FIGURE 8.16 Peroneal tenosynovitis. Note the effusion surrounding the tendons and within the lateral ankle joint.

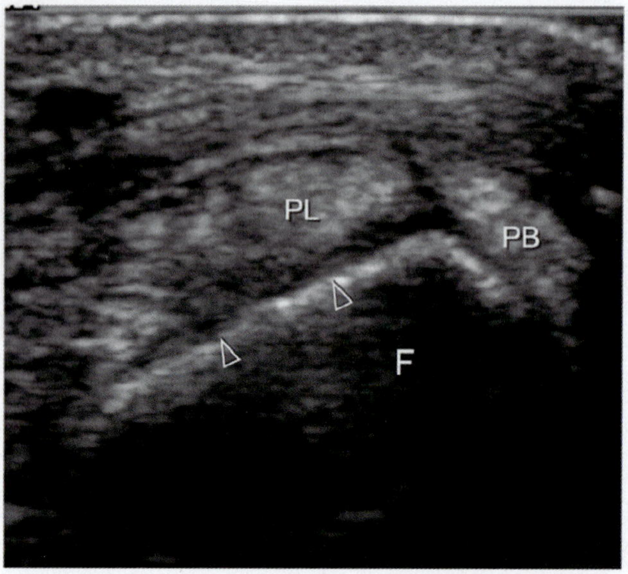

FIGURE 8.17 Peroneus brevis dislocation. Sonogram transverse to the peroneus longus tendon shows anterior dislocation of the peroneus brevis (PB) from the posterior fibula (*arrowheads*). Left side of the image is posterior. F, fibula; PL, peroneus longus tendon. (From Femino JE, Jacobson JA, Craig CL, et al. Dynamic ultrasound of the foot and ankle: Adult and pediatric applications. *Techn Foot Ankle Surg* 2007;6(1):50–61.)

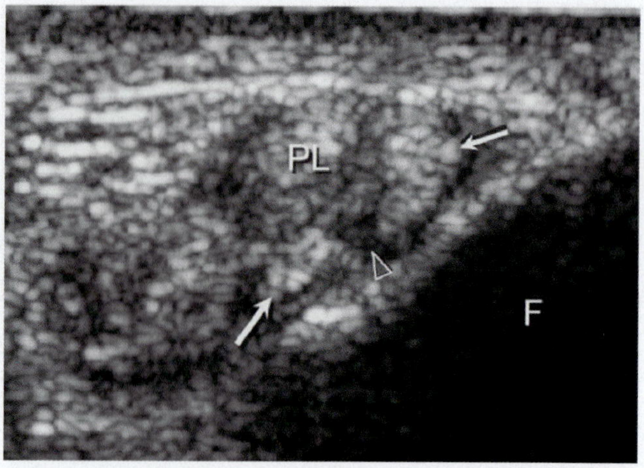

FIGURE 8.18 Peroneus brevis longitudinal split. Sonogram transverse to the peroneus longus tendon (PL) shows longitudinal split (*arrowhead*) of peroneus brevis tendon into two segments (*arrows*). Left side of the image is posterior. F, fibula. (From Femino JE, Jacobson JA, Craig CL, et al. Dynamic ultrasound of the foot and ankle: Adult and pediatric applications. *Techn Foot Ankle Surg* 2007;6(1):50–61.)

imaging is also useful in assessing the effect of implantable hardware and foreign bodies on surrounding structures (Figs. 8.25 to 8.27).

CLINICAL PEARLS

Bursitis and arthritis of the ankle and foot may coexist with peroneal tendinitis and may contribute to the patient's pain symptoms. It is important to diagnose peroneal tendonitis in a timely manner and to identify the activity and/or pathology responsible for its evolution and then initiate prompt treatment to avoid tendon rupture. Approximately 7% of patients have an accessory peroneus muscle known as the peroneus quartus muscle which lies adjacent to the peroneus longus and brevis tendons on the supramalleolar region (Fig. 8.28). This muscle and its attachments are also susceptible to trauma and may confuse the diagnosis (Fig. 8.29).

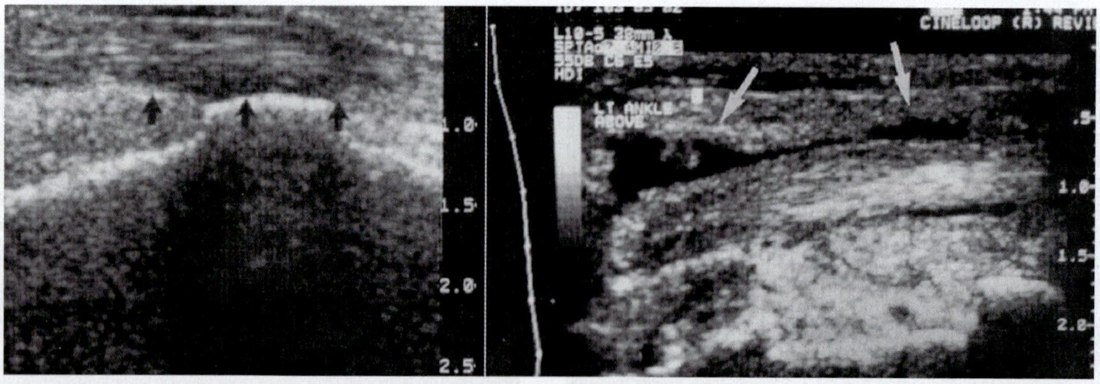

FIGURE 8.19 Longitudinal ultrasound images of two patients. Symptomatic ankles reveal a torn peroneus brevis and tibialis posterior tendon, respectively. Note the fusiform swelling (*arrows*) at the site of the tear, with disruption of the parallelism and increased hypoechoic regions. Also noted is the increased hypoechoic fluid and debris within the sheath. (From Rockett MS, Waitches G, Sudakoff G, et al. Use of ultrasonography versus magnetic resonance imaging for tendon abnormalities around the ankle. *Foot Ankle Int* 1998;19(9):604–612.)

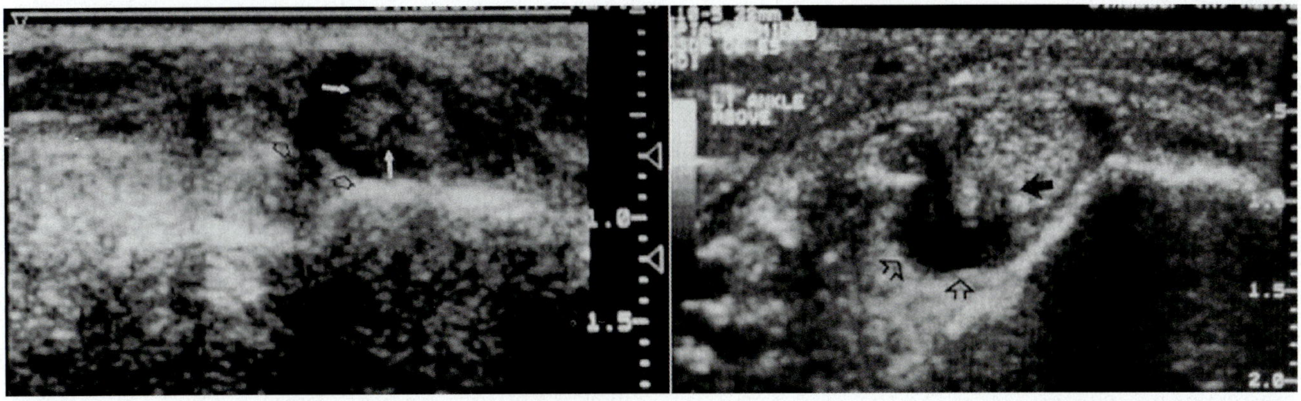

FIGURE 8.20 Transverse ultrasound images of the peroneus longus and brevis tendons. Demonstrated in both tendons is a hypoechoic line that extends from the periphery into the tendon substance (*solid arrows*). The tendons are again surrounded by fluid with echoic debris (*open arrows*). (From Rockett MS, Waitches G, Sudakoff G, et al. Use of ultrasonography versus magnetic resonance imaging for tendon abnormalities around the ankle. *Foot Ankle Int* 1998;19(9):604–612.)

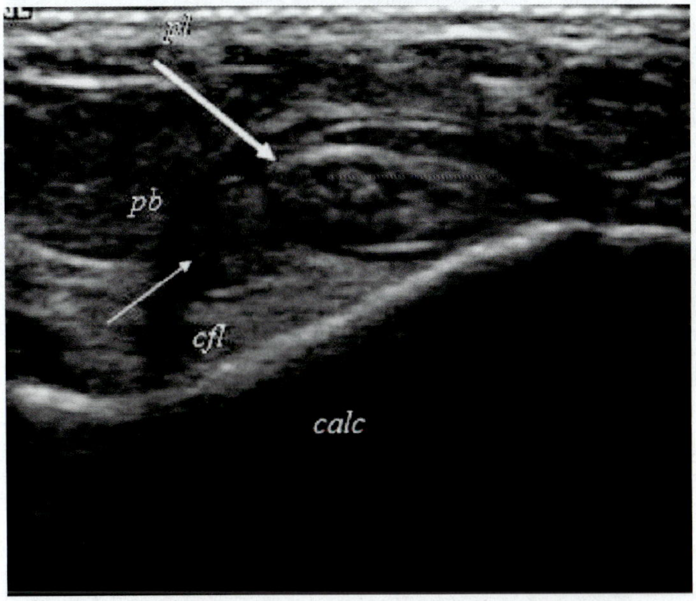

FIGURE 8.21 Subtle areas of tendinosis are best appreciated in short axis as illustrated in this image of the peroneal tendons (labeled), which was obtained at the level of the calcaneofibular ligament (cfl). The peroneus brevis (pb) is mildly inhomogeneous, and the peroneus longus (pl) contains thin intrasubstance hypoechoic clefts. The calcaneus (calc) is indicated. (From Adler R, Sofka CM, Positano RG. *Atlas of Foot and Ankle Sonography.* Philadelphia, PA: Lippincott Williams & Wilkins; 2004.)

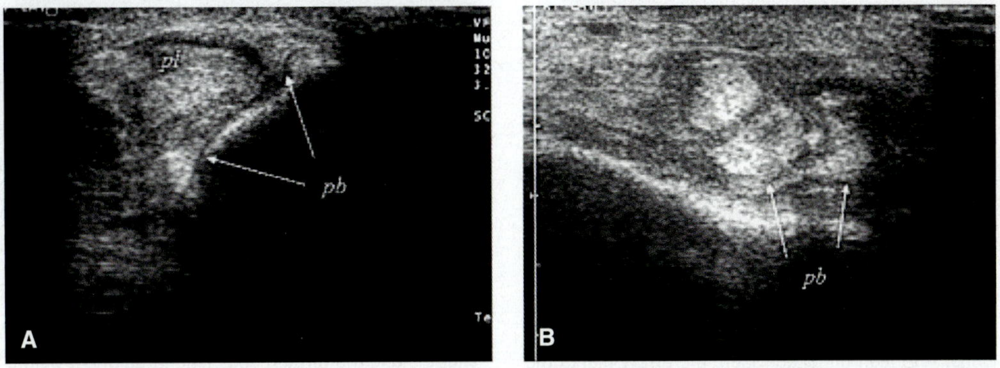

FIGURE 8.22 Short-axis views of the peroneal tendons at the level of the lateral peroneal sulcus **(A)** and calcaneofibular ligament **(B)**. Both tendons are enlarged, containing longitudinal split tears. There is a wide separation of the peroneus brevis fragments (*arrows*) in **(A)**, which are in closer apposition distally **(B)**. (From Adler R, Sofka CM, Positano RG. *Atlas of Foot and Ankle Sonography.* Philadelphia, PA: Lippincott Williams & Wilkins; 2004.)

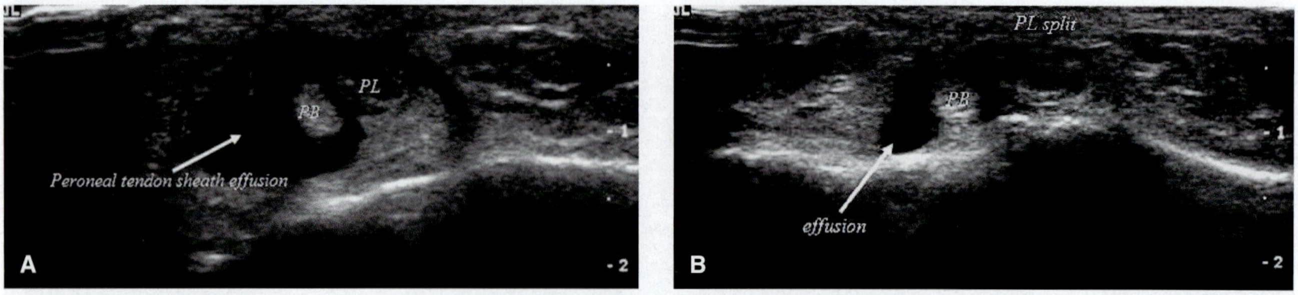

FIGURE 8.23 **A:** Short-axis ultrasound image along the lateral aspect of the ankle demonstrate tendinosis of the peroneus brevis (PB) and longus (PL) tendons. Moreover, there is a large amount of anechoic fluid surrounding the tendon, consistent with a tendon sheath effusion (effusion). **B:** A slightly more caudal image in the same patient shows a split in the peroneus longus tendon at the level of the peroneal tubercle. (From Adler R, Sofka CM, Positano RG. *Atlas of Foot and Ankle Sonography*. Philadelphia, PA: Lippincott Williams & Wilkins; 2004.)

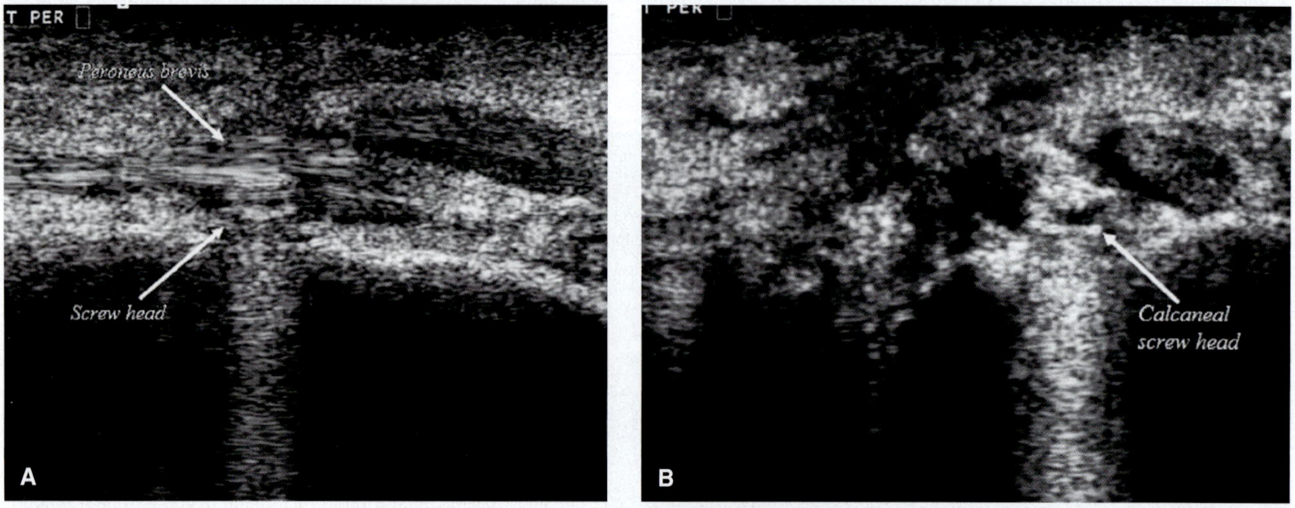

FIGURE 8.24 **A,B:** Transverse image along the lateral joint in the same patient demonstrates the relationship of the screw head to the deep fibers of the peroneus brevis (*arrow*). The patient described pain localized to the site of screw placement. (From Adler R, Sofka CM, Positano RG. *Atlas of Foot and Ankle Sonography*. Philadelphia, PA: Lippincott Williams & Wilkins; 2004.)

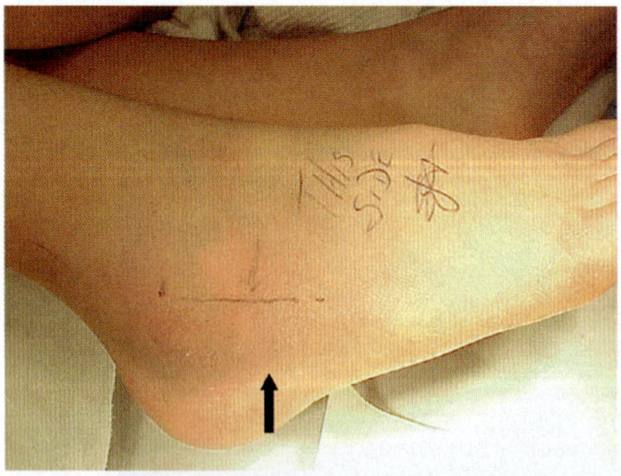

FIGURE 8.25 Edema and erythema are seen over the courses of the peroneal tendons. Although no longer seen, the arrow marks the approximate point of the puncture wound. (From Harris EJ. Retained Hawthorne fragment in a child's foot complicated by infection: diagnosis and excision aided by localization with ultrasound. *J Foot Ankle Surg* 2010;49(2):161–165.)

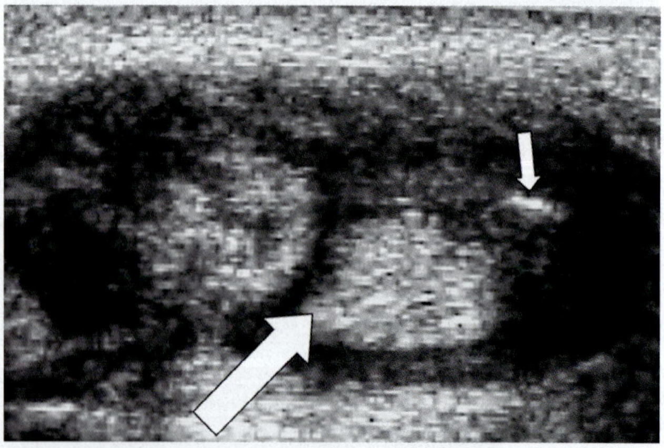

FIGURE 8.26 Ultrasound image showing the peroneal tendon sheaths and the foreign body. The large arrow points to peroneus brevis and the small arrow to the foreign body. (From Harris EJ. Retained Hawthorne fragment in a child's foot complicated by infection: diagnosis and excision aided by localization with ultrasound. *J Foot Ankle Surg* 2010;49(2):161–165.)

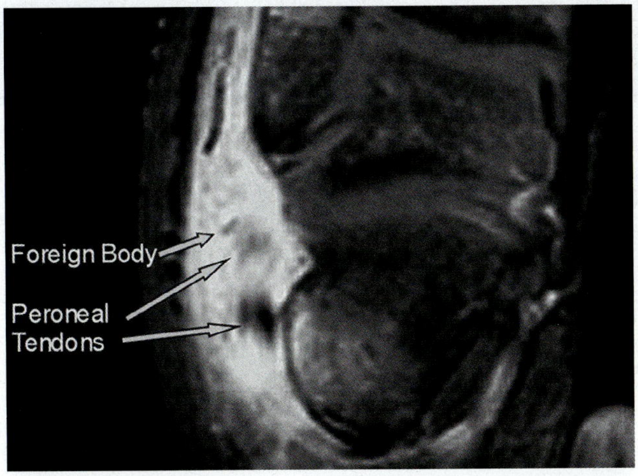

FIGURE 8.27 The MRI shows the foreign body within the sheath of peroneus brevis. There is extensive edema in the area. (From Harris EJ. Retained Hawthorne fragment in a child's foot complicated by infection: diagnosis and excision aided by localization with ultrasound. *J Foot Ankle Surg* 2010;49(2):161–165.)

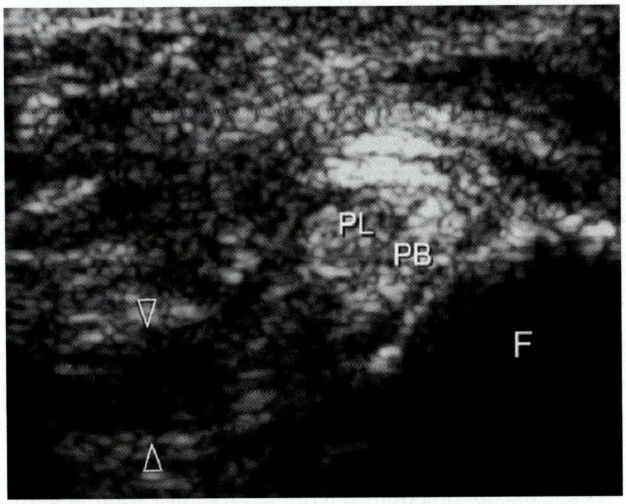

FIGURE 8.28 Peroneus quartus. Ultrasound transverse to the peroneus longus and peroneus brevis tendons shows hypoechoic peroneus quartus muscle (*arrowheads*). Left side of the image is posterior. F, fibula; PB, peroneus brevis tendon; PL, peroneus longus tendon. (From Femino JE, Jacobson JA, Craig CL, et al. Dynamic ultrasound of the foot and ankle: adult and pediatric applications. *Techn Foot Ankle Surg* 2007;6(1):50–61.)

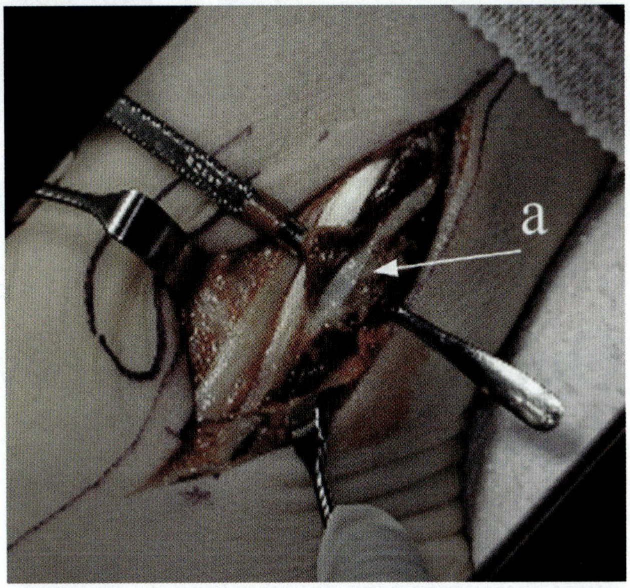

FIGURE 8.29 Peroneus quartus tendon with large muscle belly (a). (From Femino JE, Jacobson JA, Craig CL, et al. Dynamic ultrasound of the foot and ankle: adult and pediatric applications. *Techn Foot Ankle Surg* 2007;6(1):50–61.)

Suggested Readings

Bowring B, Chockalingam N. Conservative treatment of tibialis posterior tendon dysfunction: a review. *Foot(Edinb)* 2010;20(1):18–26.

Edwards MR, Jack C, Singh SK. Tibialis posterior dysfunction. *Curr Orthop* 2008;22(3):185–192.

Shibuya N, Ramanujam CL, Garcia GM. Association of tibialis posterior tendon pathology with other radiographic findings in the foot: a case-control study. *J Foot Ankle Surg* 2008;47(6):546–553.

Waldman SD. Peroneal tendinitis. In: *Atlas of Uncommon Pain Syndromes.* 2nd ed. Philadelphia, PA: Saunders; 2009:300–304.

Waldman SD. Peroneal tendinitis. In: *Pain Review.* Philadelphia, PA: Saunders; 2009:325.

Waldman SD. Injection technique for peroneal tendinitis. In: *Atlas of Pain Management Injection Techniques.* 3rd ed. Philadelphia, PA: Saunders; 2012:662–663.

Waldman SD, Campbell RSD. Peroneal tendon rupture. In: *Imaging of Pain.* Philadelphia, PA: Saunders; 2011:435–436.

CHAPTER 9

Anterior Tarsal Tunnel Syndrome and Other Abnormalities of the Deep Peroneal Nerve

ANATOMIC CONSIDERATIONS

The common peroneal nerve is one of the two major continuations of the sciatic nerve, the other being the tibial nerve (Fig. 9.1). The common peroneal nerve, which is also known as the common fibular nerve, provides sensory innervation to the inferior portion of the knee joint and the posterior and lateral skin of the upper calf. The common peroneal nerve is derived from the posterior branches of the L4, L5, and S1 and S2 nerve roots. The nerve splits from the sciatic nerve at the superior margin of the popliteal fossa and descends laterally behind the head of the fibula (Fig. 9.2). The common peroneal nerve is subject to compression at this point by circumstances such as improperly applied casts and tourniquets (Fig. 9.3). The nerve is also subject to compression as it continues its lateral course, winding around the fibula through the fibular tunnel, which is made up of the posterior border of the tendinous insertion of the peroneus longus muscle and the fibula itself. Just distal to the fibular tunnel, the nerve divides into its two terminal branches, the superficial and the deep peroneal nerves (Fig. 9.4). Each of these branches is subject to trauma and may be blocked individually as a diagnostic and therapeutic maneuver.

The deep branch continues down the leg in conjunction with the tibial artery and vein to provide sensory innervation to the web space of the first and second toes and adjacent dorsum of the foot (Figs. 9.5 and 9.6). Although this distribution of sensory fibers is small, this area is often the site of Morton's neuroma surgery and thus is important to the regional anesthesiologist. The deep peroneal nerve provides motor innervation to all of the toe extensors and the anterior tibialis muscles. The deep peroneal nerve passes beneath the dense superficial fascia of the ankle, where it is subject to an entrapment syndrome known as the anterior tarsal tunnel syndrome (Figs. 9.7 and 9.8).

CLINICAL CORRELATES

An uncommon cause of dorsal foot pain, anterior tarsal tunnel syndrome is caused by entrapment and compression of the deep peroneal nerve as it passes beneath the superficial fascia of the ankle (Figs. 9.7 and 9.8). Patients suffering from anterior tarsal tunnel syndrome complain of pain, dysesthesias, and numbness of the dorsum of the foot that radiate into the first dorsal web space. The pain associated with anterior tarsal tunnel syndrome may also radiate into the anterior ankle. There is no motor involvement unless the distal lateral division of the deep peroneal nerve is involved. Patients suffering from anterior tarsal tunnel syndrome often report nocturnal foot pain analogous to the nocturnal pain seen in carpal tunnel syndrome sufferers. The patient may report that holding the foot in the everted position may decrease the pain and paresthesia of anterior tarsal tunnel syndrome.

Severe, acute plantar flexion of the foot has been implicated in anterior tarsal tunnel syndrome, as has the wearing of overly tight shoes or squatting and bending forward, as when planting flowers. Tumor, osteophyte, ganglion, and synovitis that have in common their ability to impinge on the deep peroneal nerve such as can cause anterior tarsal tunnel syndrome (Fig. 9.9). Anterior tarsal tunnel syndrome is much less common than posterior tarsal tunnel syndrome.

Patients suffering from anterior tarsal tunnel syndrome will exhibit tenderness on palpation of the deep peroneal nerve at the dorsum of the foot. A positive Tinel's sign just medial to the dorsalis pedis pulse over the deep peroneal nerve as it passes beneath the fascia usually is present (Fig. 9.10). The pain of anterior tarsal tunnel syndrome may be elicited by active plantar flexion of the affected foot. Weakness of the extensor digitorum brevis may be identified if the lateral branch of the deep peroneal nerve is affected.

Anterior tarsal tunnel syndrome is frequently misdiagnosed as lumbar radiculopathy or diabetic neuropathy or is attributed to primary ankle pathology leading to both diagnostic and therapeutic misadventures. Plain radiographs of the ankle will help identify primary ankle pathology and electromyography will help distinguish the compromise of deep peroneal nerve associated with anterior tarsal tunnel syndrome from radiculopathy (Fig. 9.11). Most patients who suffer from lumbar radiculopathy have back pain associated with reflex, motor, and sensory changes that are associated with back pain, whereas patients with anterior tarsal tunnel syndrome have no

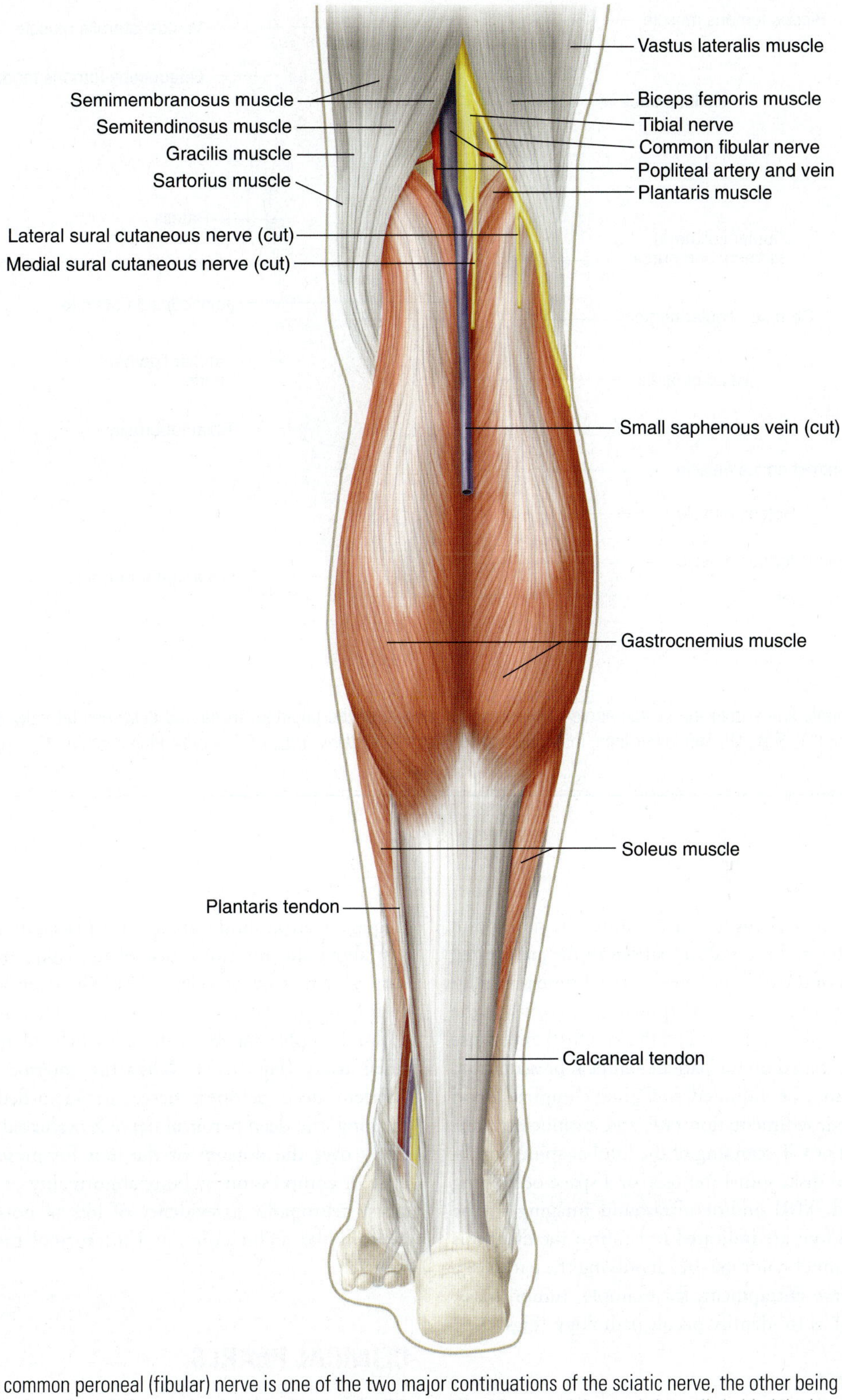

FIGURE 9.1 The common peroneal (fibular) nerve is one of the two major continuations of the sciatic nerve, the other being the tibial nerve. The peroneal nerve splits from the sciatic nerve at the superior margin of the popliteal fossa and descends laterally behind the head of the fibula. (From Tank PW, Gest TR. The lower limb. In: *Lippincott Williams & Wilkins Atlas of Anatomy*. Philadelphia, PA: Lippincott Williams & Wilkins; 2009:119.)

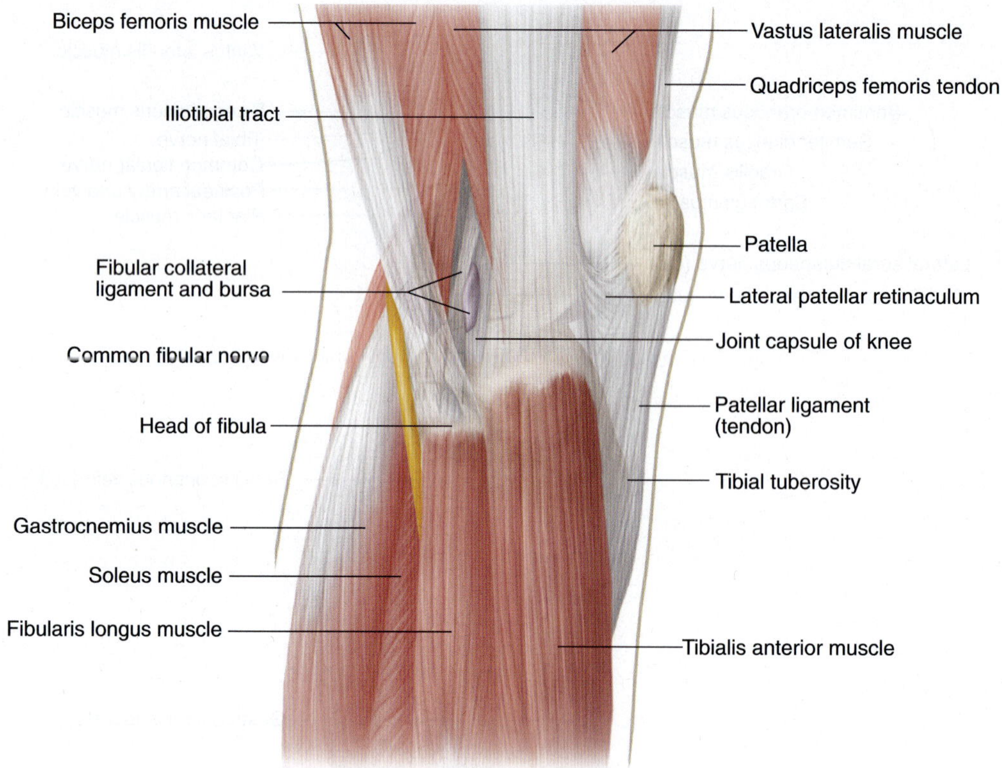

FIGURE 9.2 The nerve splits from the sciatic nerve at the superior margin of the popliteal fossa and descends laterally behind the head of the fibula. (From Tank PW, Gest TR. The lower limb. In: *Lippincott Williams & Wilkins Atlas of Anatomy*. Philadelphia, PA: Lippincott Williams & Wilkins; 2009:143.)

back pain and no reflex changes. Furthermore, the motor and sensory changes of anterior tarsal tunnel syndrome are limited to the distribution of the deep peroneal nerve. Lumbar radiculopathy and deep peroneal nerve entrapment may coexist as the so-called "double crush" syndrome and this can further confuse the clinical picture. Based on the patient's clinical presentation, additional testing may be indicated, including complete blood cell count, uric acid, sedimentation rate, and antinuclear antibody testing. MRI or CT scanning of the lumbar spine is indicated if a herniated disk, spinal stenosis, or a space-occupying lesion is suspected. MRI and/or ultrasound imaging of the anterior ankle and foot are indicated to confirm the diagnosis of anterior tarsal tunnel syndrome by identifying the pathology responsible for nerve entrapment, for example, tumor, mass, osteophyte, as well as to identify occult pathology (Figs. 9.12 to 9.14).

ULTRASOUND TECHNIQUE

To perform ultrasound evaluation of the deep peroneal nerve at the ankle, the patient is placed in the supine position with the arms resting comfortably along the patient's chest and the affected lower extremity in neutral position. A linear high frequency ultrasound transducer is placed in a transverse plane just above the anterior crease of the ankle and an ultrasound survey scan is taken (Fig. 9.15). The deep peroneal nerve is seen lying just lateral to the anterior tibial artery (Fig. 9.16). Color Doppler can be utilized to help identify the anterior tibial artery (Fig. 9.17). When the anterior tibial artery and adjacent deep peroneal nerve are identified on ultrasound imaging, the deep peroneal nerve is evaluated as it passes inferiorly over the dorsum of the foot for presence of compromise or compression by bony abnormality or soft tissue mass, cysts, neuropathy as evidence of loss of normal sonographic neurofibular architecture, and intraneural tumors (Figs. 9.18 to 9.22).

CLINICAL PEARLS

The key to performing successful ultrasound evaluation of the deep peroneal nerve at the ankle is the proper identification of the sonographic anatomy and in particular the ability to properly identify the etiology and site of deep peroneal nerve entrapment. The use of multiple imaging modalities will increase the accuracy of diagnosis and improve clinical outcomes (Fig. 9.23).

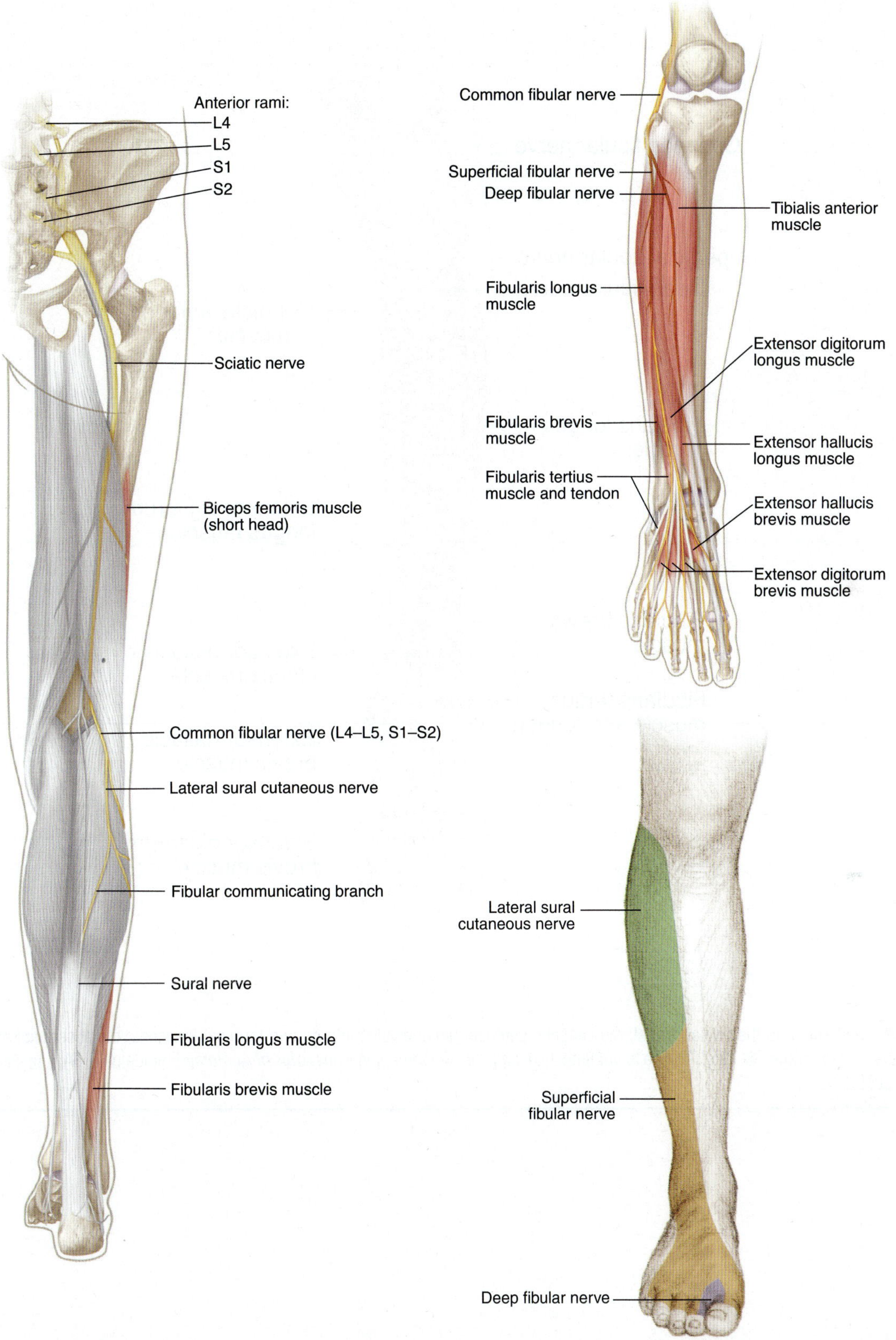

FIGURE 9.3 The common peroneal (common fibular) nerve is subject to compression at this point by circumstances such as improperly applied casts and tourniquets. The nerve is also subject to compression as it continues its lateral course, winding around the fibula through the fibular tunnel, which is made up of the posterior border of the tendinous insertion of the peroneus longus muscle and the fibula itself. Just distal to the fibular tunnel, the nerve divides into its two terminal branches, the superficial and the deep peroneal nerves. (From Tank PW, Gest TR. The lower limb. In: *Lippincott Williams & Wilkins Atlas of Anatomy*. Philadelphia, PA: Lippincott Williams & Wilkins; 2009.)

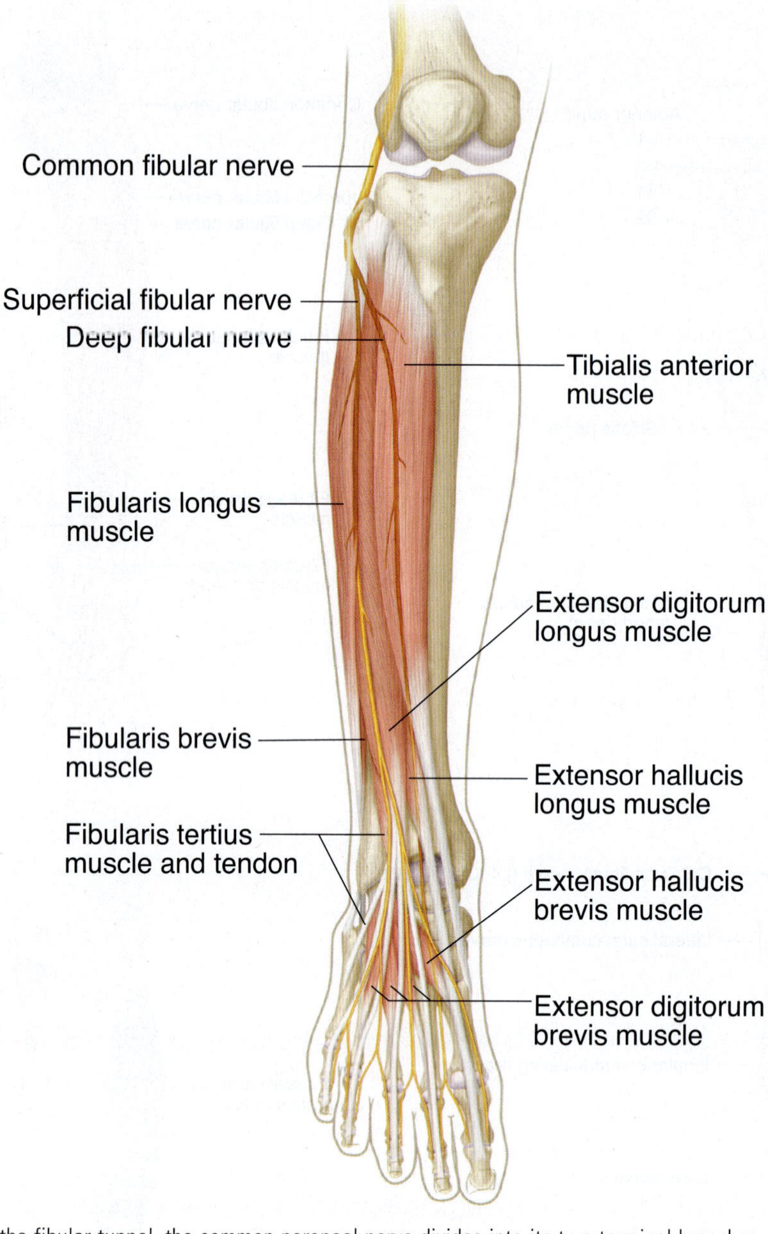

FIGURE 9.4 Just distal to the fibular tunnel, the common peroneal nerve divides into its two terminal branches, the superficial and the deep peroneal nerves. (From Tank PW, Gest TR. The lower limb. In: *Lippincott Williams & Wilkins Atlas of Anatomy*. Philadelphia, PA: Lippincott Williams & Wilkins; 2009:151.)

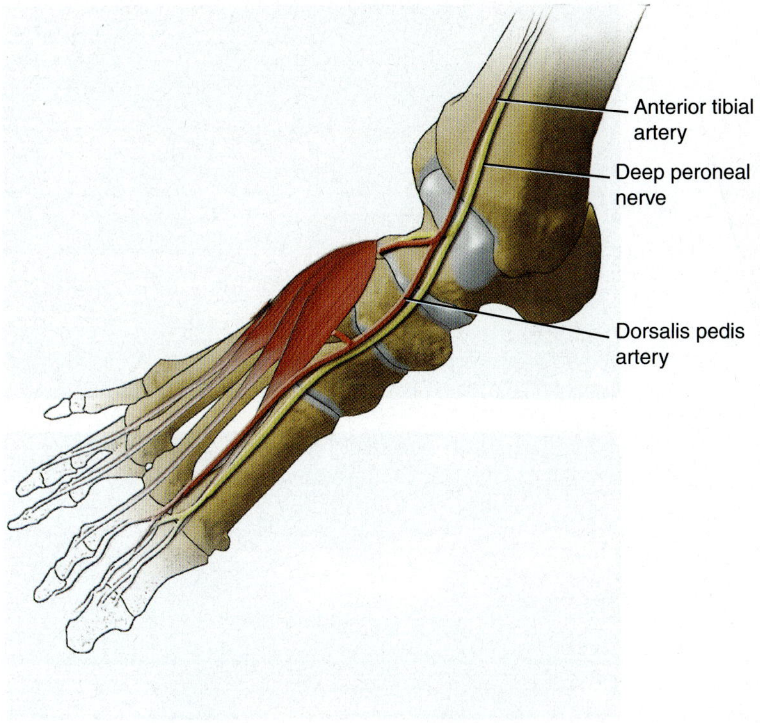

FIGURE 9.5 The anatomy of the distal deep peroneal nerve. Note the relations ankle of the nerve to the deep peroneal vein.

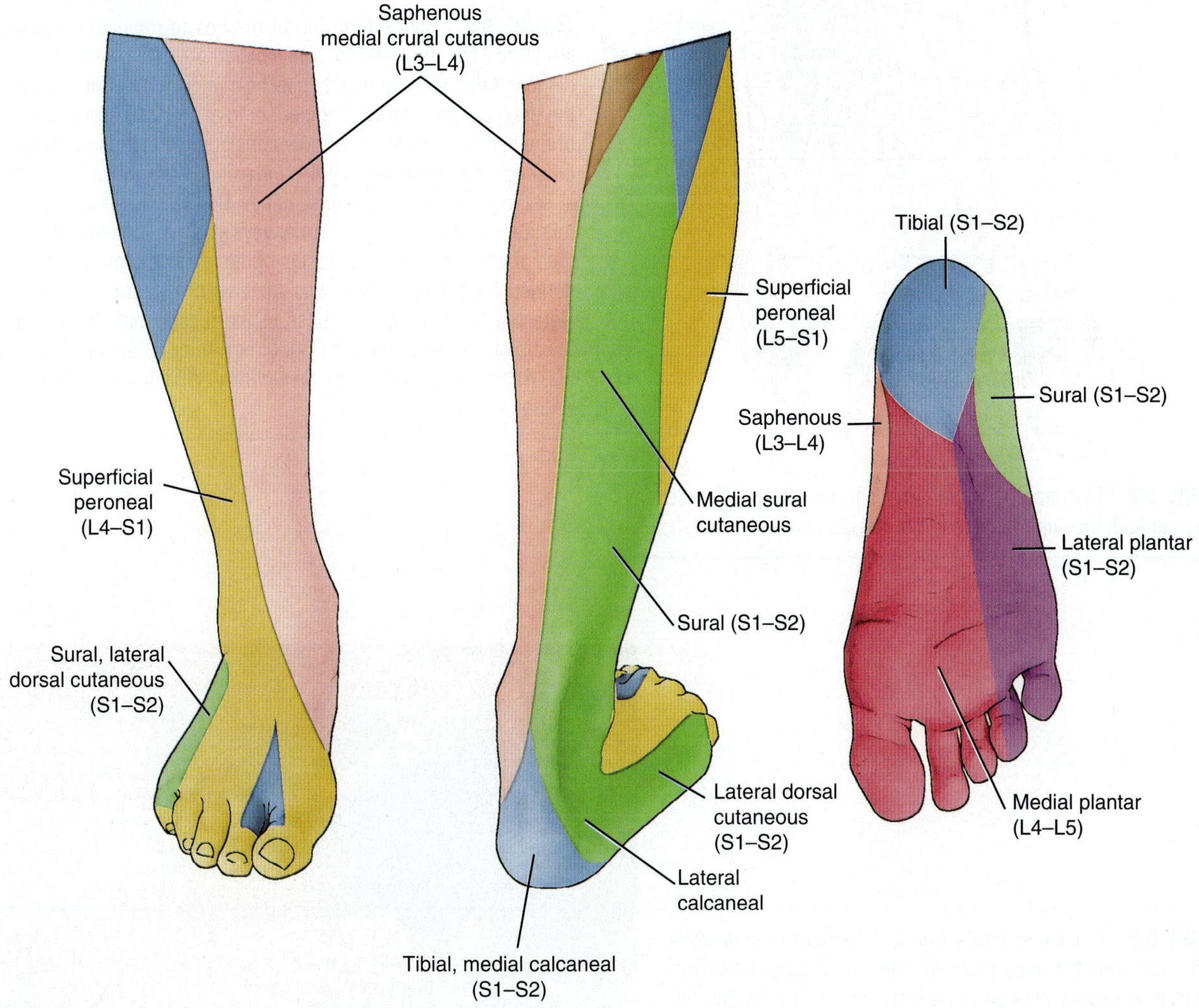

FIGURE 9.6 Sensory distribution of the distal deep peroneal nerve.

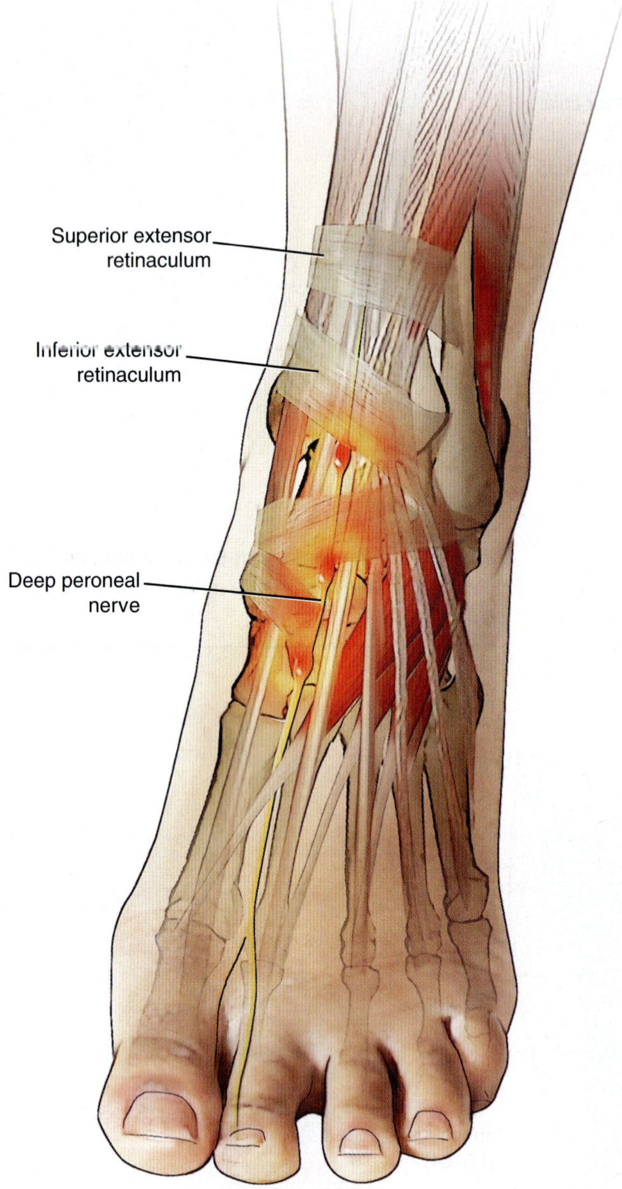

FIGURE 9.7 The deep peroneal nerve can be entrapped at several points beneath the superficial fascia of the dorsum of the foot.

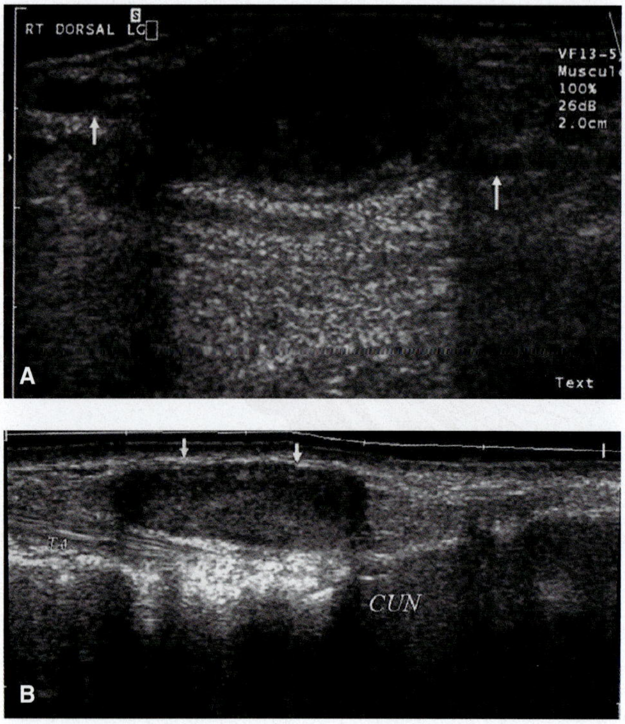

FIGURE 9.8 The relationship of masses to regional neurovascular structures can be defined with sonography. **A:** Longitudinal image demonstrates well-defined hypoechoic mass within the substance of the deep peroneal nerve (the more normal proximal and distal aspects of the nerve can be seen (*arrows*) consistent with a neurofibroma. The presence of a nerve having entry and exit points relative to such a mass is pathognomonic for a neural tumor. **B:** The presence of a nerve in relation to a neural tumor is not always evident. Longitudinal extended field of view image of the dorsum of the midfoot demonstrates a well-defined hypoechoic mass consistent with a neurofibroma (*arrows*). Note the proximity of the mass to the medial cuneiform (CUN) and the tibialis anterior tendon (TA). (From Adler R, Sofka CM, Positano RG. *Atlas of Foot and Ankle Sonography*. Philadelphia, PA: Lippincott Williams & Wilkins; 2004.)

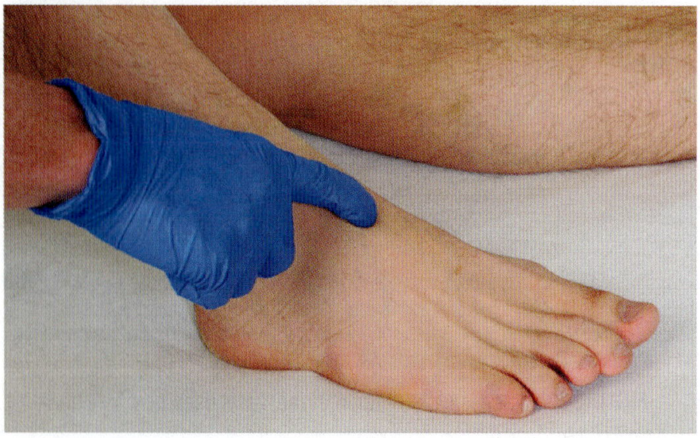

FIGURE 9.9 A positive Tinel's sign just medial to the dorsalis pedis pulse over the deep peroneal nerve as it passes beneath the fascia is usually present in patient's suffering from anterior tarsal tunnel syndrome.

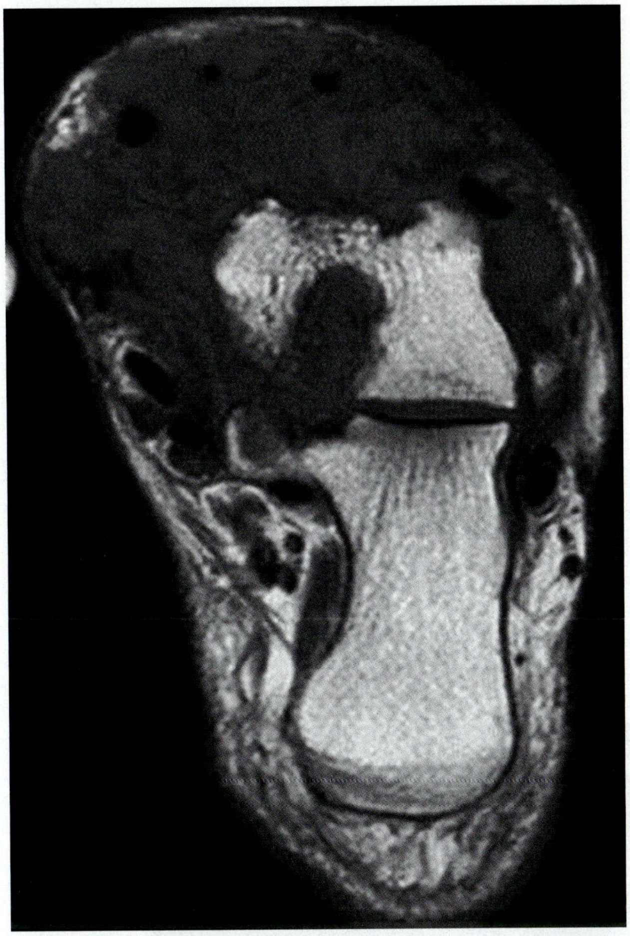

FIGURE 9.10 MRI of the anterior ankle in a patient with sympotms of anterior tarsal tunnel syndrome demonstrating a mass which is consistent with villonodular synovitis.

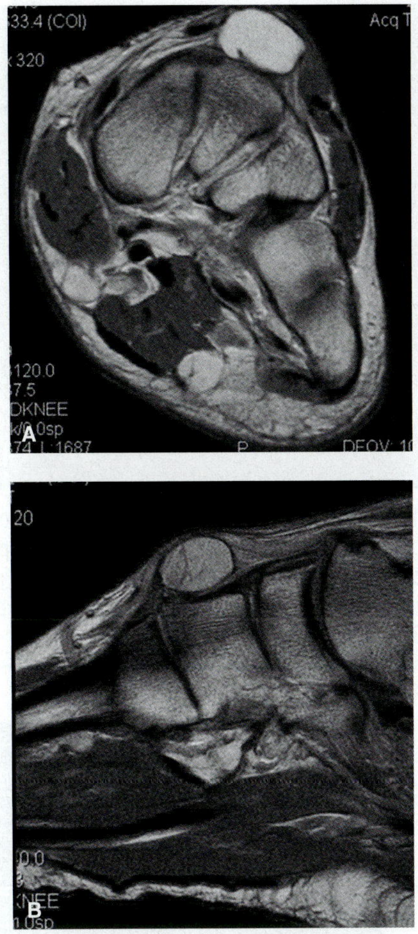

FIGURE 9.12 Midfoot ganglion compressing the medial branch of the deep peroneal nerve. Coronal **(A)** and sagittal **(B)** PD MR images. (From Simmons DN, Lisle DA, Linklater JM. Imaging of peripheral nerve lesions in the lower limb. *Top Magn Reson Imaging* 2010;21(1):51–62.)

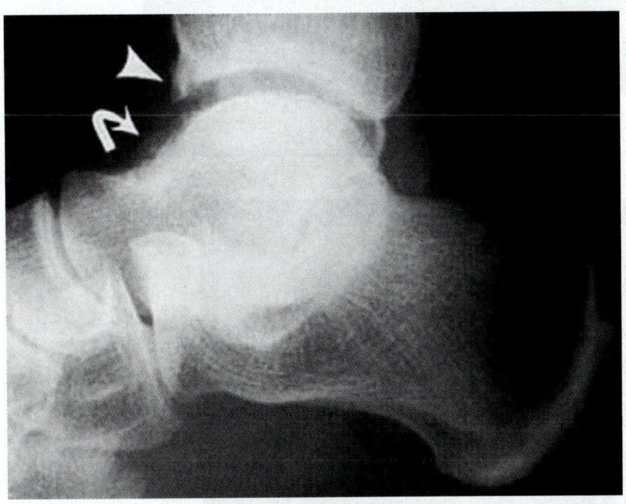

FIGURE 9.11 Lateral ankle radiograph demonstrates anterior impingement spurs arising from the anterior margin of the tibial plafond (*white arrowhead*) and the apposed margin of the anterior talar dome (*curved white arrow*). Note the preservation of tibiotalar cartilage space. (From Umans H. Ankle impingement syndromes. *Semin Musculoskelet Radiol* 2002;6(2):133–139.)

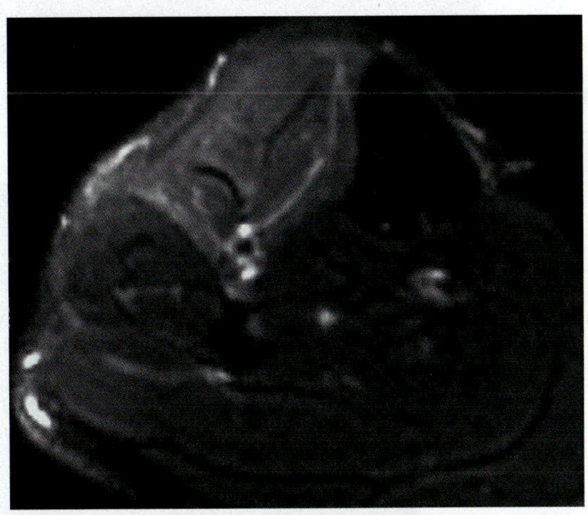

FIGURE 9.13 Deep peroneal nerve distribution subacute denervation effect involving the muscles of the anterior compartment (tibialis anterior, extensor digitorum longus, and extensor hallucis longus), manifests as edema-like signal on an axial fat-suppressed PD MR image. (From Simmons DN, Lisle DA, Linklater JM. Imaging of peripheral nerve lesions in the lower limb. *Top Magn Reson Imaging* 2010;21(1):51–62.)

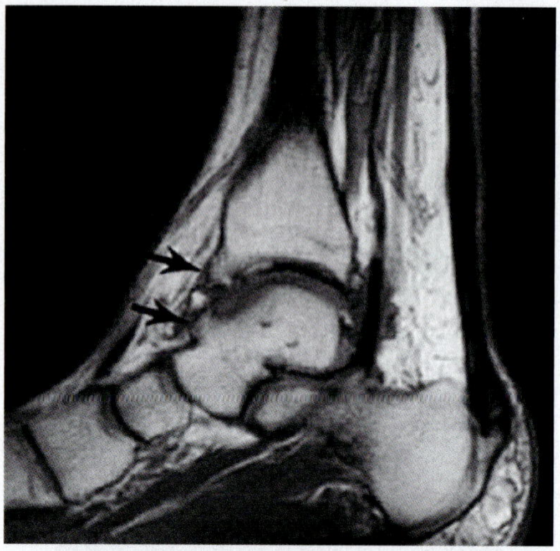

FIGURE 9.14 Sagittal T1-weighted spin echo image of an ankle with anterior impingement spurs at the margin of tibial plafond and intracapsular talus, proximal to the talar neck (*arrows*). (From Umans H. Ankle impingement syndromes. *Semin Musculoskelet Radiol* 2002;6(2):133–139. Courtesy of Mark E. Schweitzer, MD.)

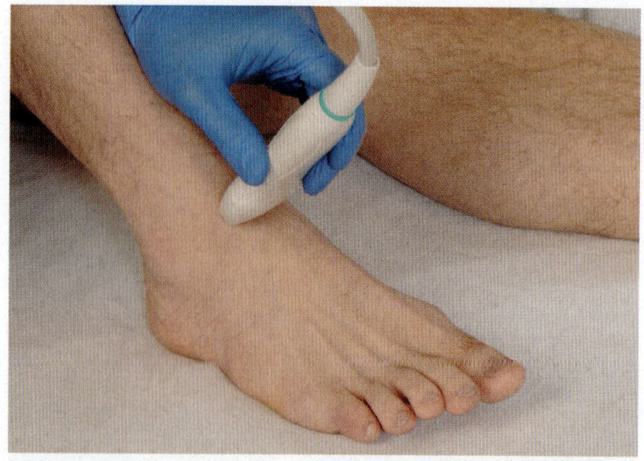

FIGURE 9.15 Proper transverse position of the ultrasound transducer for ultrasound evaluation of the deep peroneal nerve at the ankle.

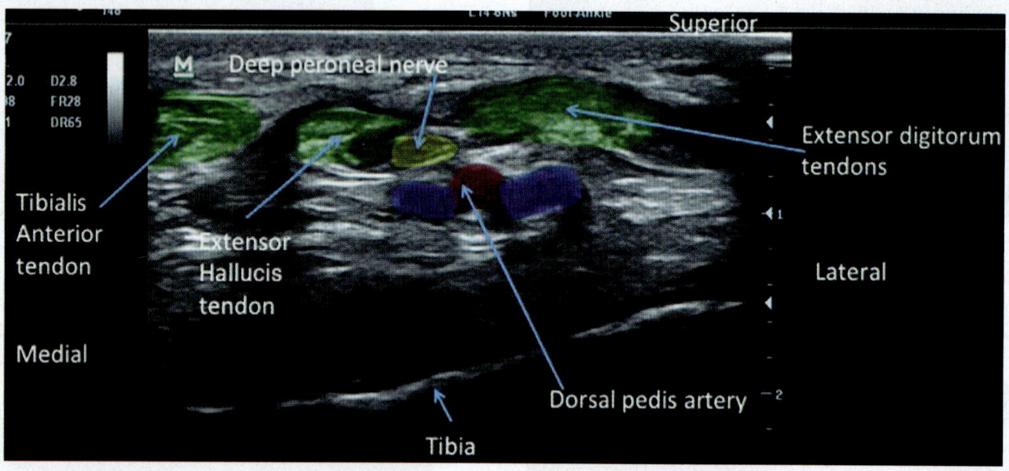

FIGURE 9.16 Transverse ultrasound image demonstrating the tibial artery and vein and the deep peroneal nerve just above and lateral to the vein.

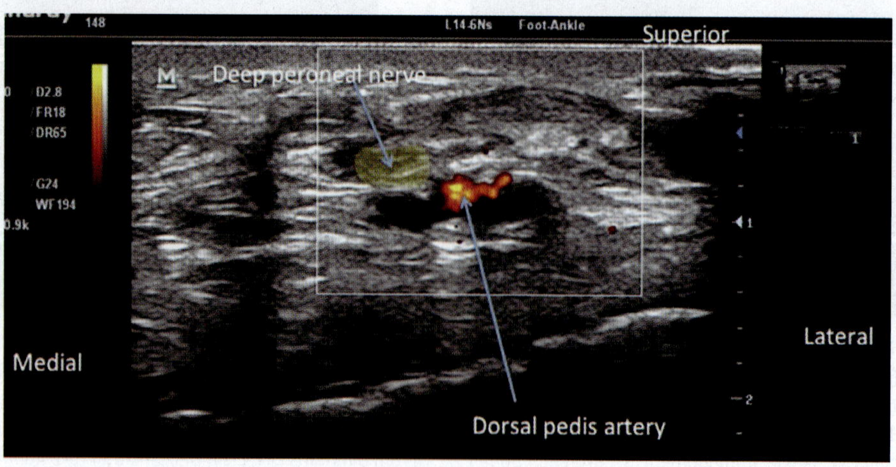

FIGURE 9.17 Transverse color Doppler image demonstrating the popliteal vein and artery, and the relationship of the vein to the deep peroneal nerve.

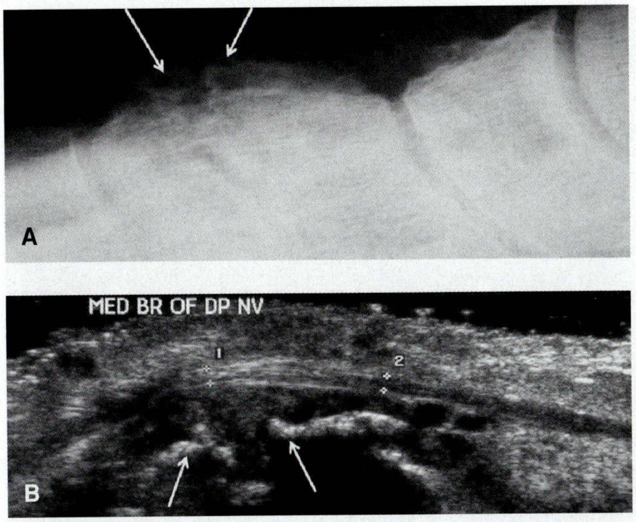

FIGURE 9.18 **A:** Dorsal tarsometatarsal joint osteophytes demonstrated on a lateral radiograph (*arrows*). **B:** Corresponding longitudinal ultrasound image of the medial branch of deep peroneal nerve illustrating displacement of the nerve by the TMT joint osteophytes and distended capsule. (From Simmons DN, Lisle DA, Linklater JM. Imaging of peripheral nerve lesions in the lower limb. *Topics Magn Reson Imaging* 2010;21(1):51–62.)

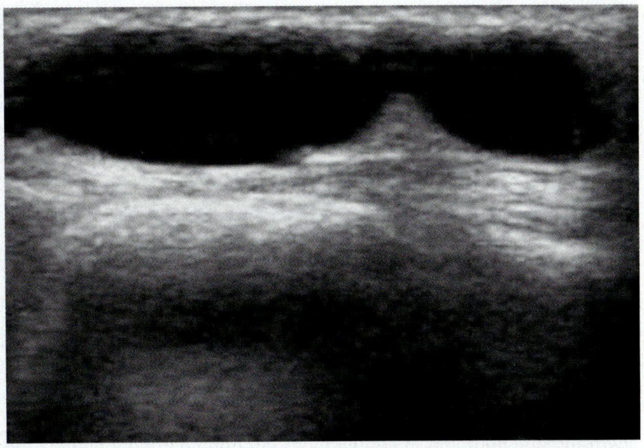

FIGURE 9.19 Ultrasound showing anechoic bilobed ganglion cyst in the foot compressing the deep peroneal nerve. (From Ahmed R, Nazarian LN. Overview of musculoskeletal sonography. *Ultrasound Q* 2010;26(1):27–35.)

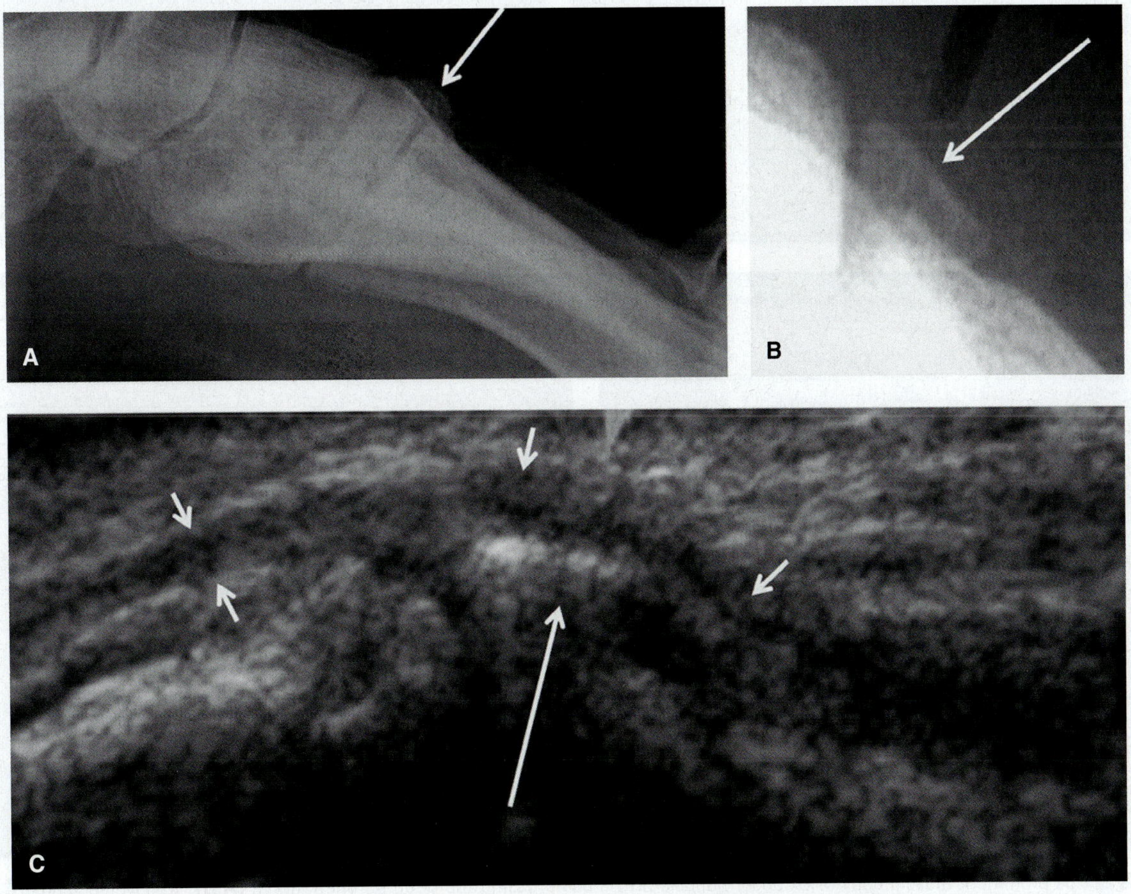

FIGURE 9.20 Os intermetatarseum shown on lateral radiograph **(A)** and magnified lateral radiograph **(B)** of the foot. Longitudinal ultrasound image (**C**) in the same position as **B** demonstrates the ossicle (*long arrow*) displacing the medial branch of the deep peroneal nerve (*short arrows*). (From Simmons DN, Lisle DA, Linklater JM. Imaging of peripheral nerve lesions in the lower limb. *Top Magn Reson Imaging* 2010;21(1):51–62.)

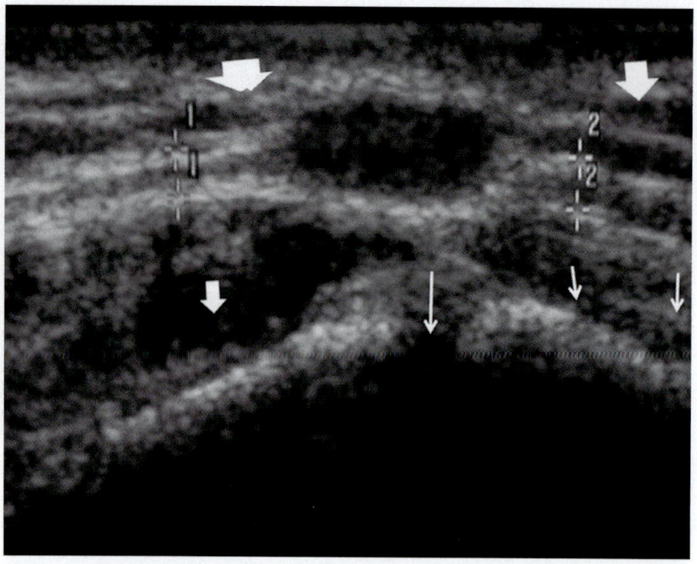

FIGURE 9.21 Longitudinal ultrasound image demonstrates a posttraumatic neuroma in continuity of the deep peroneal nerve at midfoot level secondary to tight footwear. (From Simmons DN, Lisle DA, Linklater JM. Imaging of peripheral nerve lesions in the lower limb. *Top Magn Reson Imaging* 2010;21(1):51–62.)

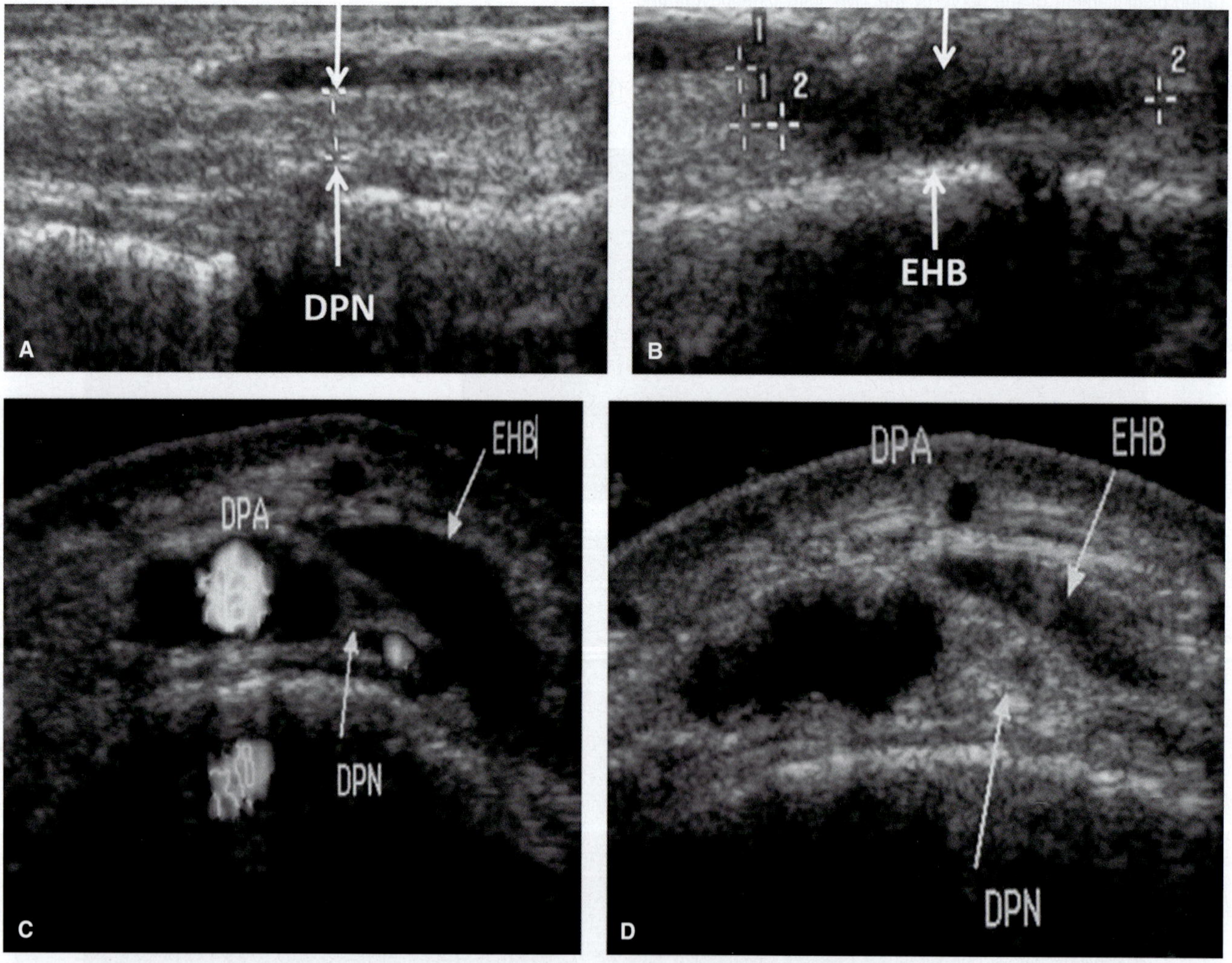

FIGURE 9.22 A prominent muscle belly of extensor hallucis brevis compressing the deep peroneal nerve **(A,B)**. Transverse scans **(C,D)** illustrate the compression of the nerve by the muscle. Surgical confirmation. DPA, dorsalis pedis artery; EHB, extensor hallucis brevis; DPN, deep peroneal nerve. (From Simmons DN, Lisle DA, Linklater JM. Imaging of peripheral nerve lesions in the lower limb. *Top Magn Reson Imaging* 2010;21(1):51–62.)

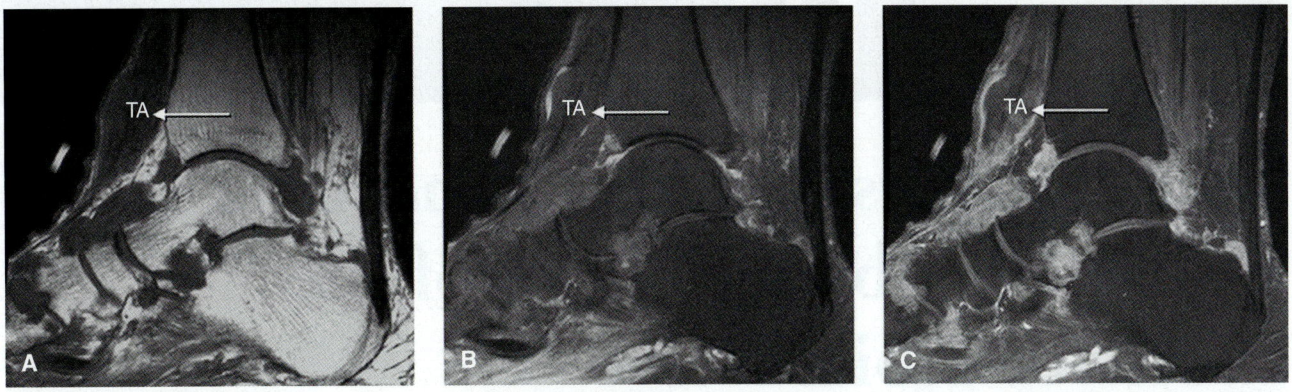

FIGURE 9.23 Sagittal FSE-T1 **(A)**, fs-FSE-T2 **(B)**, and post-Gd fs-SPGR **(C)** images in a patient with known crystalline arthropathy who presented with a clinically palpable anterior ankle mass. There is marked fusiform thickening of the tenosynovial compartment of the tibialis anterior (TA) tendon (*long arrows*) compatible with extensive deposition of tophaceous gout with extension and infiltration into the degenerated and partially torn underlying tendon. Advanced changes of gout are also seen at scattered joints of the ankle, midfoot, and hindfoot. (From Collins MS, Felmlee JP. 3T magnetic resonance imaging of ankle and hindfoot tendon pathology. *Topics Magn Reson Imaging* 2009;20(3):175–188; Fig. 4A-C.)

Suggested Readings

DiDomenico LA, Masternick EB. Anterior tarsal tunnel syndrome. *Clin Podiatr Med Surg* 2006;23(3):611–620.

Lopez-Ben R. Imaging of nerve entrapment in the foot and ankle. *Foot Ankle Clin* 2011;16(2):213–224.

Waldman SD. Functional anatomy of the foot and ankle. In: *Pain Review.* Philadelphia, PA: Saunders; 2009:155–156.

Waldman SD. Anterior tarsal tunnel syndrome. In: *Pain Review.* Philadelphia, PA: Saunders; 2009:322–323.

Waldman SD. Anterior tarsal tunnel syndrome. In: *Atlas of Common Pain Syndromes.* 3rd ed. Philadelphia, PA: Saunders; 2012:356–358.

Waldman SD. Injection technique for anterior tarsal tunnel syndrome. In: *Atlas of Pain Management Injection Techniques.* 3rd ed. Philadelphia, PA: Saunders; 2012:431–434.

Waldman SD, Campbell RSD. Anterior tarsal tunnel syndrome. In: *Imaging of Pain.* Philadelphia, PA: Saunders; 2011:421–423.

CHAPTER 10

Posterior Tarsal Tunnel Syndrome and Other Abnormalities of the Posterior Tibial Nerve

ANATOMIC CONSIDERATIONS

The tibial nerve is one of the two major continuations of the sciatic nerve, the other being the common peroneal nerve (Fig. 10.1). The tibial nerve provides sensory innervation to the posterior portion of the calf, the heel, and the medial plantar surface. The tibial nerve splits from the sciatic nerve at the superior margin of the popliteal fossa and descends in a slightly medial course through the popliteal fossa. The tibial nerve at the ankle lies just beneath the popliteal fascia and is readily accessible for neural blockade. The tibial nerve continues its downward course, running between the two heads of the gastrocnemius muscle, passing deep into the soleus muscle (Fig. 10.2). The nerve courses medially between the Achilles tendon and the medial malleolus, where it divides into the medial and lateral plantar nerves, providing sensory innervation to the heel and medial plantar surface (Figs. 10.3 and 10.4). The tibial nerve is subject to compression at this point as the nerve passes through the posterior tarsal tunnel (Fig. 10.5). The posterior tarsal tunnel is made up of the flexor retinaculum, the bones of the ankle, and the lacunar ligament. In addition to the posterior tibial nerve, the tunnel contains the posterior tibial artery and vein as well as a number of flexor musculotendinous units.

CLINICAL CORRELATES

An uncommon cause of plantar foot pain, posterior tarsal tunnel syndrome, is caused by entrapment and compression of the posterior tibial nerve as it passes through the posterior tarsal tunnel (Fig. 10.5). The most common cause of compression of the posterior tibial nerve within the posterior tarsal tunnel location is trauma to the ankle, including fracture, dislocation, and crush injuries (Fig. 10.6). The boundaries of the posterior tarsal tunnel are the flexor retinaculum, the bones of the ankle, and the lacunate ligament. The posterior tarsal tunnel contains the posterior tibial nerve, vein and artery, tibialis posterior, flexor digitorum longus, and flexor hallucis longus musculotendinous units. These musculotendinous units are subject to the development of tenosynovitis, while the posterior tibial artery is subject to the development of aneurysms and posterior tibial vein is subject to the development of thrombophlebitis and varicosities (Fig. 10.7). Patients with rheumatoid arthritis have a higher incidence of posterior tarsal tunnel syndrome than the general population. Posterior tarsal tunnel syndrome is much more common than anterior tarsal tunnel syndrome.

Posterior tarsal tunnel syndrome presents clinically in a manner very analogous to carpal tunnel syndrome. Night-time foot pain analogous to the nocturnal pain of carpal tunnel syndrome is often present. The patient suffering from posterior tarsal tunnel will frequently complain of pain, numbness, and dysesthesias involving the plantar surface of the foot and may radiate into the medial ankle. The medial and lateral plantar divisions of the posterior tibial nerve provide motor innervation to the intrinsic muscles of the foot. The patient may note weakness of the toe flexors and instability of the foot caused by weakness of the lumbrical muscles.

Physical findings include tenderness over the posterior tibial nerve at the medial malleolus. A positive Tinel sign usually is present just below and behind the medial malleolus over the posterior tibial nerve (Fig. 10.8). Active inversion of the ankle often reproduces the symptoms of the posterior tarsal tunnel syndrome. Weakness of the flexor digitorum brevis and the lumbrical muscles may be present if the medial and lateral branches of the posterior tibial nerve are compromised.

Posterior tarsal tunnel syndrome is frequently misdiagnosed as lumbar radiculopathy or diabetic neuropathy or is attributed to primary ankle pathology leading to both diagnostic and therapeutic misadventures. Plain radiographs of the ankle will help identify primary ankle pathology and electromyography will help distinguish the compromise of posterior tibial nerve associated with posterior tarsal tunnel syndrome from radiculopathy (Fig. 10.9). Most patients who suffer from lumbar radiculopathy have back pain associated with reflex, motor, and sensory changes that are associated with back pain, whereas patients with posterior tarsal tunnel syndrome have no back pain and no reflex changes. Furthermore, the motor and sensory changes of posterior tarsal tunnel syndrome are limited to the distribution of the medial and lateral plantar divisions of

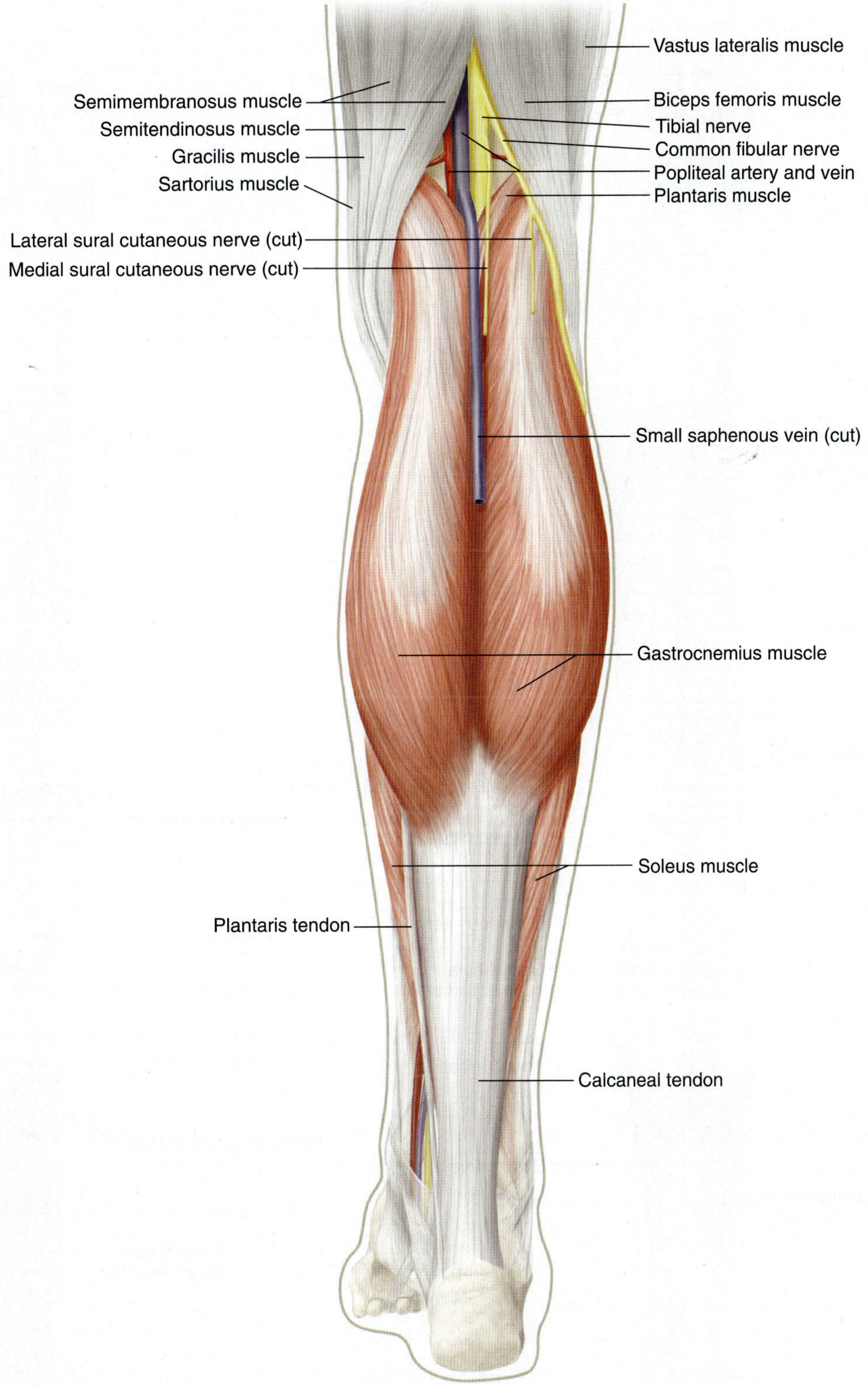

FIGURE 10.1 The tibial nerve is one of the two major continuations of the sciatic nerve, the other being the common peroneal nerve. (From Tank PW, Gest TR. The lower limb. In: *Lippincott Williams & Wilkins Atlas of Anatomy*. Philadelphia, PA: Lippincott Williams & Wilkins; 2009:119.)

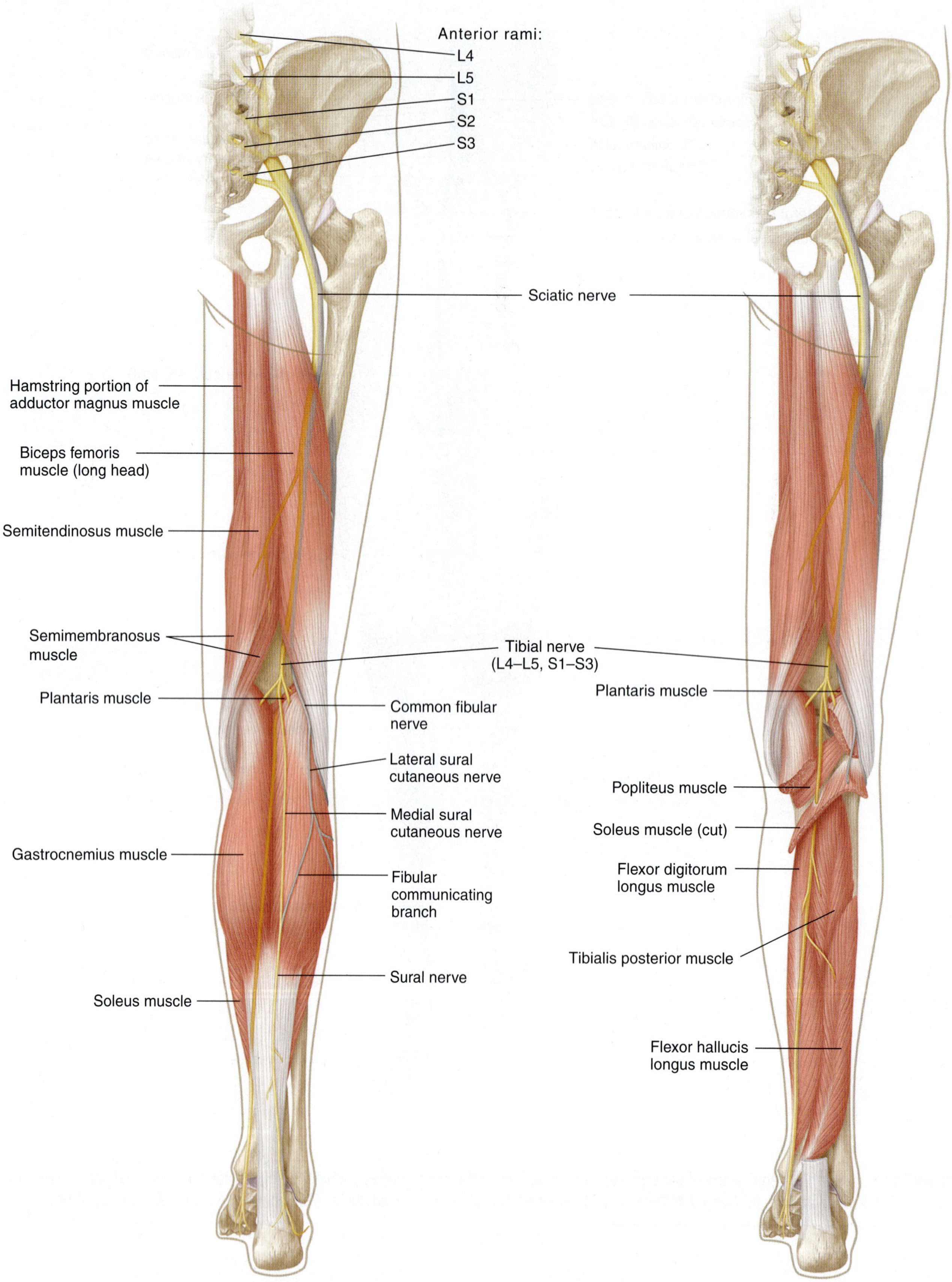

FIGURE 10.2 The anatomy of the tibial nerve. (From Tank PW, Gest TR. The lower limb. In: *Lippincott Williams & Wilkins Atlas of Anatomy*. Philadelphia, PA: Lippincott Williams & Wilkins; 2009:119.)

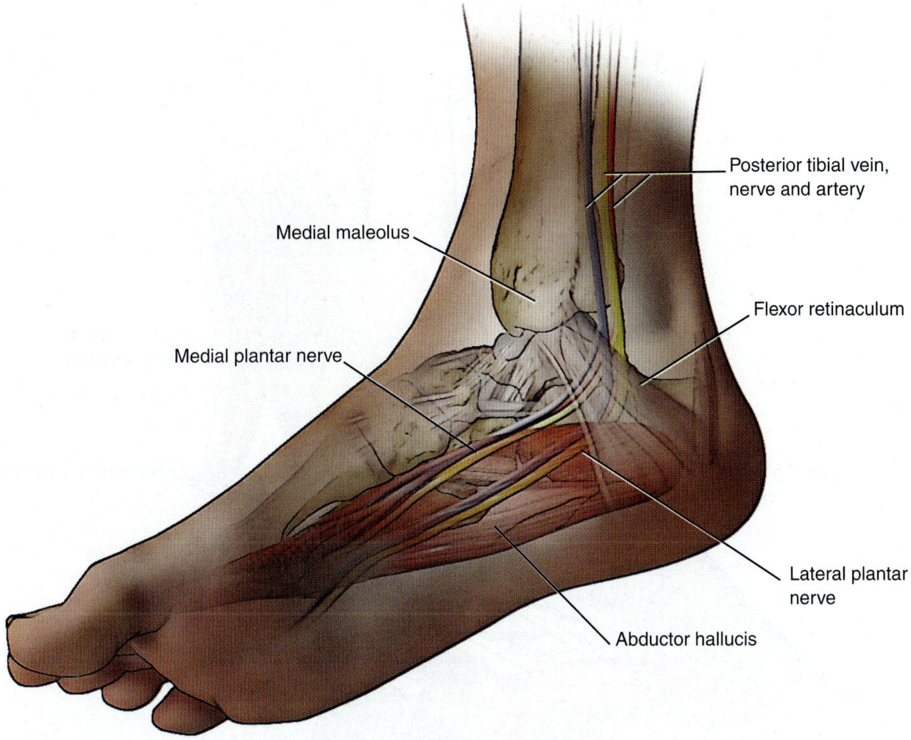

FIGURE 10.3 Relationship of the posterior tibial nerve and the tibial artery and vein.

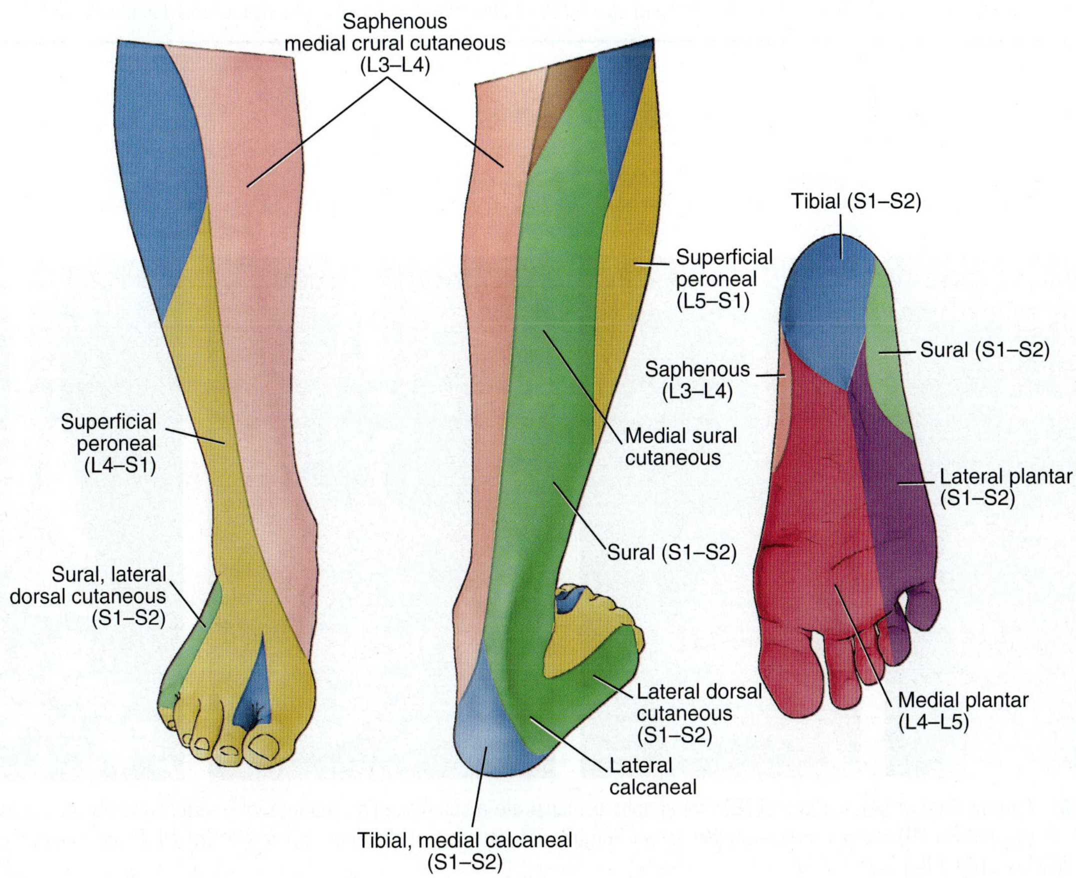

FIGURE 10.4 The posterior tibial nerve provides sensory innervation to the posterior portion of the calf, the heel, and the medial plantar surface.

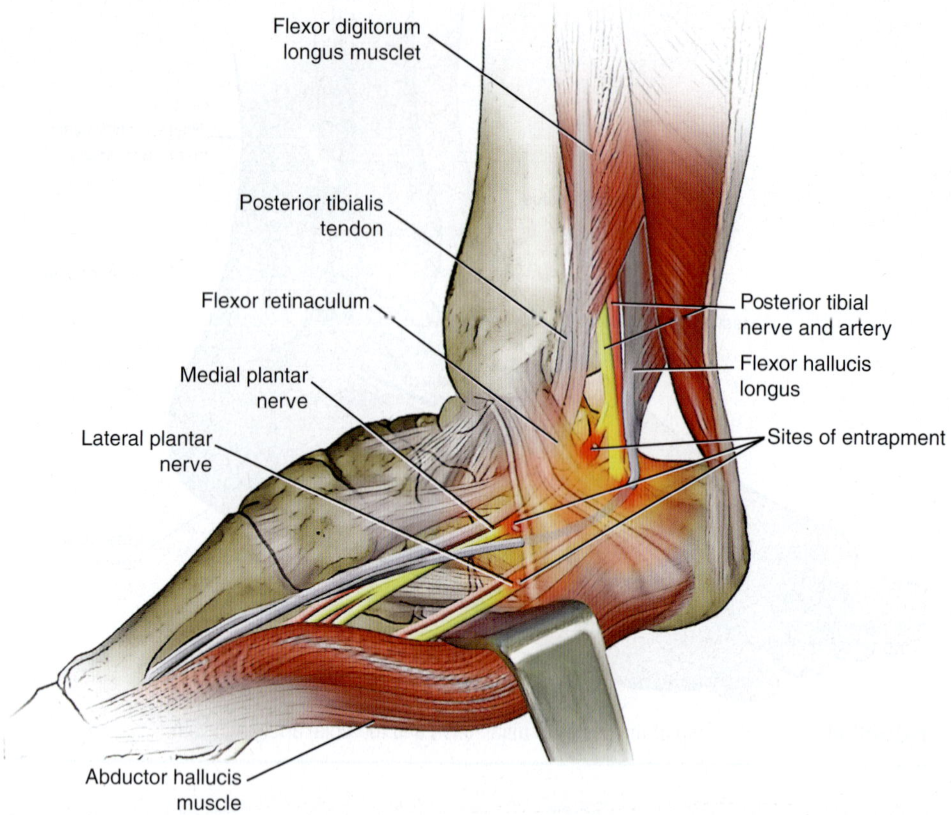

FIGURE 10.5 The posterior tibial nerve can be entrapped at several points beneath the superficial fascia of the dorsum of the foot.

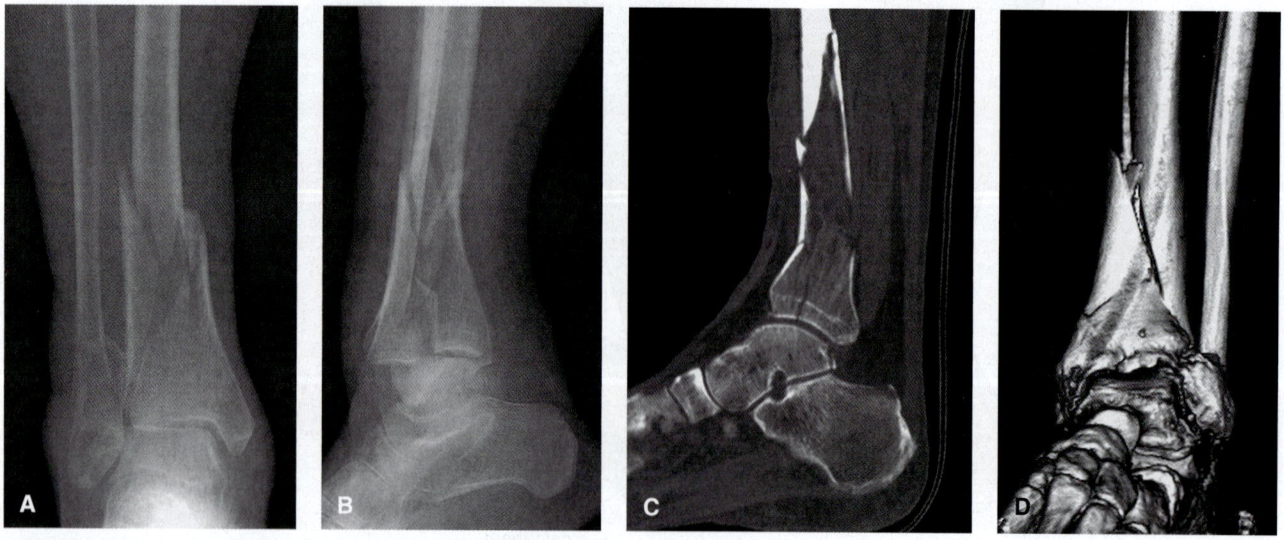

FIGURE 10.6 Anteroposterior **(A)** and lateral **(B)** radiographs demonstrate a complex pilon fracture with associated fibular fracture. Sagittal reformatted CT **(C)** and 3D **(D)** images preoperatively. (From Berquist TH. *Imaging of the Foot and Ankle*. 3rd ed. Philadelphia, PA: Lippincott Williams & Wilkins; 2011:249.)

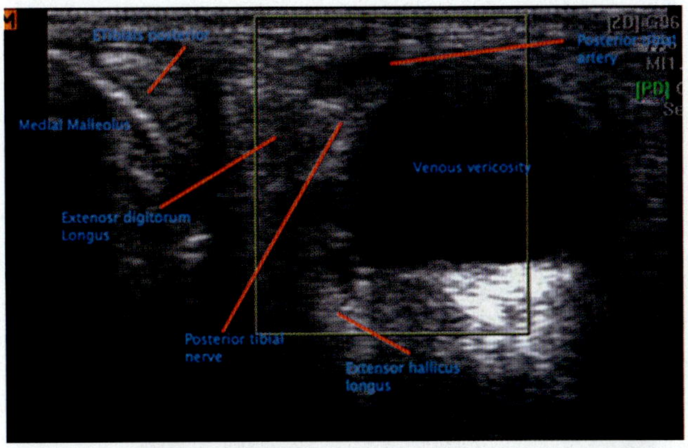

FIGURE 10.7 Ultrasound image demonstrating compression of the posterior tibial nerve by a large varicosity of the posterior tibial vein.

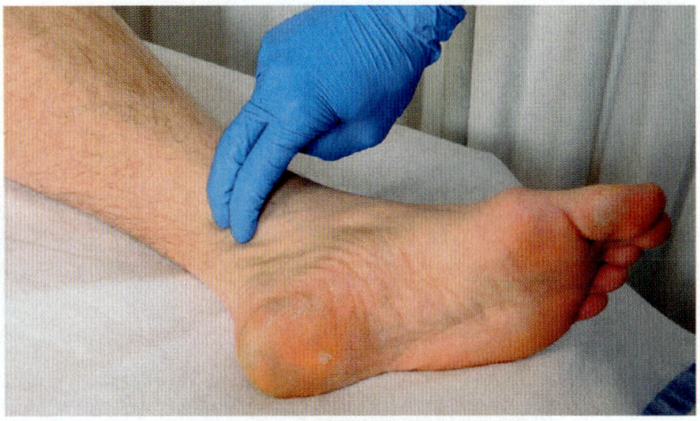

FIGURE 10.8 A positive Tinel sign just posterior to the medial malleolus over the posterior tibial nerve as it passes beneath the fascia is usually present in patient's suffering from posterior tarsal tunnel syndrome.

the posterior tibial nerve. Lumbar radiculopathy and posterior tibial nerve entrapment may coexist as the so-called "double crush" syndrome and this can further confuse the clinical picture. Based on the patient's clinical presentation, additional testing may be indicated, including complete blood cell count, uric acid, sedimentation rate, and antinuclear antibody testing. MRI or CT scanning of the lumbar spine is indicated if a herniated disk, spinal stenosis, or a space-occupying lesion is suspected. MRI and/or ultrasound imaging of the posterior ankle and foot are indicated to confirm the diagnosis of posterior tarsal tunnel syndrome by identifying the pathology responsible for nerve entrapment, for example, tumor, mass, osteophyte, as well as to identify occult pathology (Figs. 10.10 to 10.14).

ULTRASOUND TECHNIQUE

For ultrasound evaluation of the posterior tibial nerve at the ankle, the patient is placed in the supine position with the arms resting comfortably along the chest and the affected lower extremity externally rotated. The pulsation of the posterior tibial artery is then identified by palpation (Fig. 10.8). A linear high-frequency ultrasound transducer is placed in a longitudinal plane over the previously identified pulsation of the posterior tibial artery, and then the superior aspect of the transducer is rotated toward the front of the ankle with the superior aspect of the ultrasound transducer lying on the posteroinferior border of the medial malleolus and the inferior

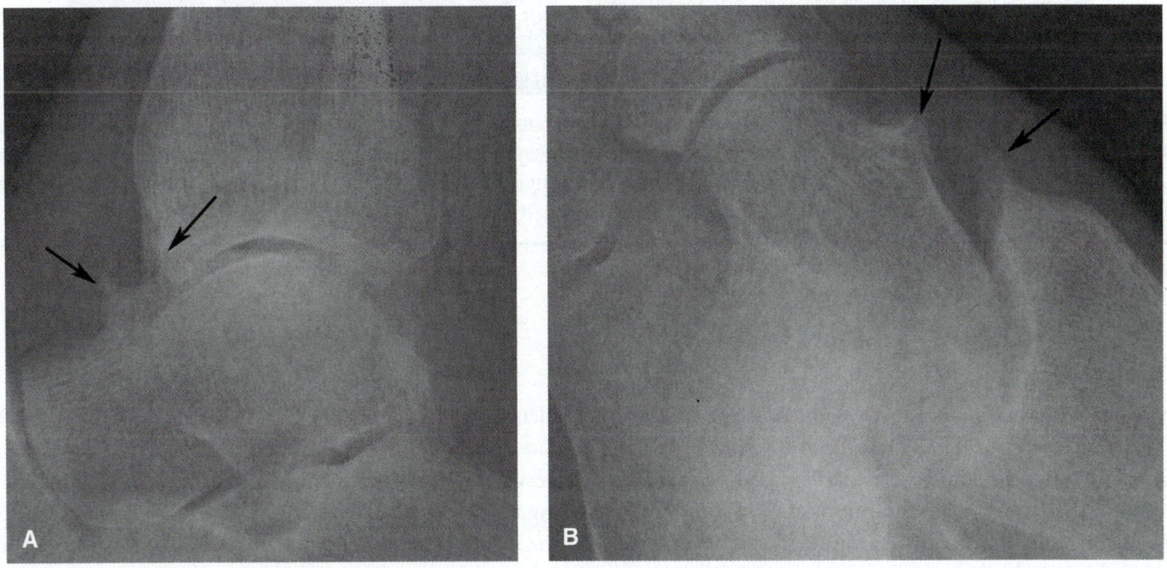

FIGURE 10.9 Anterior ankle impingement. Stage III anterior ankle impingement. Lateral **(A)** and oblique **(B)** radiographs demonstrating talar and anterior tibial osteophytes (*arrows*). (From Berquist TH. *Imaging of the Foot and Ankle*. 3rd ed. Philadelphia, PA: Lippincott Williams & Wilkins; 2011:328.)

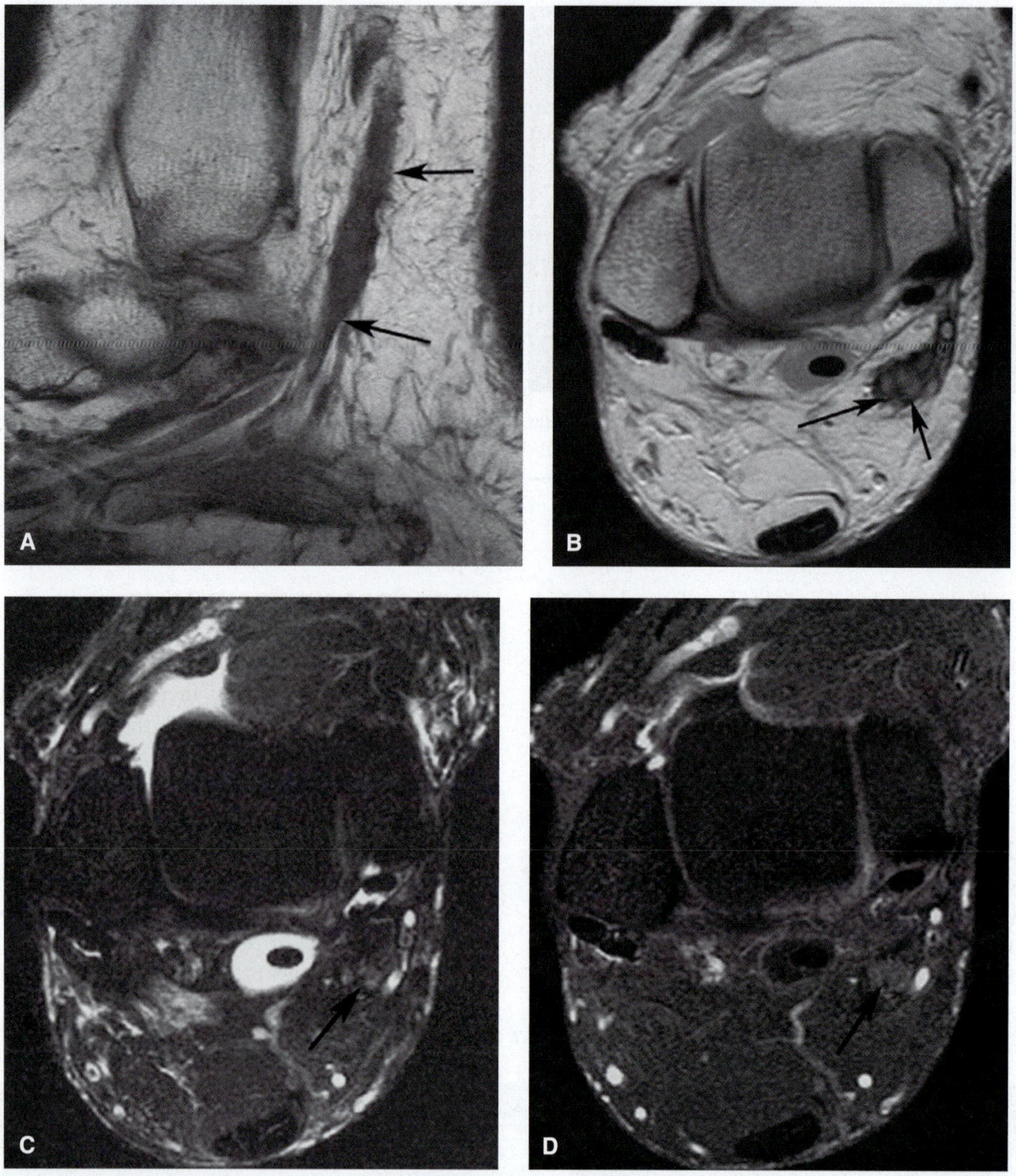

FIGURE 10.10 Tarsal tunnel syndrome. Sagittal **(A)** and axial **(B)** T1-weighted images demonstrating a neuroma of the tibial nerve (*arrows*). Axial fast spin echo T2-weighted **(C)** and postcontrast fat-suppressed T1-weighted **(D)** images demonstrate no increase in signal intensity and minimal contrast enhancement of the fibrous neural lesion (*arrow*). (From Berquist TH. Soft tissue trauma and overuse syndromes. *Imaging of the Foot and Ankle*. 3rd ed. Philadelphia, PA: Lippincott Williams & Wilkins; 2011:182.)

aspect of the ultrasound transducer pointed at the calcaneus (Fig. 10.15). This will put the ultrasound transducer perpendicular to the posterior tibial nerve, artery, and vein as they pass through the posterior tarsal tunnel. An ultrasound survey scan is taken. The posterior tibial artery and vein can be seen lying between the skin, subcutaneous tissues and flexor retinaculum, and the medial tubercle of the talus (Fig. 10.16). The posterior tibial nerve will be seen to lie just beneath the posterior tibial artery and vein. Color Doppler can be used to help identify the posterior tibial artery and vein (Fig. 10.17). When the posterior tibial artery and vein and the posterior tibial nerve lying beneath them are identified on ultrasound imaging, the posterior tibial nerve is evaluated as it passes inferiorly through the posterior tarsal tunnel for presence of compromise or compression by bony abnormality or soft tissue mass, cysts, neuropathy as evidence of loss of normal sonographic neurofibular architecture, and intraneural tumors (Figs. 10.18 to 10.23).

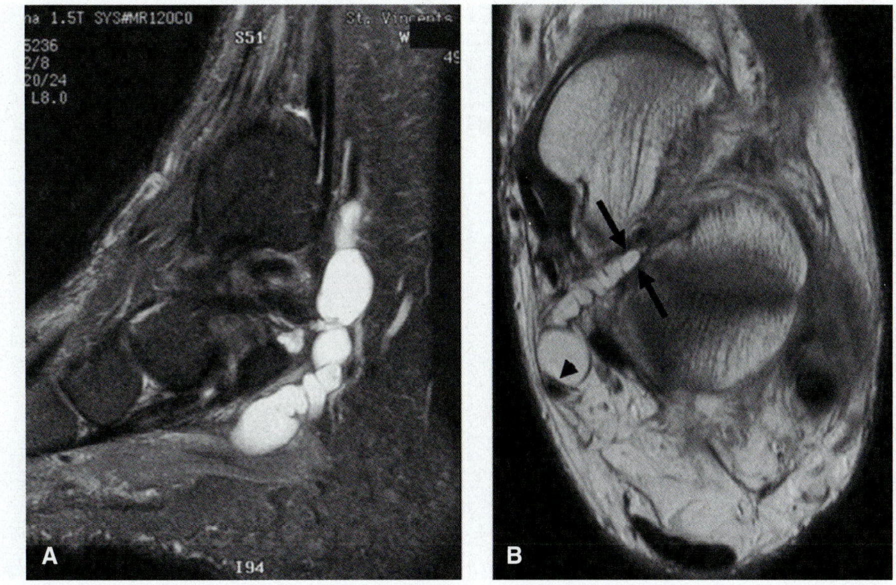

FIGURE 10.11 Tarsal tunnel ganglion. **A:** Sagittal fat-suppressed PD MR image demonstrating a large tarsal tunnel ganglion cyst arising from the sinus tarsi. **B:** Axial PD MR image demonstrating medial displacement of the MPN (*arrowhead*) by the ganglion and origin of the ganglion from the interosseous talocalcaneal ligament within the sinus tarsi (*arrows*). (From Simmons DN, Lisle DA, Linklater JM. Imaging of peripheral nerve lesions in the lower limb. *Top Magn Reson Imaging* 2010;21(1):51–62.)

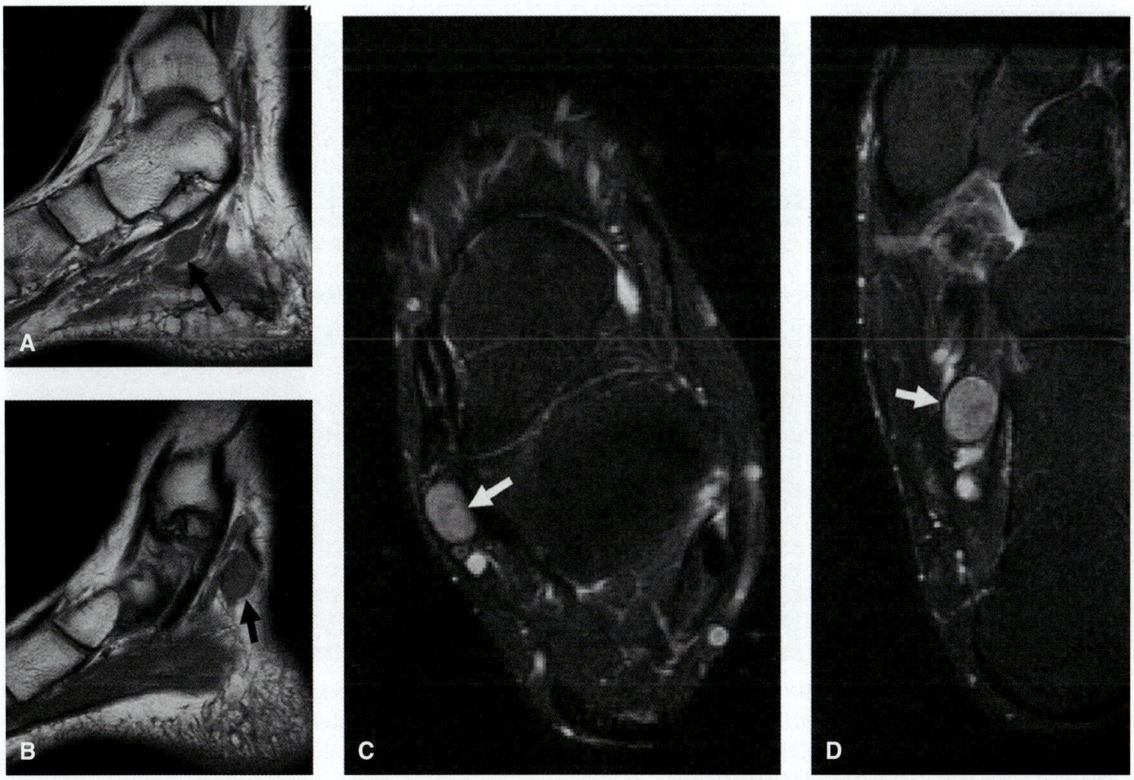

FIGURE 10.12 Two separate peripheral nerve sheath tumors (schwannomas) of the LPN (*arrows*). Sagittal T1 **(A,B)** and axial fat-suppressed PD MR **(C,D)** images demonstrating the two separate lesions. (From Simmons DN, Lisle DA, Linklater JM. Imaging of peripheral nerve lesions in the lower limb. *Top Magn Reson Imaging* 2010;21(1):51–62.)

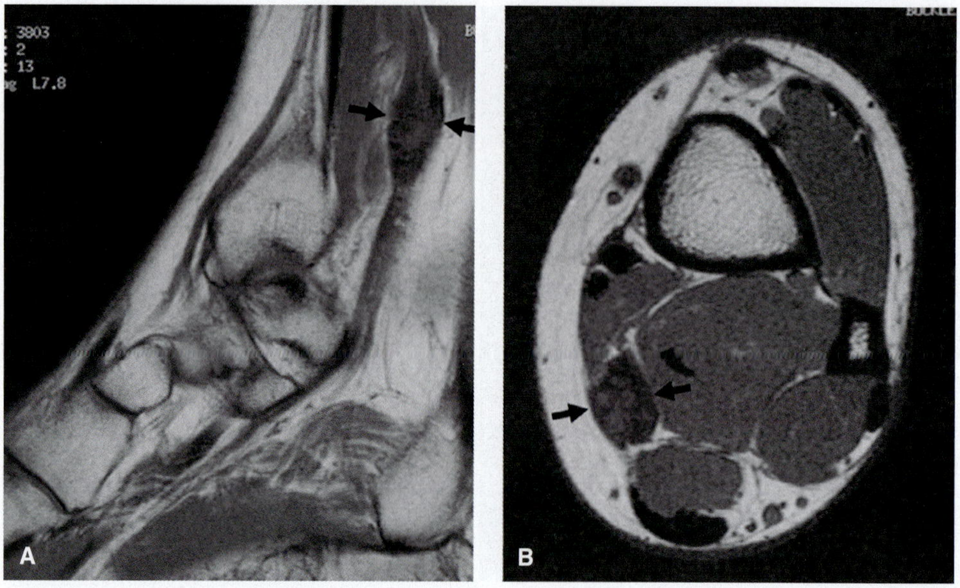

FIGURE 10.13 Posttraumatic neuroma of the tibial nerve. Sagittal **(A)** and axial **(B)** PD MR images of a posttraumatic tibial nerve neuroma (*arrows*). (From Simmons DN, Lisle DA, Linklater JM. Imaging of peripheral nerve lesions in the lower limb. *Top Magn Reson Imaging* 2010;21(1): 51–62.)

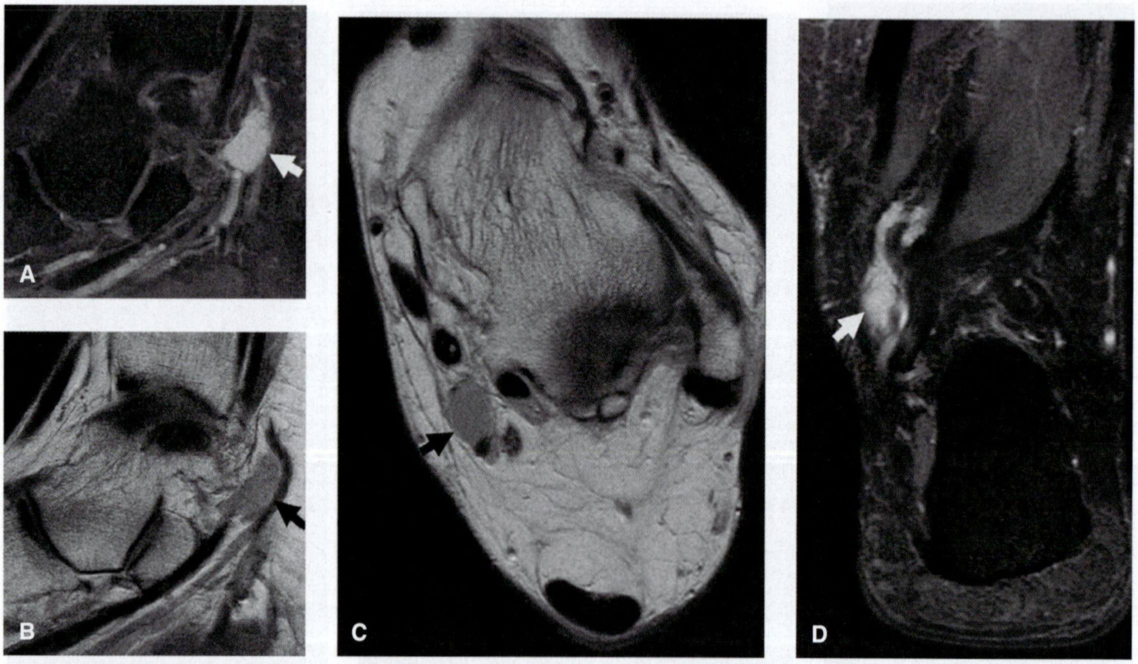

FIGURE 10.14 Low flow vascular malformation in the tarsal tunnel mimicking a ganglion cyst. **A:** Sagittal PD and fat-suppressed PD **(B)** and axial PD **(C)** and postcontrast coronal fat-suppressed **(D)** T1 MR images. Note diffuse postcontrast enhancement of the lesion **(D)**, identical to that of an adjacent vein, excluding the differential diagnosis of a ganglion. (From Simmons DN, Lisle DA, Linklater JM. Imaging of peripheral nerve lesions in the lower limb. *Top Magn Reson Imaging* 2010;21(1):51–62.)

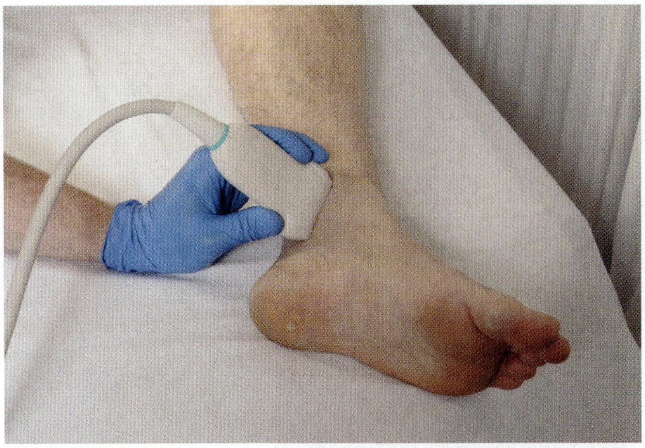

FIGURE 10.15 Proper longitudinal position of the ultrasound transducer with the superior aspect of the transducer rotated toward the anterior ankle for ultrasound evaluation of the posterior tibial nerve at the ankle.

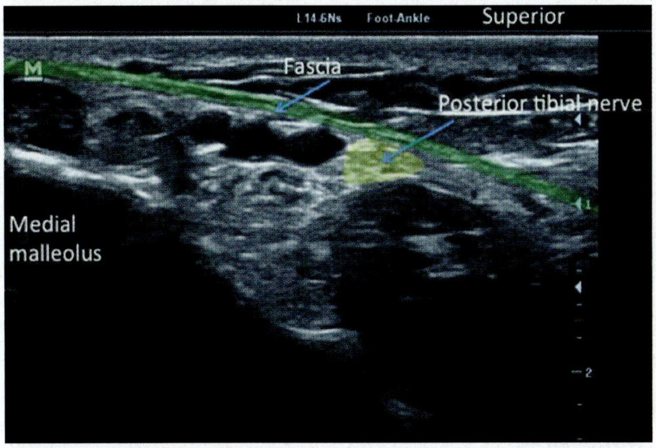

FIGURE 10.16 Transverse ultrasound image demonstrating the posterior tibial artery and vein and the posterior tibial nerve adjacent to the vein. (Posterior is to the right.)

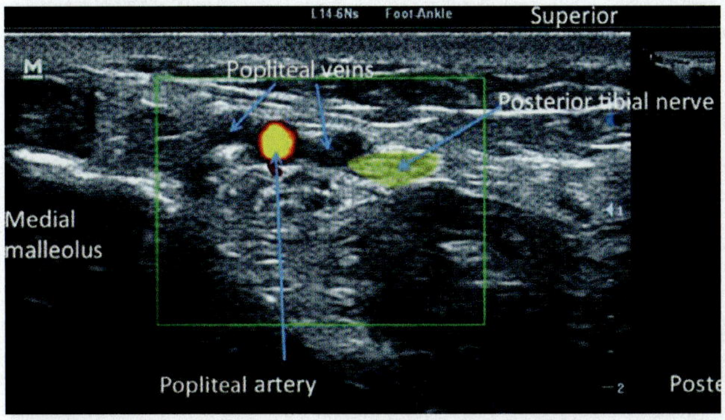

FIGURE 10.17 Transverse color Doppler image demonstrating the popliteal vein and artery and the relationship of the vein to the posterior tibial nerve.

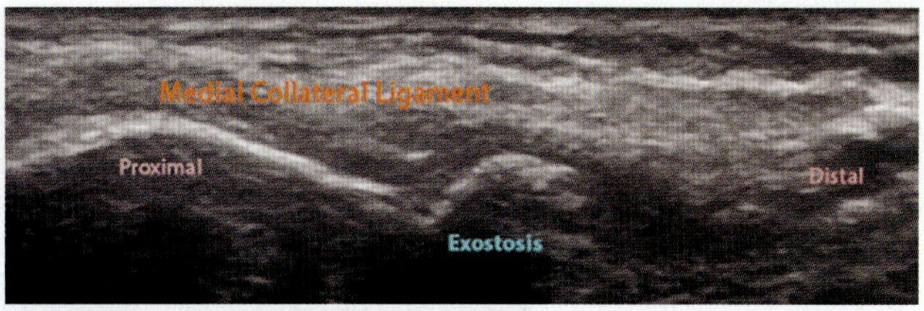

FIGURE 10.18 Longitudinal ultrasound image on the medial tibia demonstrating an exostosis.

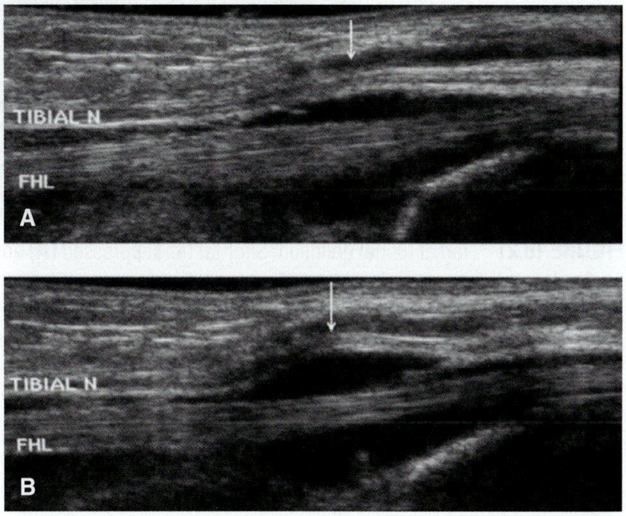

FIGURE 10.19 Tenosynovitis compressing the posterior tibial nerve. **A:** Longitudinal ultrasound image demonstrating tenosynovitis of flexor hallucis longus with an effusion in the tendon sheath. **B:** On plantar flexion of the big toe the fluid in the sheath moved proximally and displaced the tibial nerve. (From Simmons DN, Lisle DA, Linklater JM. Imaging of peripheral nerve lesions in the lower limb. *Top Magn Reson Imaging* 2010;21(1):51–62.)

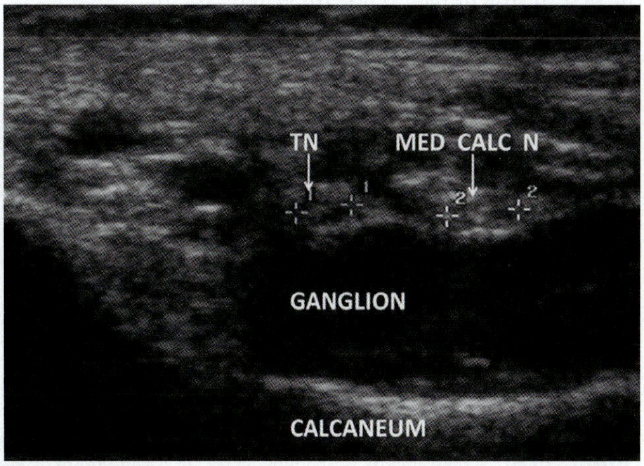

FIGURE 10.20 Transverse ultrasound image demonstrate a large tarsal tunnel ganglion cyst arising from the subtalar joint displacing the tibial nerve and MCN. tn, tibial nerve; MCN, medial calcaneal nerve. (From Simmons DN, Lisle DA, Linklater JM. Imaging of peripheral nerve lesions in the lower limb. *Top Magn Reson Imaging* 2010;21(1):51–62.)

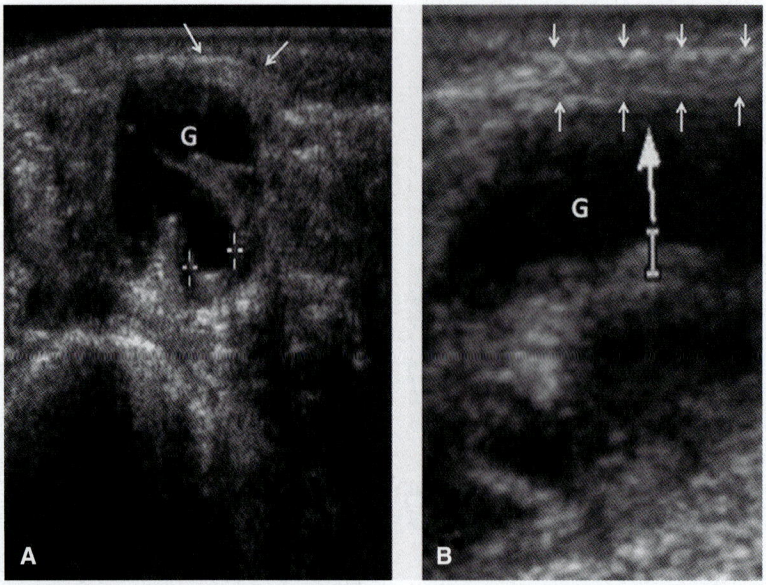

FIGURE 10.21 Tarsal tunnel ganglion. Sagittal fat-suppressed **(A)** and axial **(B)** PD MR images demonstrating a large tarsal tunnel ganglion cyst arising from an extra-articular talocalcaneal coalition (*small arrows*) compressing MPN (*large arrow*) and LPN. Note the intraosseous cystic change and bone marrow edema at the talar margin of the coalition and small ganglionic component at the apex of the sinus tarsi. g, ganglion. (From Simmons DN, Lisle DA, Linklater JM. Imaging of peripheral nerve lesions in the lower limb. *Top Magn Reson Imaging* 2010;21(1):51–62.)

CLINICAL PEARLS

The key to performing successful ultrasound injection technique for posterior tarsal tunnel syndrome is the proper identification of the sonographic anatomy and, in particular, the ability to properly identify the posterior tibial nerve at the site of nerve entrapment. This should not be a problem if the above technique is used. The judicious use of multiple imaging modalities will improve the accuracy of diagnosis by identifying coexistent occult pathology and will aid in crafting the best treatment plan (Figs. 10.24 and 10.25).

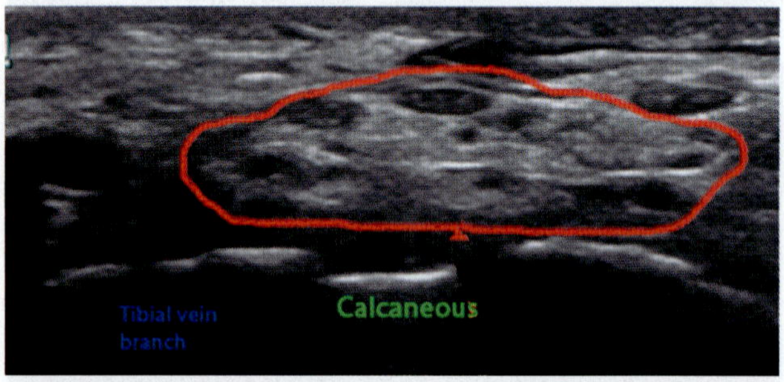

FIGURE 10.22 Transverse ultrasound image demonstrating a large neuroma of the posterior tibial nerve.

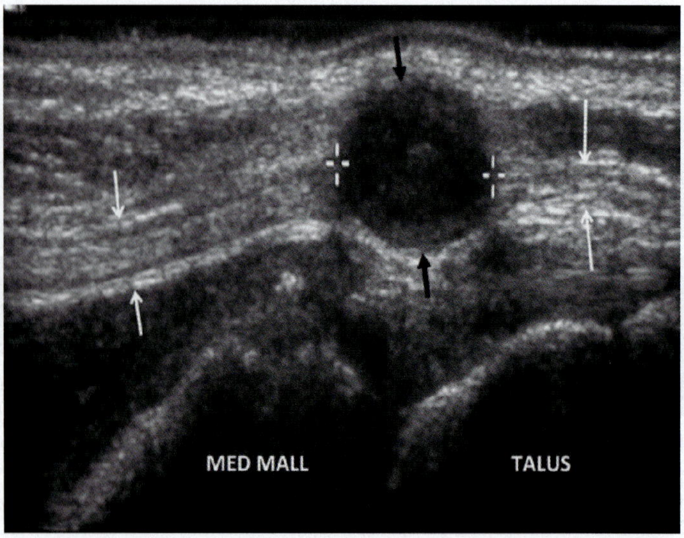

FIGURE 10.23 Longitudinal ultrasound scan of a peripheral nerve sheath tumor (*black arrows*) arising from the tibial nerve in the proximal tarsal tunnel. Normal nerve indicated by white arrows. (From Simmons DN, Lisle DA, Linklater JM. Imaging of peripheral nerve lesions in the lower limb. *Top Magn Reson Imaging* 2010;21(1):51–62.)

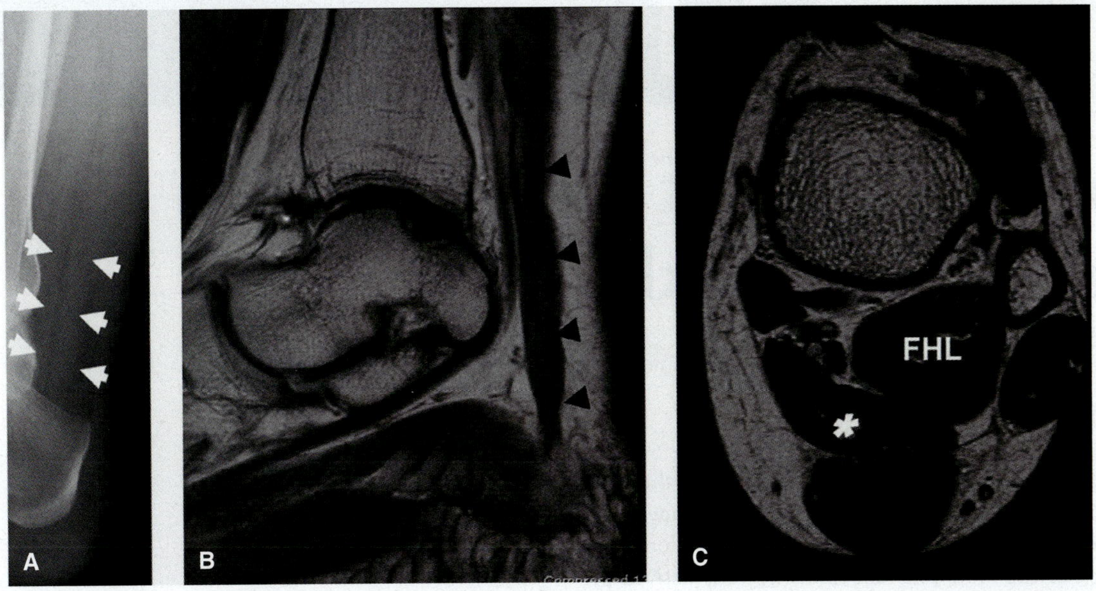

FIGURE 10.24 Accessory muscle (tibiocalcaneus internus) causing tarsal tunnel syndrome. **A:** Lateral radiograph of the ankle demonstrating the soft tissue outline of the accessory muscle (*arrows*). Sagittal **(B)** and axial **(C)** PD MR images demonstrating the accessory muscle lying beneath the deep fascia (*arrowheads* and *asterisk*). (From Simmons DN, Lisle DA, Linklater JM. Imaging of peripheral nerve lesions in the lower limb. *Top Magn Reson Imaging* 2010;21(1):51–62.)

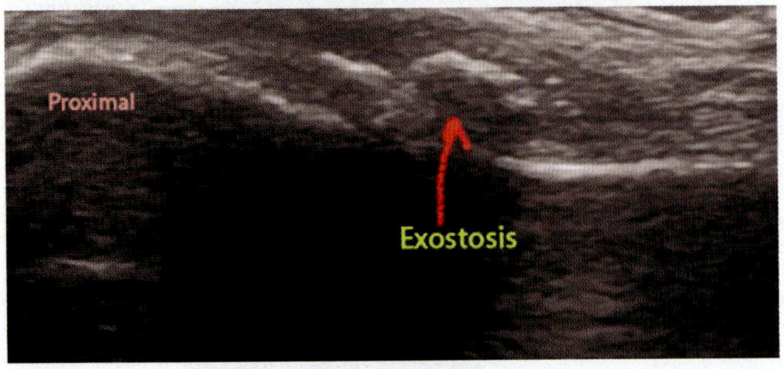

FIGURE 10.25 Longitudinal ultrasound image of the medial aspect of the tibia demonstrating an exostosis.

Suggested Readings

Cancilleri F, Ippolito M, Amato C, et al. Tarsal tunnel syndrome: four uncommon cases. *Foot Ankle Surg* 2007;13(4):214–217.

Fujita I, Matsumoto K, Minami T, et al. Tarsal tunnel syndrome caused by epineural ganglion of the posterior tibial nerve: report of 2 cases and review of the literature. *J Foot Ankle Surg* 2004;43(3):185–190.

Mezrow CK, Sanger JR, Matloub HS. Acute tarsal tunnel syndrome following partial avulsion of the flexor hallucis longus muscle: a case report. *J Foot Ankle Surg* 2002;41(4):243–246.

Waldman SD. Functional anatomy of the foot and ankle. In: *Pain Review.* Philadelphia, PA: Saunders; 2009:155–156.

Waldman SD. Posterior tarsal tunnel syndrome. In: *Pain Review.* Philadelphia, PA: Saunders; 2009:323–324.

Waldman SD. Injection technique for posterior tarsal tunnel syndrome. In: *Atlas of Pain Management Injection Techniques.* 3rd ed. Philadelphia, PA: Saunders; 2012:435–436.

Waldman SD. Posterior tarsal tunnel syndrome. In: *Atlas of Common Pain Syndromes.* 3rd ed. Philadelphia, PA: Saunders; 2012:359–361.

Waldman SD, Campbell RSD. Posterior tarsal tunnel syndrome. In: *Imaging of Pain.* Philadelphia, PA: Saunders; 2011:425–426.

CHAPTER 11

Abnormalities of the Saphenous Nerve at the Ankle

ANATOMIC CONSIDERATIONS

The saphenous nerve is the largest sensory branch of the femoral nerve. The saphenous nerve provides sensory innervation to the medial malleolus, the medial calf, and a portion of the medial arch of the foot. The saphenous nerve is derived primarily from the fibers of the L3 and L4 nerve roots. The nerve travels along with the femoral artery through Hunter's canal and moves superficially as it approaches the ankle (Fig. 11.1). It passes over the medial malleolus of the tibia, splitting into terminal sensory branches (Figs. 11.2 and 11.3). The saphenous nerve is subject to trauma or compression anywhere along its course. The nerve is frequently traumatized during vein harvest for coronary artery bypass grafting procedures. The saphenous nerve is also subject to compression as it passes over the medial condyle of the femur. Less commonly, the nerve is damaged or compressed distally as it passes beneath the fascia of the dorsum of the foot.

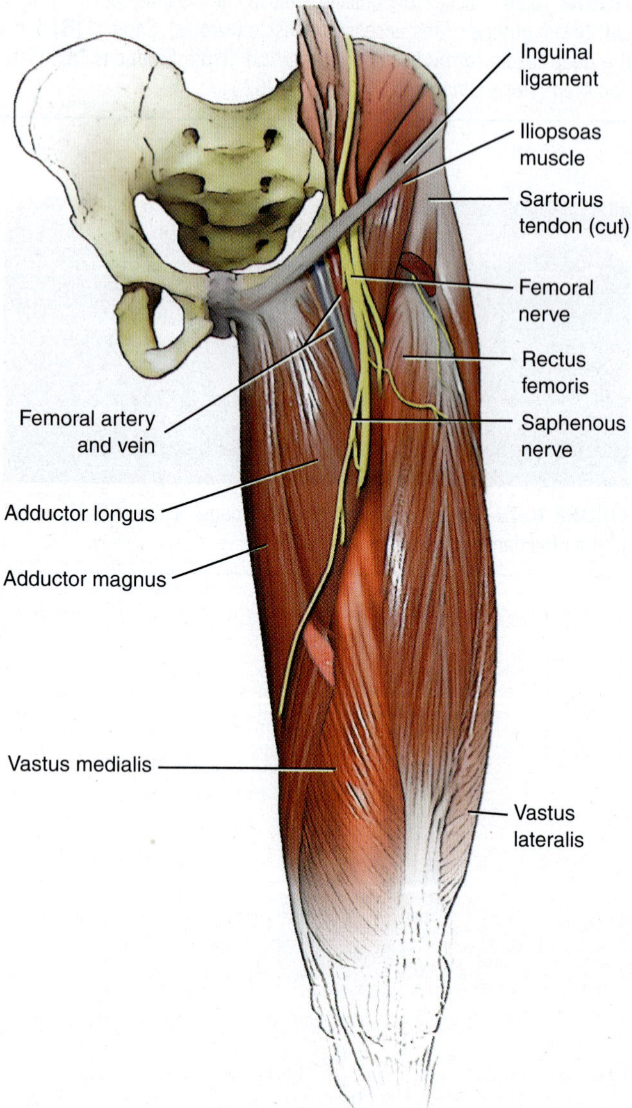

FIGURE 11.1 The anatomy of the proximal saphenous nerve.

CLINICAL CORRELATES

Saphenous neuralgia is caused by entrapment and compression of the saphenous nerve anywhere along its course, with compromise of the nerve most common as it passes through Hunter's canal, at the medial condyle of the femur, and as it passes beneath the fascia of the dorsum of the foot (Fig. 11.1). The saphenous nerve is frequently traumatized during vein stripping and harvest procedures, with the infrapatellar branch of the saphenous nerve frequently damaged during total knee arthroplasty (Fig. 11.4). The nerve can also be damaged by trauma to the ankle, including fracture, dislocation, and crush injuries (Figs. 11.5 and 11.6). The musculotendinous units of the tibialis muscles are subject to the development of tenosynovitis which may also compromise the nerve.

Electrodiagnostic testing should be considered in all patients who suffer from saphenous nerve dysfunction to provide both neuroanatomic and neurophysiologic information regarding nerve function. Magnetic resonance imaging and ultrasound imaging of the popliteal fossa as well as anywhere along the course of the saphenous nerve are also useful in determining the cause of saphenous nerve compromise.

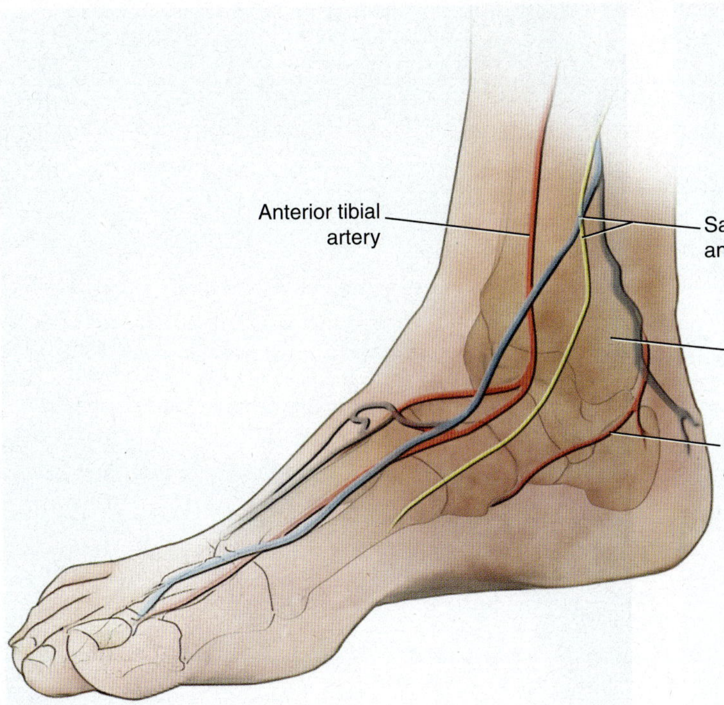

FIGURE 11.2 The anatomy of the distal saphenous nerve. Note the relationship of the nerve to the saphenous vein.

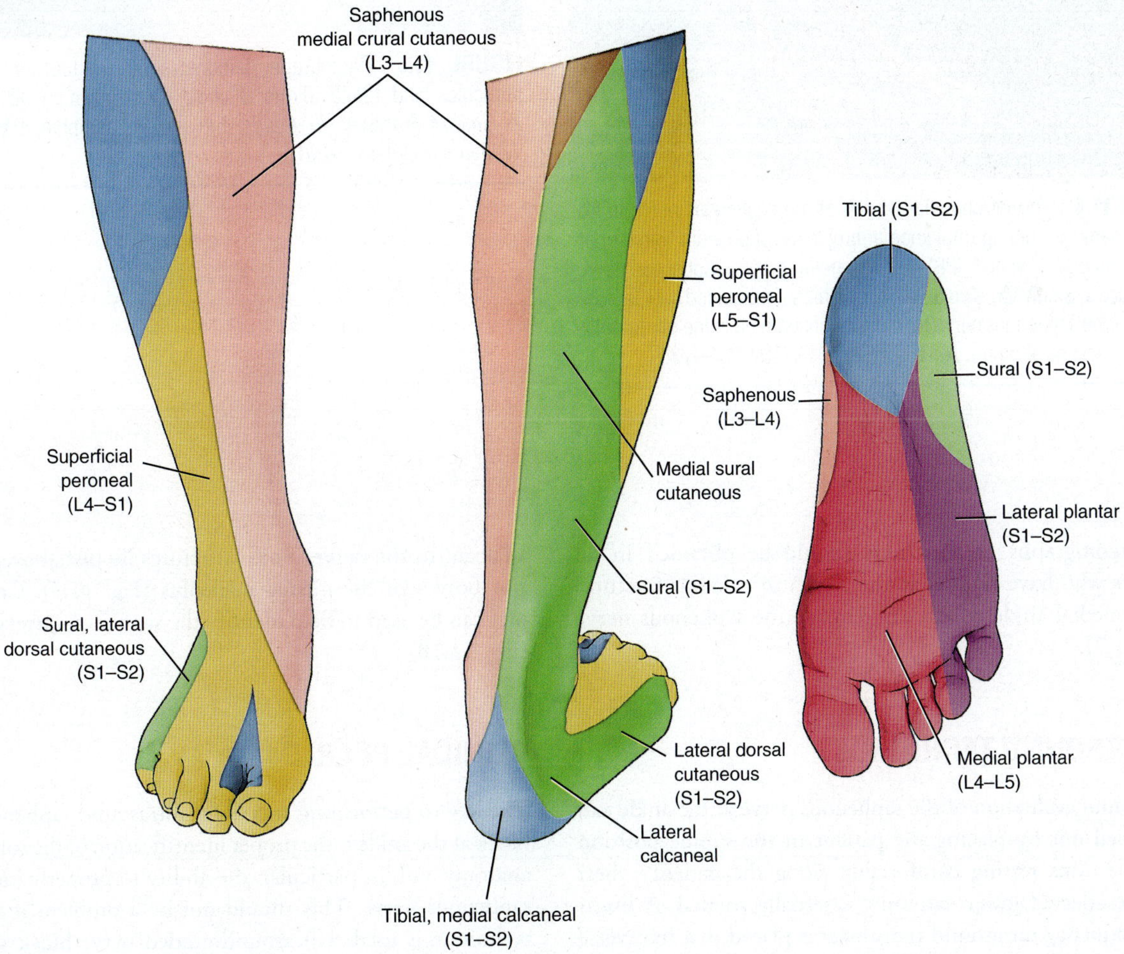

FIGURE 11.3 Sensory distribution of the distal saphenous nerve.

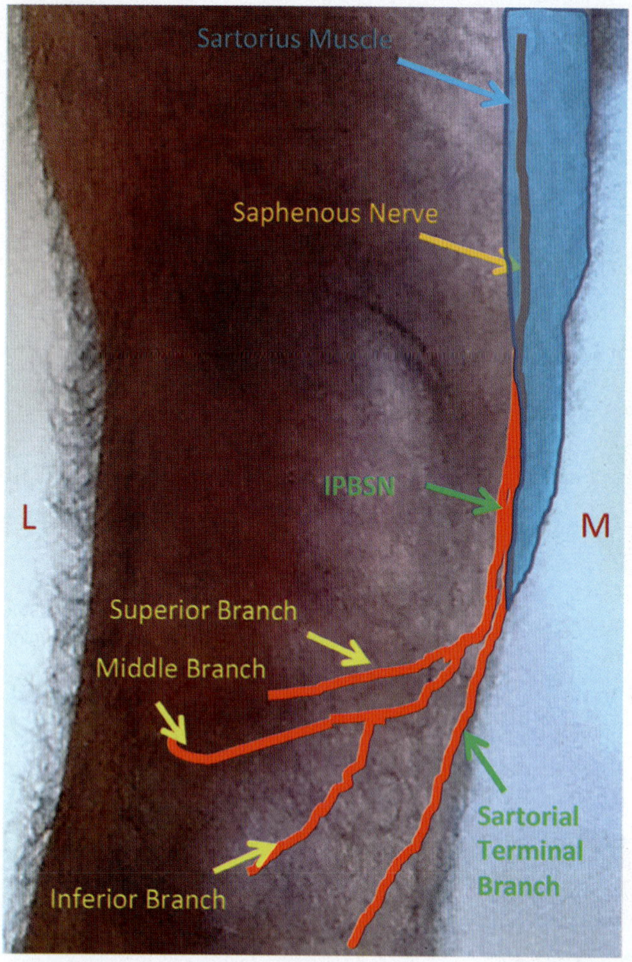

FIGURE 11.4 The infrapatellar branch of the saphenous nerve is frequently damaged during total knee arthroplasty. Saphenous nerve anatomy. M, medial; L, lateral; IPBSN, infrapatellar branch saphenous nerve. (From Jose J, Smith MK, Kaplan LD, et al. Ultrasound-guided needle localization of the saphenous nerve for removal of neuroma in the infrapatellar branches: technical report. *Neurosurgery* 2014;75(6):717–722.)

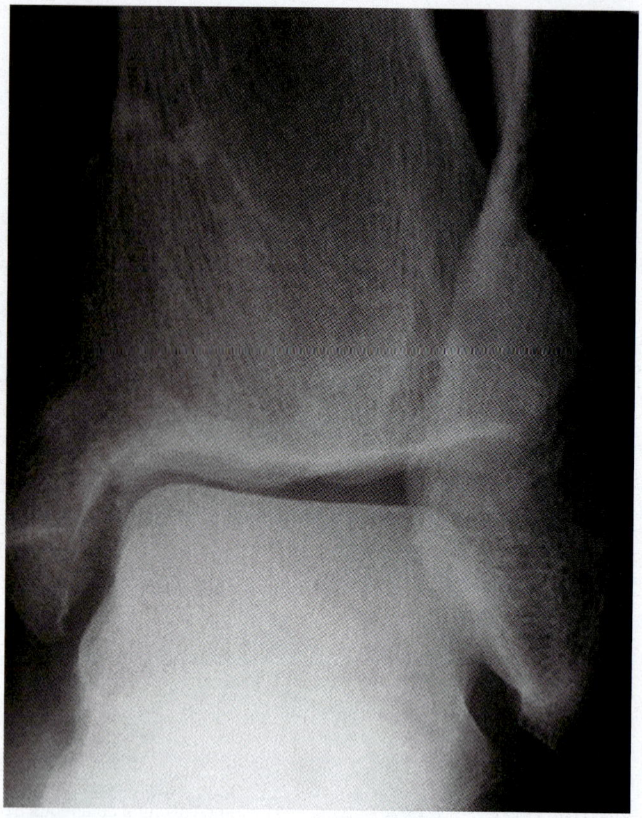

FIGURE 11.5 Radiograph demonstrating fracture of the medial malleolus and fibula. (From Bucholz RW, Heckman JD. *Rockwood & Green's Fractures in Adults*. 5th ed. Philadelphia, PA: Lippincott Williams & Wilkins; 2001.)

Plain radiographs of the ankle should be obtained in all patients who have trauma to the ankle, to rule out fractures of the medial ankle which can damage the saphenous nerve (Fig. 11.7).

ULTRASOUND TECHNIQUE

Ultrasound evaluation of the saphenous nerve at the ankle can be carried out by placing the patient in the supine position with the arms resting comfortably along the patient's chest and the affected lower extremity externally rotated. A linear high-frequency ultrasound transducer is placed in a transverse plane just above and slightly in front of the medial malleolus (Fig. 11.8). The compressible saphenous vein is seen lying just adjacent to the nerve. Both structures lie just above the anterior border of the medial malleolus (Fig. 11.9). Color Doppler can be used to help identify the saphenous artery and vein (Fig. 11.10).

CLINICAL PEARLS

The key to performing successful ultrasound saphenous nerve block at the ankle is the proper identification of the sonographic anatomy and, in particular, the ability to properly identify the saphenous nerve. This should not be a problem if the above technique is used. Ultrasound-guided nerve block with local anesthetic can serve as a diagnostic maneuver in patient with unexplained ankle pain.

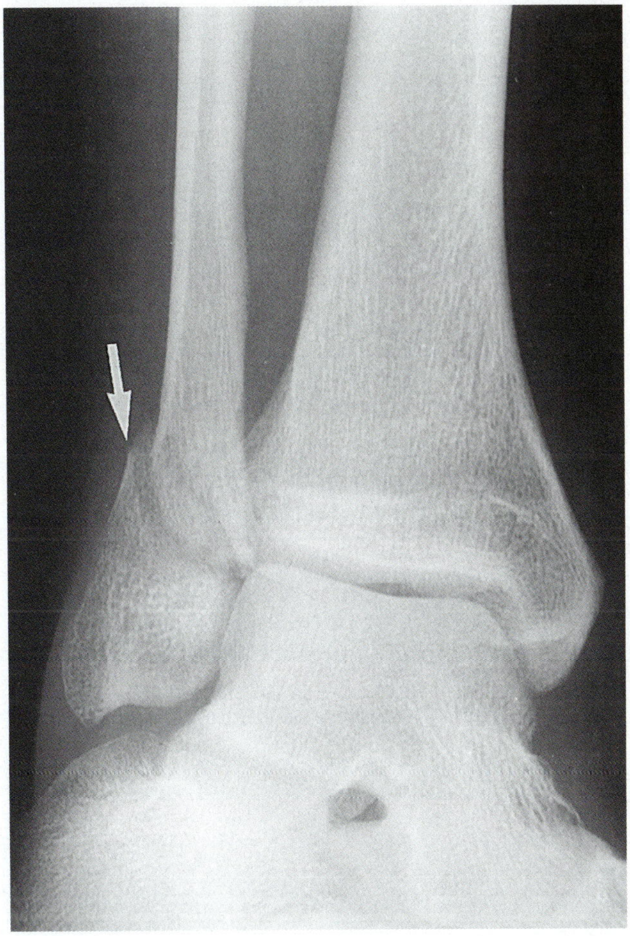

FIGURE 11.6 Distal fibula fracture. Medial oblique ankle. Note the most common fracture of the lateral malleolus is an oblique fracture extending upward (*arrow*). This fracture is best seen on the medial oblique projection. (From Rowe LJ, Yochum TR, Maola CJ. Trauma. Arthritic disorders. In: *Yochum and Rowes' Essentials of Skeletal Radiology*. 3rd ed. Vol. 1. Philadelphia, PA: Lippincott Williams & Wilkins; 2005:875.)

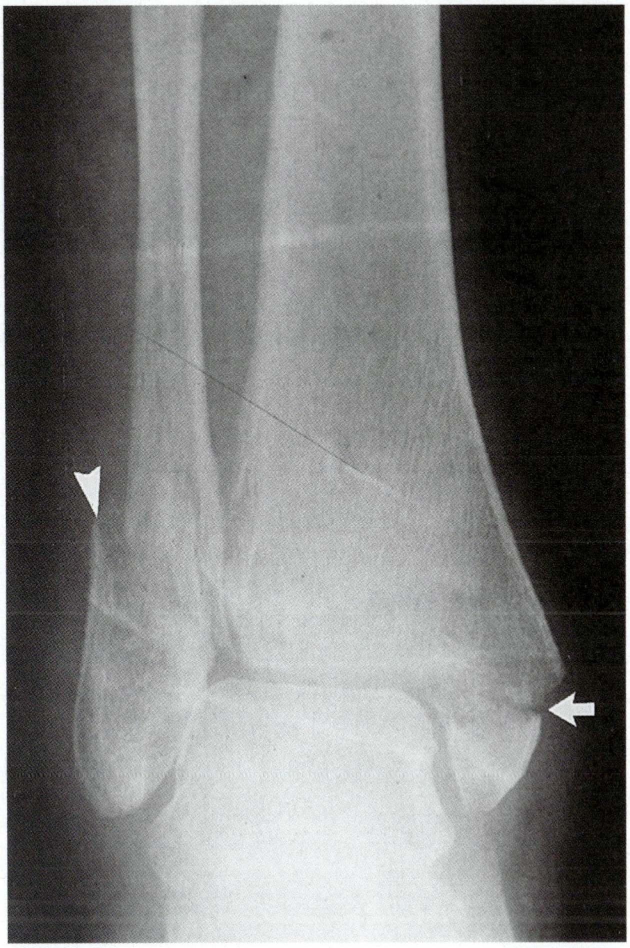

FIGURE 11.7 Bimalleolar fracture. AP ankle. Note the characteristic transverse fracture through the medial malleolus (*arrow*), along with a spiral fracture of the lateral malleolus (*arrowhead*). (From Rowe LJ, Yochum TR, Maola CJ. Trauma. Arthritic disorders. In: *Yochum and Rowes' Essentials of Skeletal Radiology*. 3rd ed. Vol. 1. Philadelphia, PA: Lippincott Williams & Wilkins; 2005:875.)

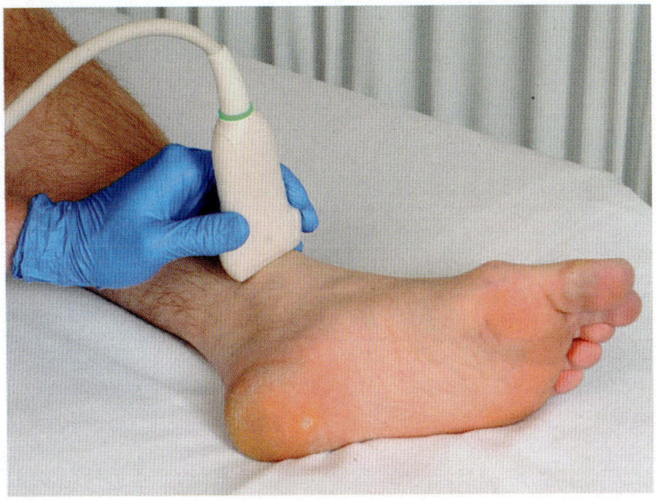

FIGURE 11.8 Proper transverse position of the ultrasound transducer for ultrasound-guided saphenous nerve block at the ankle.

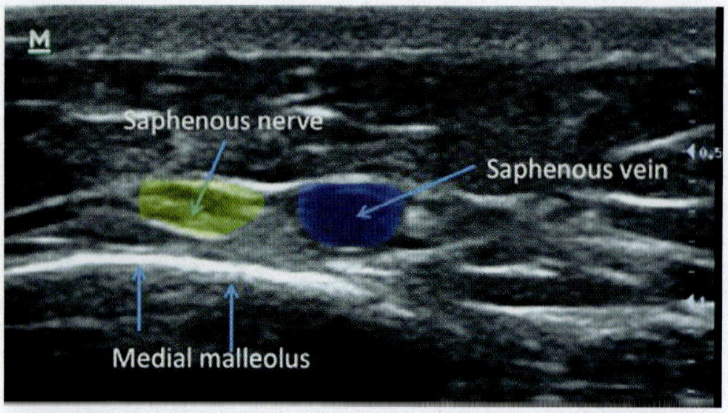

FIGURE 11.9 Transverse ultrasound image demonstrating the saphenous vein and the saphenous nerve just above and lateral to the vein. (Anterior is to the left, posterior to the right.)

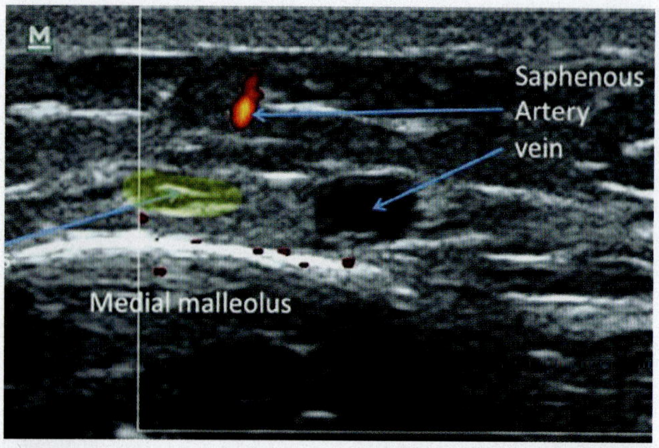

FIGURE 11.10 Transverse color Doppler image demonstrating the popliteal vein and artery and the relationship of the vein to the saphenous nerve (shaded yellow).

Suggested Readings

Cho KH, Wansaicheong GKL. Ultrasound of the foot and ankle. *Ultrasound Clin* 2012;7(4):487–503.

Lopez-Ben R. Imaging of nerve entrapment in the foot and ankle. *Foot Ankle Clin* 2011;16(2):213–224.

Sanders B, Rolf R, McClelland W, et al. Prevalence of saphenous nerve injury after autogenous hamstring harvest: an anatomic and clinical study of sartorial branch injury. *Arthroscopy* 2007;23(9):956–963.

Waldman SD. Saphenous nerve block at the ankle. In: *Atlas of Interventional Pain Management.* 3rd ed. Philadelphia, PA: Saunders; 2009:555–558.

CHAPTER 12

Abnormalities of the Superficial Peroneal Nerve at the Ankle

ANATOMIC CONSIDERATIONS

The common peroneal nerve is one of the two major continuations of the sciatic nerve, the other being the tibial nerve. The common peroneal nerve, which is also known as the common fibular nerve, provides sensory innervation to the inferior portion of the knee joint, and the posterior and lateral skin of the upper calf. The common peroneal nerve is derived from the posterior branches of the L4, L5, and S1 and S2 nerve roots. The nerve splits from the sciatic nerve at the superior margin of the popliteal fossa and descends laterally behind the head of the fibula (Fig. 12.1). The common peroneal nerve is subject to compression at this point by circumstances such as improperly applied casts and tourniquets. The nerve is also subject to compression as it continues its lateral course, winding around the fibula through the fibular tunnel, which is made up of the posterior border of the tendinous insertion of the peroneus longus muscle and the fibula itself. Just distal to the fibular tunnel, the nerve divides into its two terminal branches, the superficial and the deep peroneal nerves (Fig. 12.2). These branches are also known as the superficial and the deep fibular nerves. Each of these branches is subject to trauma and may be blocked individually with local anesthetic as a diagnostic and therapeutic maneuver.

The deep branch continues down the leg in conjunction with the tibial artery and vein to provide sensory innervation to the web space of the first and second toes and adjacent dorsum of the foot (Fig. 12.3). Although this distribution of sensory fibers is small, this area is often the site of Morton's neuroma surgery and thus is important to the regional anesthesiologist. The superficial peroneal nerve provides motor innervation to

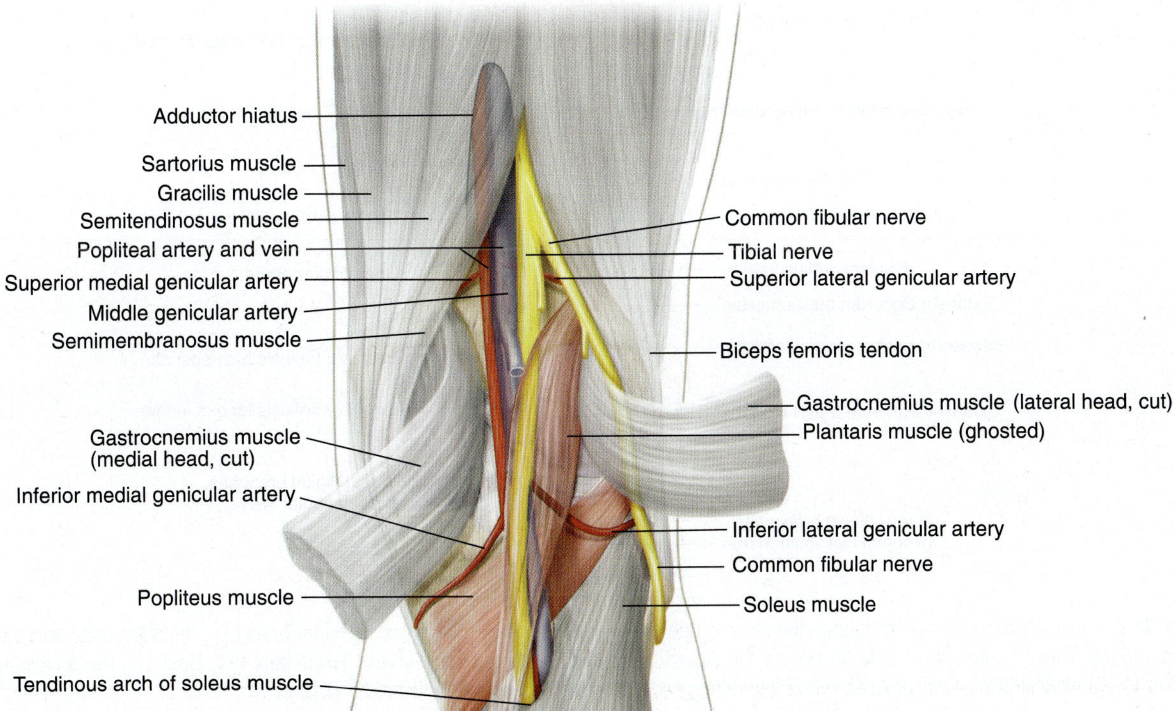

FIGURE 12.1 The common peroneal nerve is one of the two major continuations of the sciatic nerve, the other being the tibial nerve. (From Tank PW, Gest TR. The lower limb. In: *Lippincott Williams & Wilkins Atlas of Anatomy*. Philadelphia, PA: Lippincott Williams & Wilkins; 2009:117.)

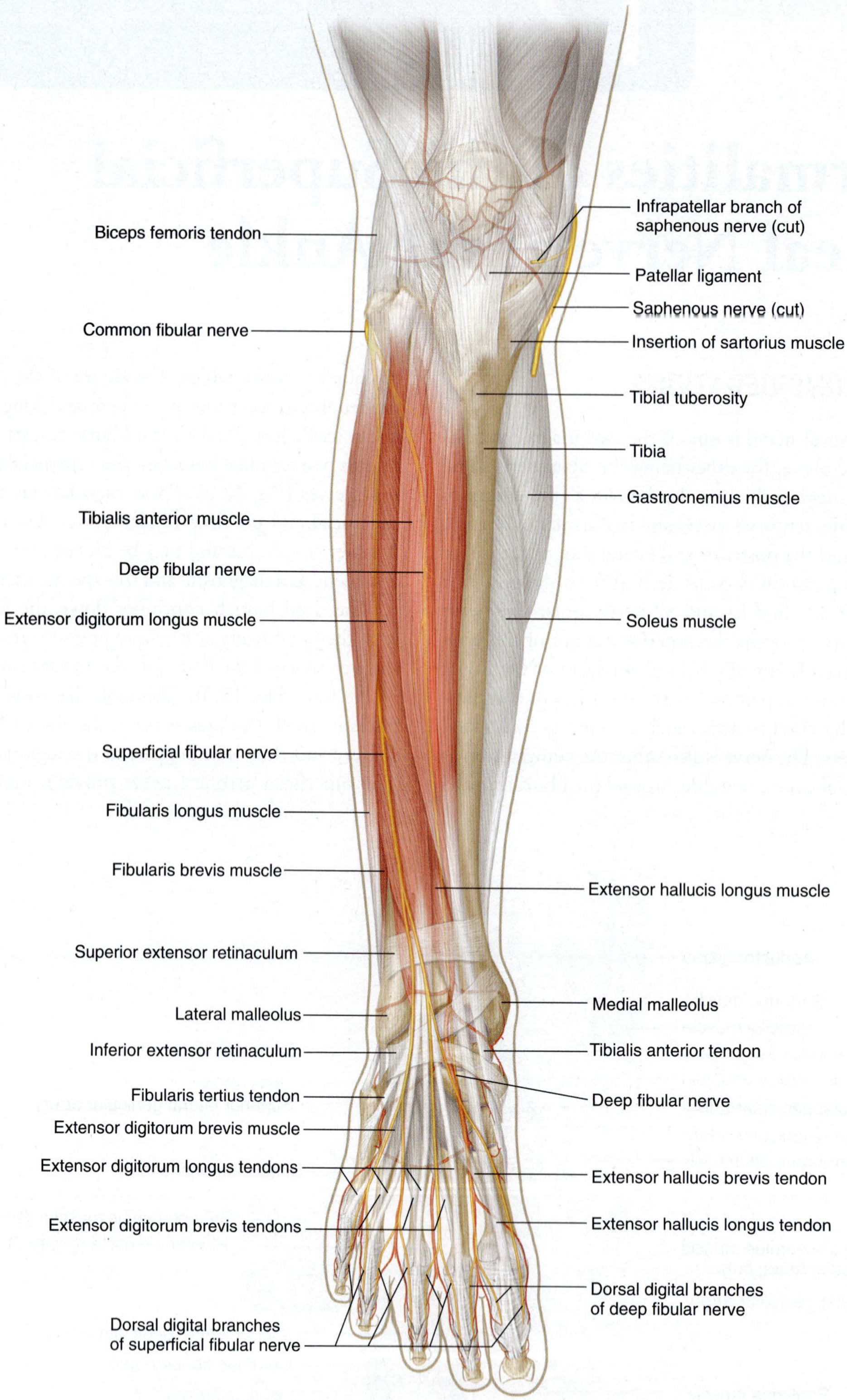

FIGURE 12.2 Just distal to the fibular tunnel, the common peroneal nerve divides into its two terminal branches, the superficial and the deep peroneal nerves. These branches are also known as the superficial and the deep fibular nerves. (From Tank PW, Gest TR. The lower limb. In: *Lippincott Williams & Wilkins Atlas of Anatomy*. Philadelphia, PA: Lippincott Williams & Wilkins; 2009:125.)

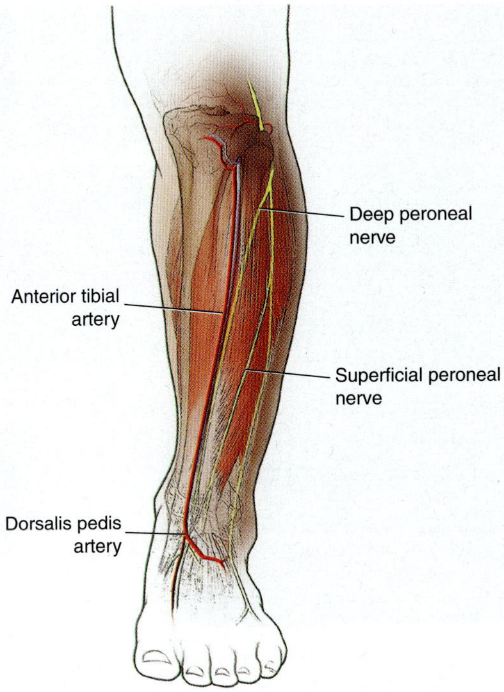

FIGURE 12.3 The anatomy of the distal superficial peroneal nerve. Note the relationship of the nerve to the superficial peroneal vein.

all of the toe extensors and the anterior tibialis muscles. The superficial peroneal nerve passes beneath the dense superficial fascia of the ankle, where it is subject to an entrapment syndrome known as the anterior tarsal tunnel syndrome. The superficial peroneal nerve also provides sensory innervation to the toes except for the area between the first and second toe, which is supplied by the deep peroneal nerve (Fig. 12.4).

CLINICAL CORRELATES

The superficial peroneal nerve and its branches are the most commonly injured nerves of the ankle and foot with the average age of patients suffering from this problem being 28 years. Occurring equally in males and females, superficial peroneal neuropathy and entrapment is most commonly seen in runners, hockey, tennis, and racquetball players. Tight ice skates and ski boots have also been implicated in the evolution of this common sports injury. Other common causes of superficial peroneal neuropathy include compression and/or injury by ganglion cysts, tumors, fibular fractures, tenosynovitis, aberrant muscles, penetrating injuries, compartment syndromes, ankle edema, and ankle sprains (Figs. 12.5 and 12.6). The nerve is occasionally injured during ankle arthroscopy.

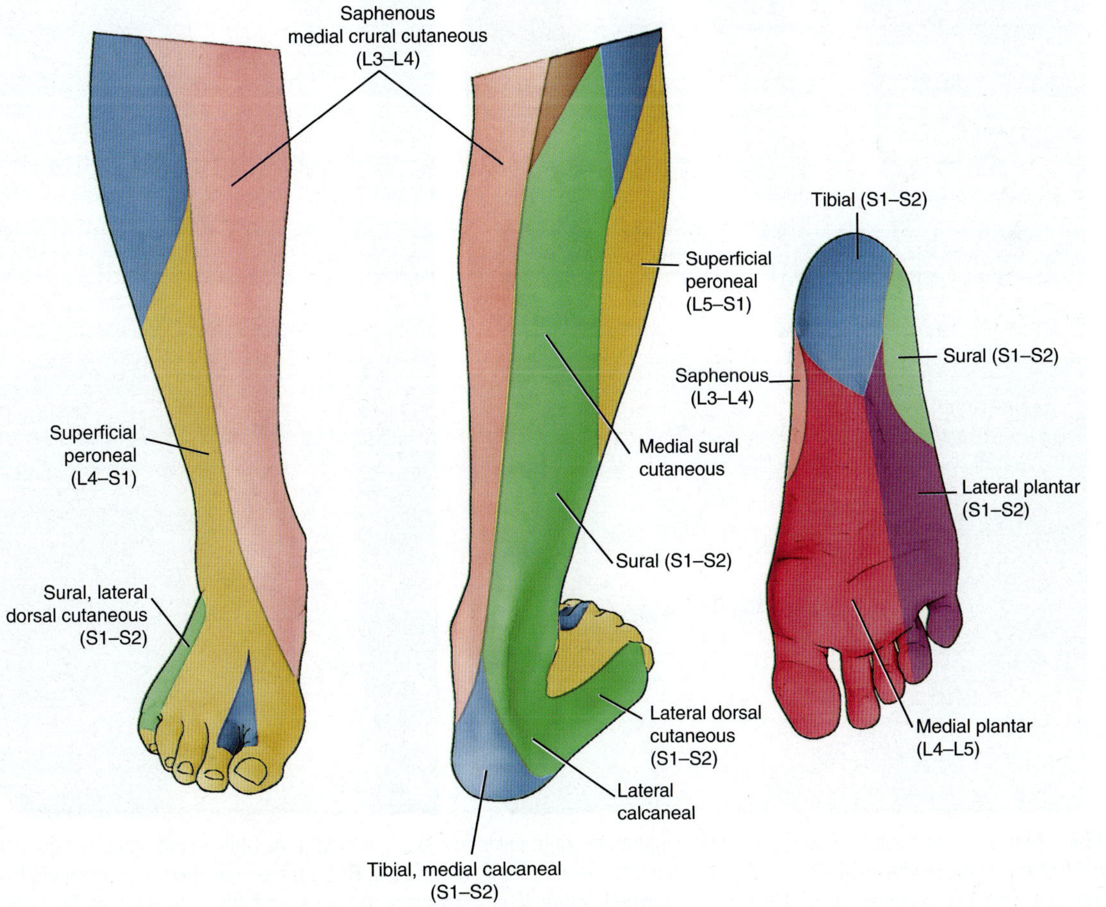

FIGURE 12.4 Sensory distribution of the distal superficial peroneal nerve.

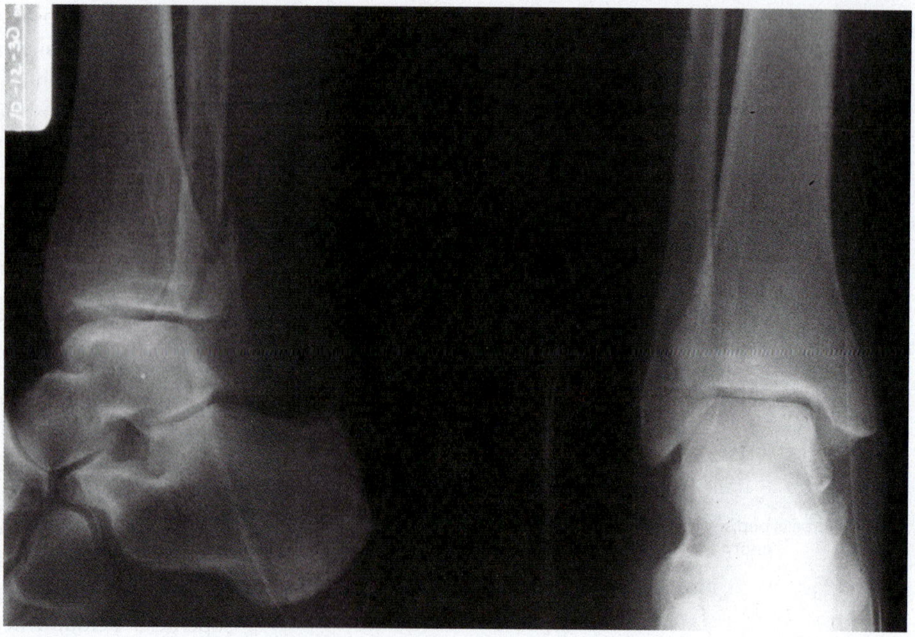

FIGURE 12.5 Radiographs demonstrating a fracture of the distal fibula. (From Bucholz RW, Heckman JD. *Rockwood & Green's Fractures in Adults*. 5th ed. Philadelphia, PA: Lippincott Williams & Wilkins; 2001.)

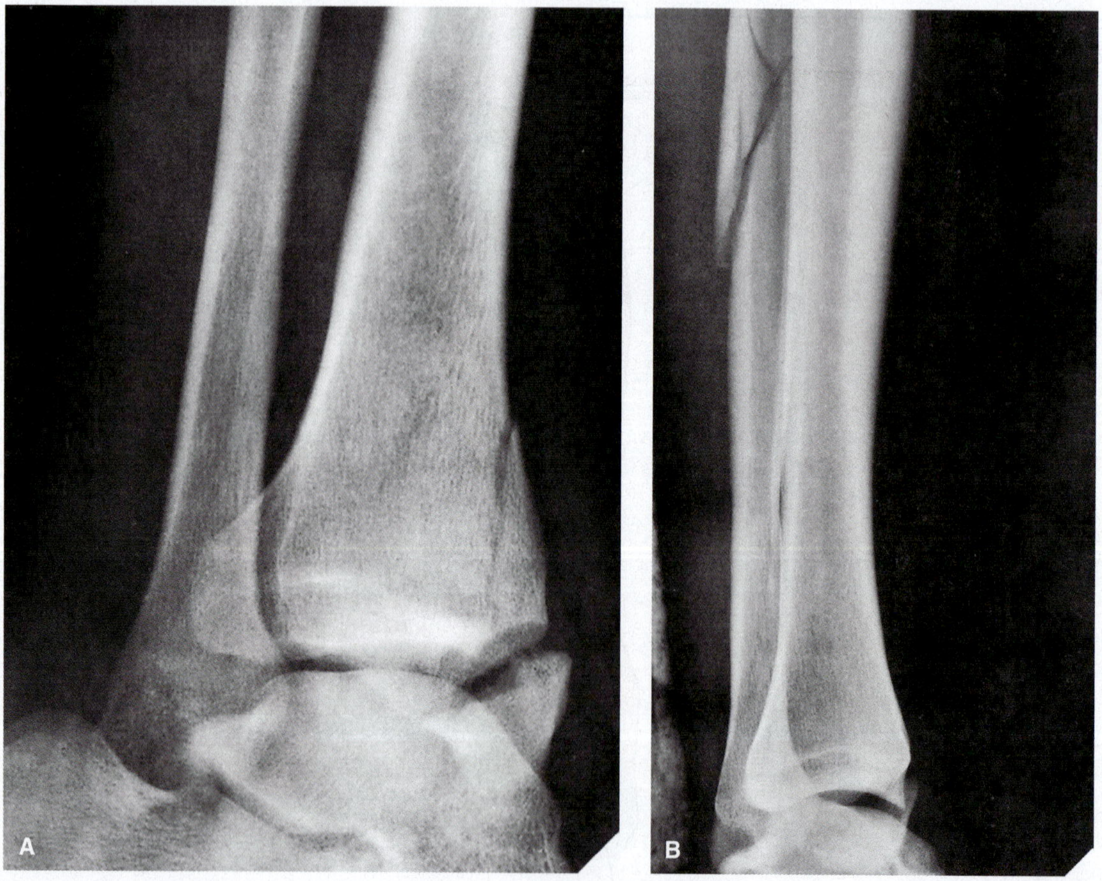

FIGURE 12.6 Maisonneuve fracture. A 22-year-old man injured his right ankle in a skiing accident. **A:** Oblique radiograph of the ankle shows a comminuted fracture of the medial malleolus, with extension into the anterior lip of the tibia. **B:** On the lateral view, a comminuted fracture of the fibula is apparent. This is a characteristic of a Maisonneuve-type fracture. (From Greenspan A. Lower limb III: ankle and foot. In: *Orthopedic Imaging: A Practical Approach*. 5th ed. Philadelphia, PA: Lippincott Williams & Wilkins; 2011:340.)

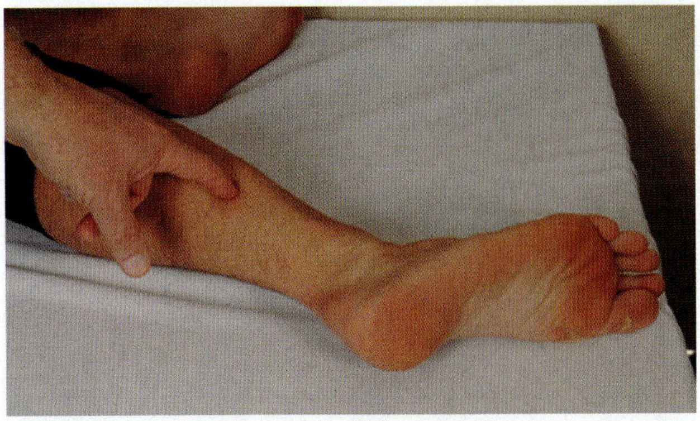

FIGURE 12.7 The most common site of entrapment of the superficial peroneal nerve is the point at which it exits from the deep fascia. Impingement by the edge of the fascia alone or in combination with muscle herniation from beneath the edge of the fascia is responsible for compromise of the nerve. There will often be point tenderness as this point lies 9 to 12 cm above the most distal portion of the fibula.

The most common site of entrapment of the superficial peroneal nerve is the point at which it exits from the deep fascia. Impingement by the edge of the fascia alone or in combination with muscle herniation from beneath the edge of the fascia, is responsible for compromise of the nerve. There will often be point tenderness as this point lies 9 to 12 cm above the most distal portion of the fibula (Fig. 12.7). A Tinel's sign may be present. Physical examination may also identify a fascial defect, especially in the presence of trauma. The pain may be made worse by having the patient actively dorsiflex and evert the foot against resistance.

Patients suffering from compromise of the superficial tibial nerve will complain of pain over the lateral calf which radiates into the dorsum of the ankle and foot. If there is significant nerve compromise, the patient may also complain of paresthesias and numbness into this same distribution. Swelling may be noted, with the pain made worse with squatting, walking, and running. Unlike other nerve entrapment syndromes, night pain is uncommon because of mobilization of lower extremity fluid when assuming the supine position, resulting in decreased intracompartmental pressures.

Electrodiagnostic testing should be considered in all patients who suffer from superficial peroneal nerve dysfunction to provide both neuroanatomic and neurophysiologic information regarding nerve function. Magnetic resonance imaging and ultrasound imaging anywhere along the course of the superficial peroneal nerve are also useful in determining the cause of superficial peroneal nerve compromise (Fig. 12.8). Plain radiographs and/or computerized tomography of the ankle should

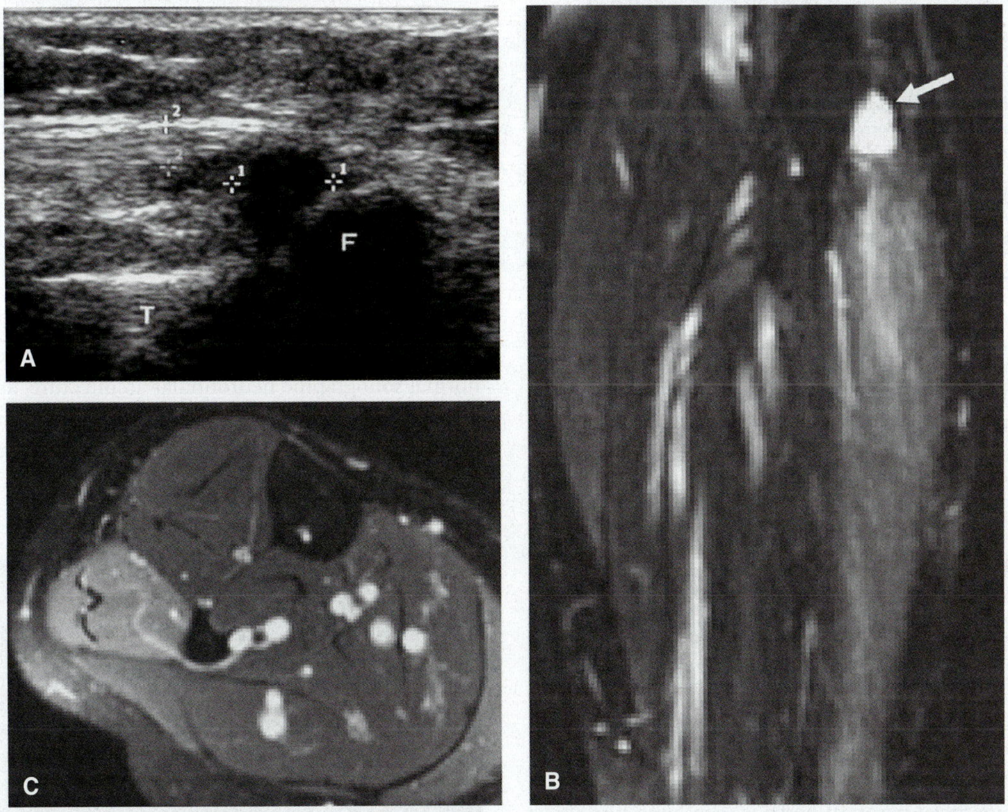

FIGURE 12.8 **A:** Transverse ultrasound image of the lateral knee demonstrating a proximal tibiofibular joint ganglion cyst, displacing and compressing the adjacent superficial peroneal nerve. **B:** Coronal STIR MR image demonstrating edema in the peroneus longus and brevis muscles consistent with subacute denervation effect due to compression of the SPN because of an adjacent proximal tibiofibular joint ganglion cyst (*arrow*). **C:** Axial fat-suppressed PD MR image demonstrating edema-like signal in the peroneus longus and brevis muscles, consistent with subacute denervation effect. (From Simmons DN, Lisle DA, Linklater JM. Imaging of peripheral nerve lesions in the lower limb. *Top Magn Reson Imaging* 2010;21(1):51–62.)

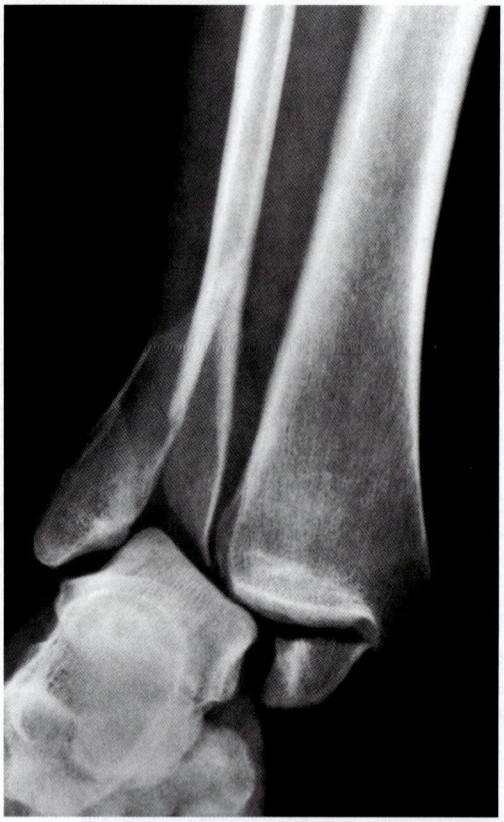

FIGURE 12.9 Anteroposterior radiograph of the ankle demonstrates a spiral fracture of the fibula beginning at the level of the tibiofibular syndesmosis with consequent tear of the inferoposterior portion of the syndesmotic complex; the interosseous membrane is intact. The site of the fracture of the medial malleolus suggests that the deltoid ligament may be intact. (From Greenspan A. Lower limb III: ankle and foot. In: *Orthopedic Imaging: A Practical Approach*. 5th ed. Philadelphia, PA: Lippincott Williams & Wilkins; 2011:342.)

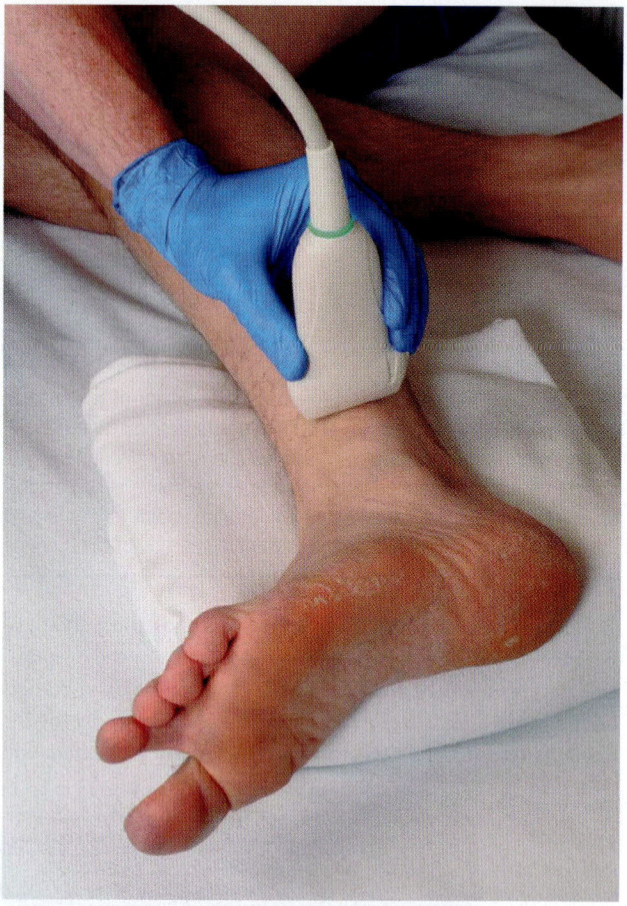

FIGURE 12.10 Proper transverse position of the ultrasound transducer for ultrasound evaluation of the superficial peroneal nerve at the ankle.

be obtained in all patients who have trauma to the ankle to rule out fractures of the medial ankle which can damage the superficial peroneal nerve (Fig. 12.9).

ULTRASOUND TECHNIQUE

Ultrasound evaluation of the superficial peroneal nerve is carried out by placing the patient in the lateral curled up position with the affected leg positioned up on a folded blanket. A linear high-frequency ultrasound transducer is placed in a transverse plane approximately 8 cm above the lateral malleolus of the ankle and an ultrasound survey scan is taken (Fig. 12.10). The superficial peroneal nerve is seen lying just above the fibula and peroneal muscles (Fig. 12.11). Color Doppler imaging can help identify the anterior tibial artery with the superficial peroneal nerve lying just above it (Fig. 12.12). When the superficial peroneal nerve is identified on ultrasound imaging, the nerve is evaluated as it passes inferiorly for presence of compromise or compression by bony abnormality or soft tissue mass, cysts, neuropathy as evidence of loss of normal sonographic neurofibular architecture, and intraneural tumors (Figs. 12.13 to 12.17). Color Doppler may help clarify the diagnosis by identifying areas of increased blood flow (Fig. 12.18).

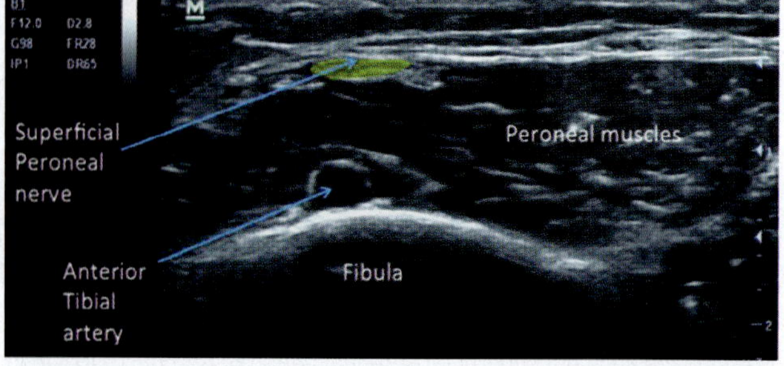

FIGURE 12.11 Transverse ultrasound image demonstrating the tibial artery and vein and the superficial peroneal nerve just above and lateral to the vein.

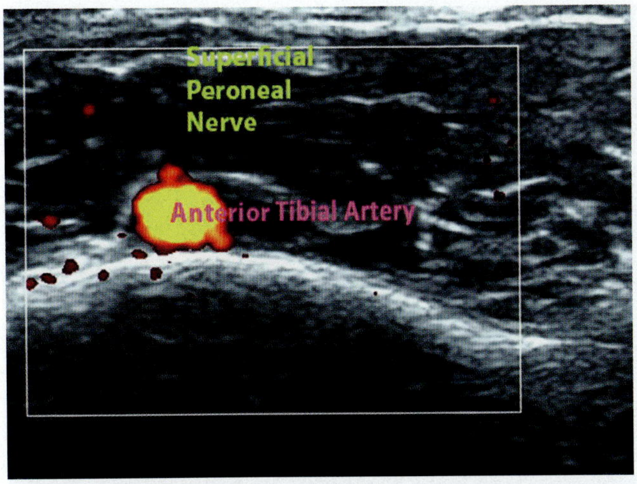

FIGURE 12.12 Color Doppler imaging can help identify the anterior tibial artery with the superficial peroneal nerve lying just above it.

CLINICAL PEARLS

The key to performing successful ultrasound evaluation of the superficial peroneal nerve block at the ankle is the proper identification of the sonographic anatomy and, in particular, the ability to properly identify the superficial peroneal nerve. This should not be a problem if the above technique is used. The use of ultrasound-guided block of the superficial peroneal nerve may serve as both a diagnostic and a therapeutic maneuver (Fig. 12.19).

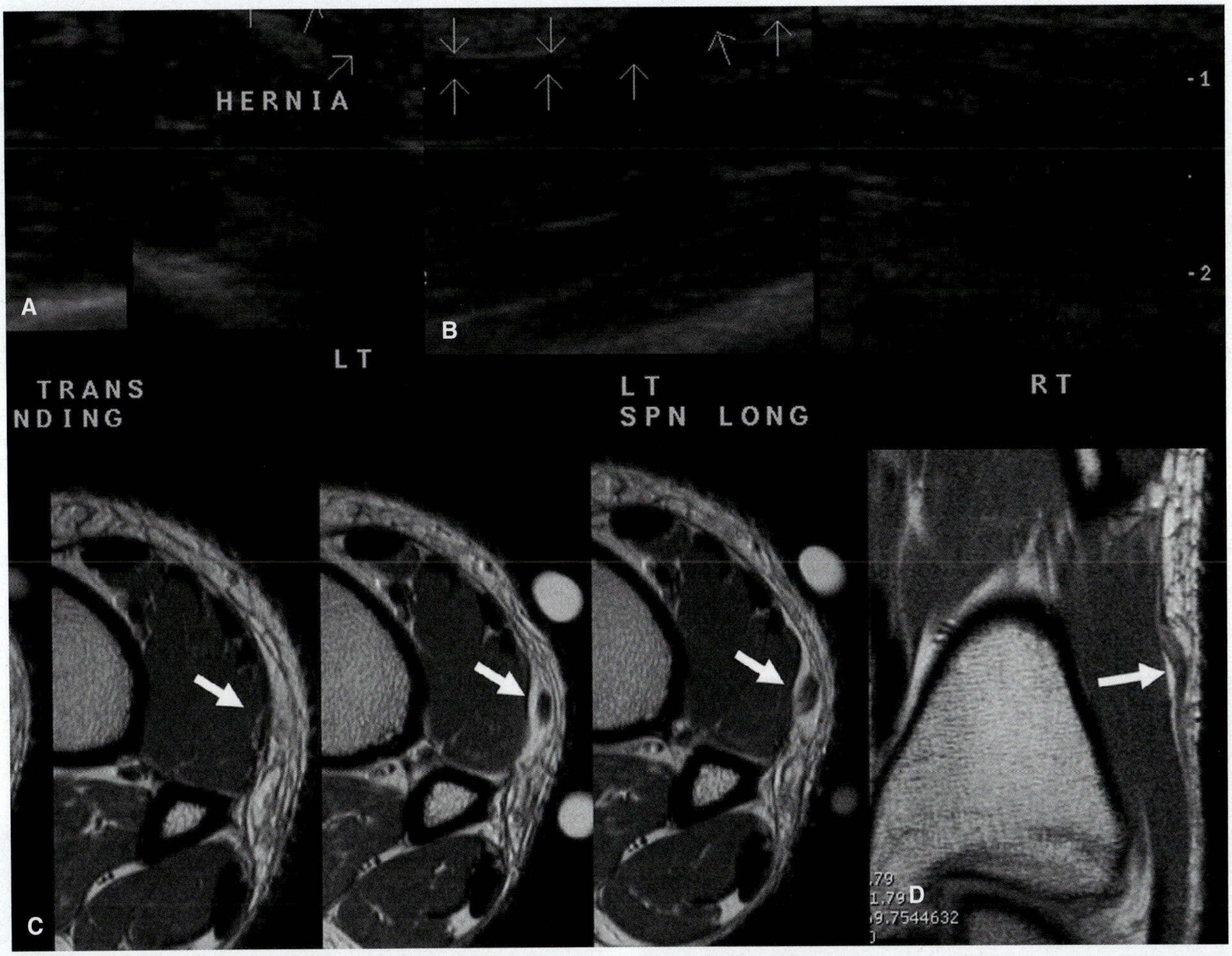

FIGURE 12.13 Superficial peroneal nerve (SPN) entrapment at the point of piercing the deep fascia in the lower leg. Transverse **(A)** and longitudinal **(B)** ultrasound images of the symptomatic left SPN and asymptomatic right SPN demonstrating thickening of the SPN just distal to the point where it pierces the deep fascia, with incipient muscle hernia at this level on dynamic ultrasound in the transverse plane with the patient standing **(A)**. Corresponding axial **(C)** and longitudinal **(D)** magnetic resonance images demonstrate focal thickening of the SPN (*arrows*). Note the use of skin markers to highlight the symptomatic area. (From Simmons DN, Lisle DA, Linklater JM. Imaging of peripheral nerve lesions in the lower limb. *Top Magn Reson Imaging* 2010;21(1):51–62.)

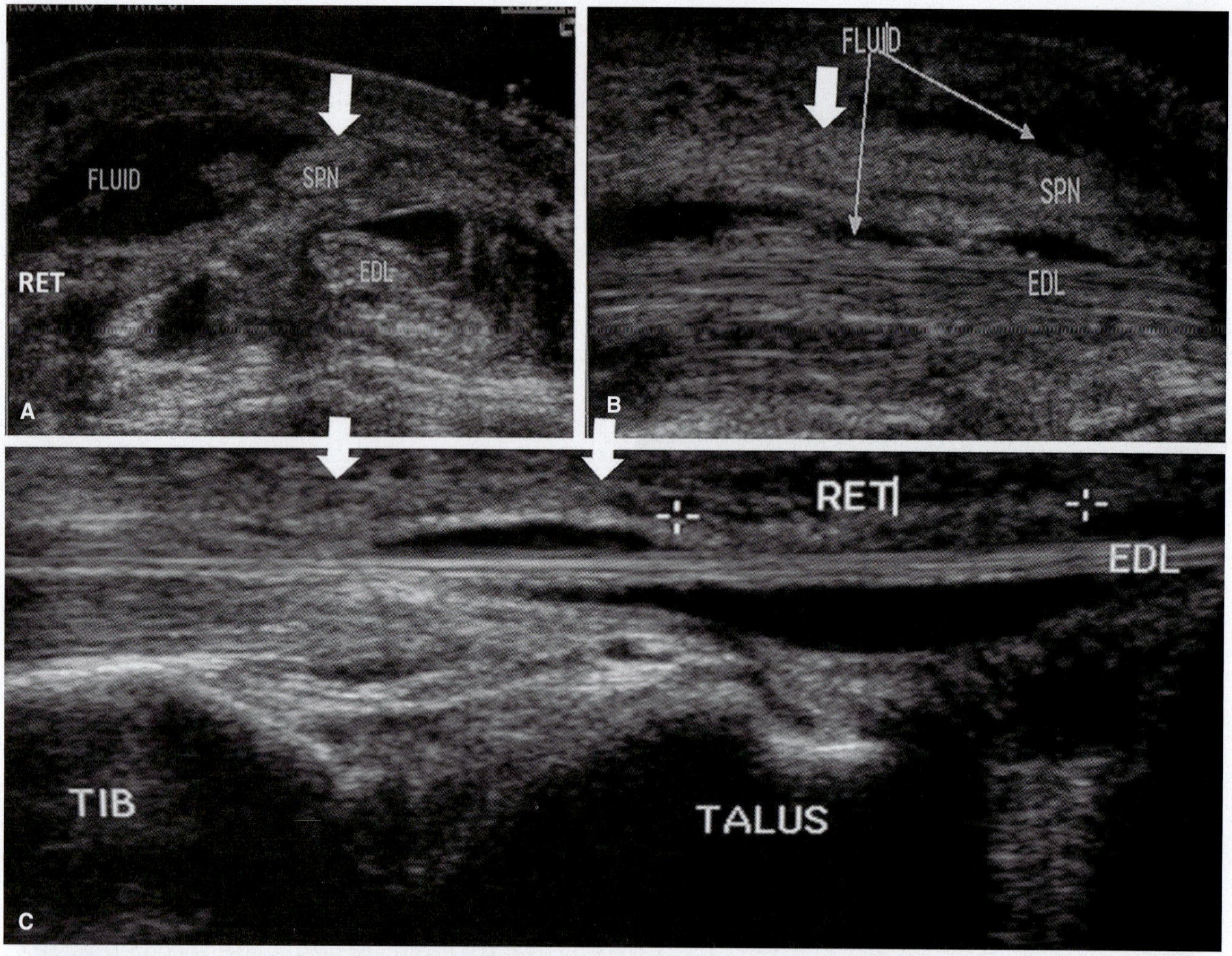

FIGURE 12.14 Compression of the superficial peroneal nerve by fluid from tenosynovitis. Ultrasound demonstration of an effusion in the extensor digitorum longus tendon sheath on transverse **(A)** and longitudinal **(B,C)** images with extensive edema in the overlying subcutaneous tissues. The SPN (*broad arrows*) lies superficial to the extensor retinaculum and is partially surrounded by the fluid. There were clinical features of SPN neural irritation. (From Simmons DN, Lisle DA, Linklater JM. Imaging of peripheral nerve lesions in the lower limb. *Top Magn Reson Imaging* 2010;21(1):51–62.)

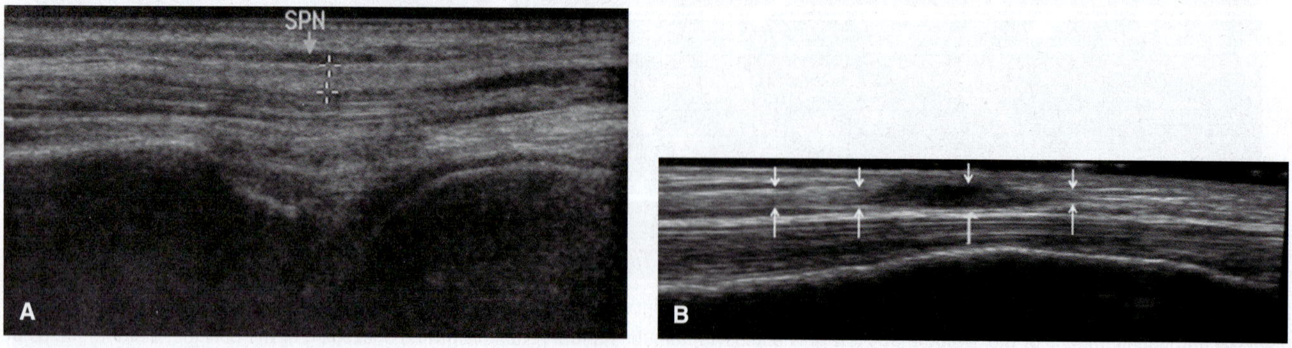

FIGURE 12.15 **A:** Ultrasound appearance of normal superficial peroneal nerve at the ankle joint level (*arrows*). **B:** This contrasts with focal thickening and hypoechoic echotextural change in the superficial peroneal nerve more proximally at the distal tibial level, reflecting an area of posttraumatic neuroma in continuity (*arrows*). (From Simmons DN, Lisle DA, Linklater JM. Imaging of peripheral nerve lesions in the lower limb. *Top Magn Reson Imaging* 2010;21(1):51–62.)

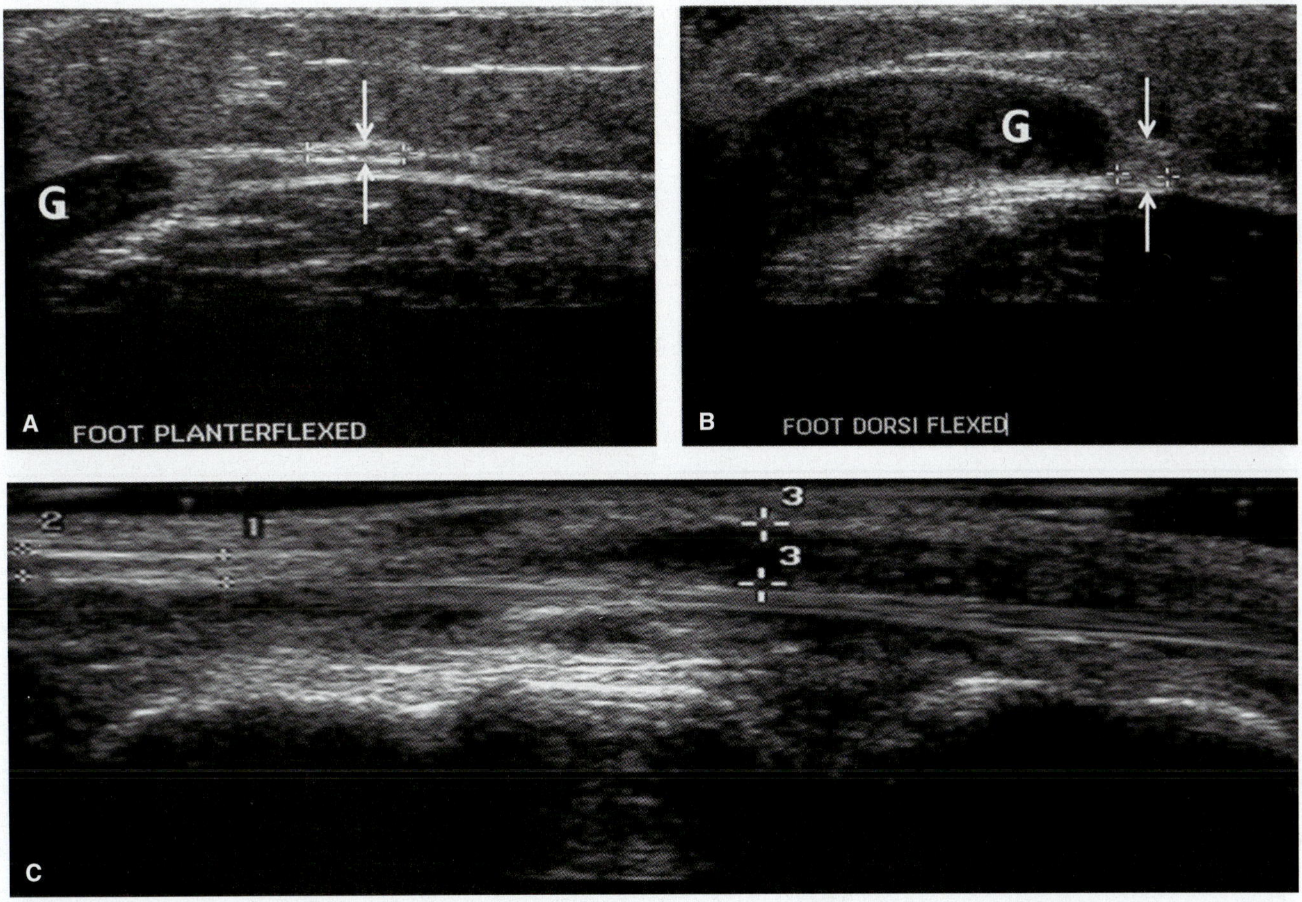

FIGURE 12.16 **A:** Superficial peroneal nerve (*arrows*) appears normal with the ankle in neutral flexion. **B:** On dorsiflexion of the foot, a large ganglion from the lateral side of the ankle bulged up and compressed the SPN. **C:** Longitudinal ultrasound image demonstrating swelling of the superficial peroneal nerve in an area of contusion. (From Simmons DN, Lisle DA, Linklater JM. Imaging of peripheral nerve lesions in the lower limb. *Top Magn Reson Imaging* 2010;21(1):51–62.)

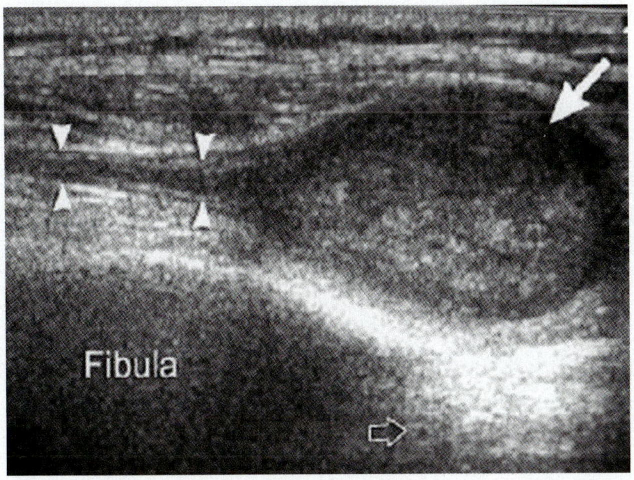

FIGURE 12.17 Schwannoma of superficial peroneal nerve branch. Sonogram longitudinal to the intermediate dorsal cutaneous nerve shows the predominately hypoechoic schwannoma (*arrow*) with posterior acoustic enhancement (*open arrow*). Note the continuity with entering nerve (*arrowheads*). (From Jacobson JA. Musculoskeletal ultrasound and MRI: Which do I choose? *Semin Musculoskelet Radiol* 2005;9(2):135–149; Fig. 5.)

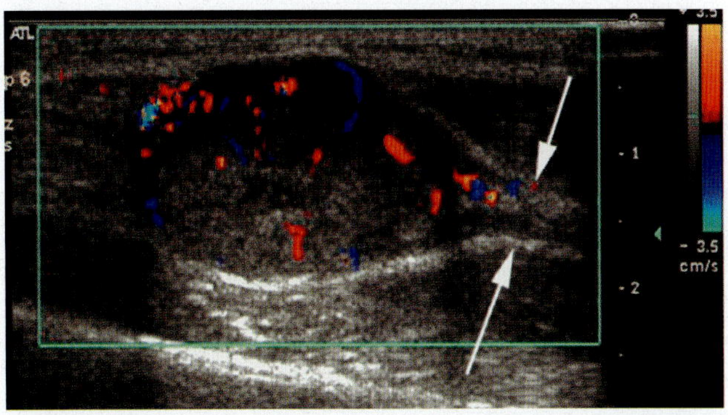

FIGURE 12.18 Color Doppler shows a nerve sheath tumor. Note the large, characteristically hypoechoic mass with posterior enhancement and increased blood flow. Distally, the nerve resumes its normal size and echotexture (*arrows*). (From Thain LM, Downey DB. Sonography of peripheral nerves: technique, anatomy, and pathology. *Ultrasound Q* 2002;18(4):225–245;Fig. 7.)

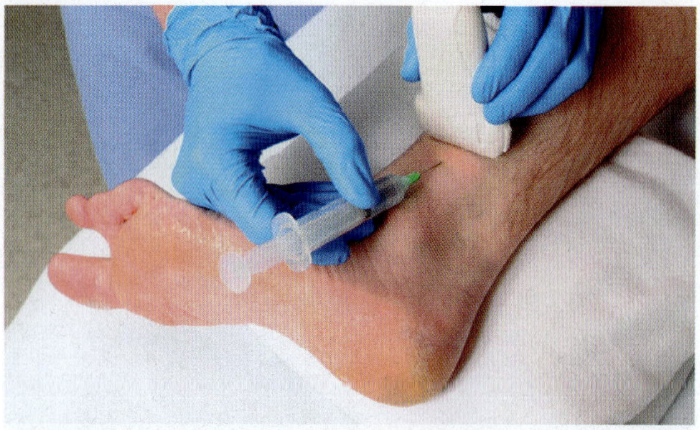

FIGURE 12.19 Proper out-of-plane needle position for performing superficial peroneal nerve block at the ankle.

Suggested Readings

Barrett SL, Dellon AL, Rosson GD, et al. Superficial peroneal nerve (superficial fibularis nerve): the clinical implications of anatomic variability. *J Foot Ankle Surg* 2006;45(3)L174–L176.

Cho KH, Wansaicheong GKL. Ultrasound of the foot and ankle. *Ultrasound Clin* 2012;7(4):487–503.

Lopez-Ben R. Imaging of nerve entrapment in the foot and ankle. *Foot Ankle Clin* 2011;16(2):213–224.

Şayli U, Tekdemyr Y, Çubuk HE, et al. The course of the superficial peroneal nerve: an anatomical cadaver study. *Foot Ankle Surg* 1998;4(2):63–69.

Waldman SD. Superficial peroneal nerve block at the ankle. In: *Atlas of Interventional Pain Management.* 3rd ed. Philadelphia, PA: Saunders; 2009:567–569.

Waldman SD. Superficial peroneal nerve block at the ankle. In: *Pain Review.* Philadelphia, PA: Saunders; 2009:578–579.

Waldman SD. Anterior tarsal tunnel syndrome. In: *Pain Review.* Philadelphia, PA: Saunders; 2009:322–323.

CHAPTER 13

Abnormalities of the Sural Nerve at the Ankle

ANATOMIC CONSIDERATIONS

The sural nerve is a branch of the posterior tibial nerve (Fig. 13.1). The sural nerve passes from the posterior calf around the lateral malleolus to provide sensory innervation of the posterior lateral aspect of the calf and the lateral surface of the foot and fifth toe and the plantar surface of the heel (Figs. 13.2 and 13.3). The sural nerve is subject to compression at the ankle and is known as boot syndrome because it is associated with compression of the nerve by boots that are too tight. Because the sural nerve is a pure sensory nerve, it is commonly sacrificed when a nerve biopsy is needed to diagnose peripheral neuropathies (Fig. 13.4).

CLINICAL CORRELATES

Saphenous neuralgia is caused by entrapment and compression of the saphenous nerve anywhere along its course, with compromise of the nerve most commonly caused by ganglion cysts and tenosynovitis arising from the peroneal tendon sheaths as well as ganglion cysts arising from the calcaneocuboidal joint (Fig. 13.5). The saphenous nerve is frequently traumatized during vein stripping and harvest procedures, with the infrapatellar branch of the saphenous nerve frequently damaged during total knee arthroplasty (Fig. 13.4). The nerve can also be damaged by trauma to the ankle, including sprain, fracture of the fibula, fracture of the base of the fifth metatarsal, dislocation,

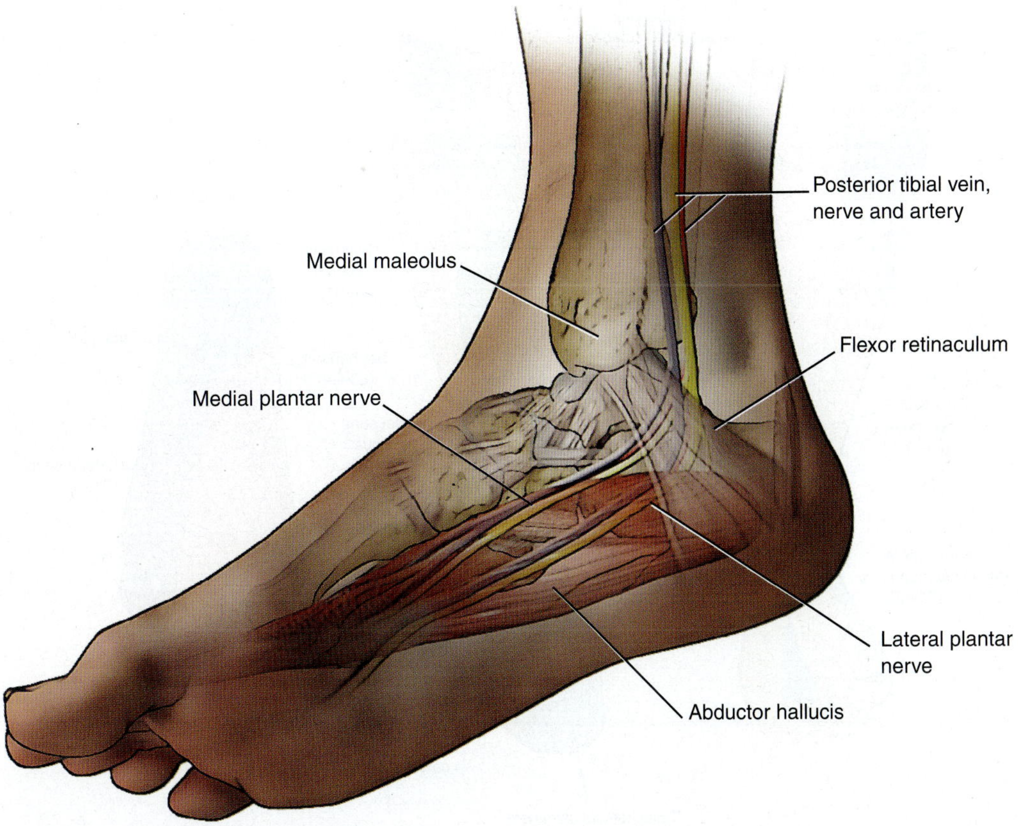

FIGURE 13.1 The relationship of the posterior tibial nerve and the tibial artery and vein.

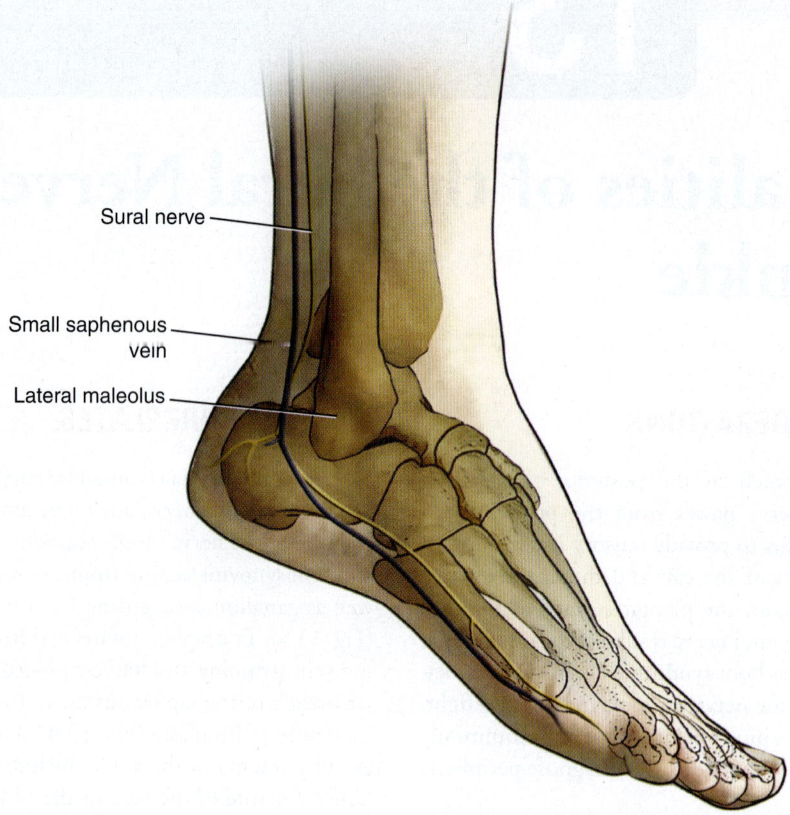

FIGURE 13.2 The anatomy of the sural nerve.

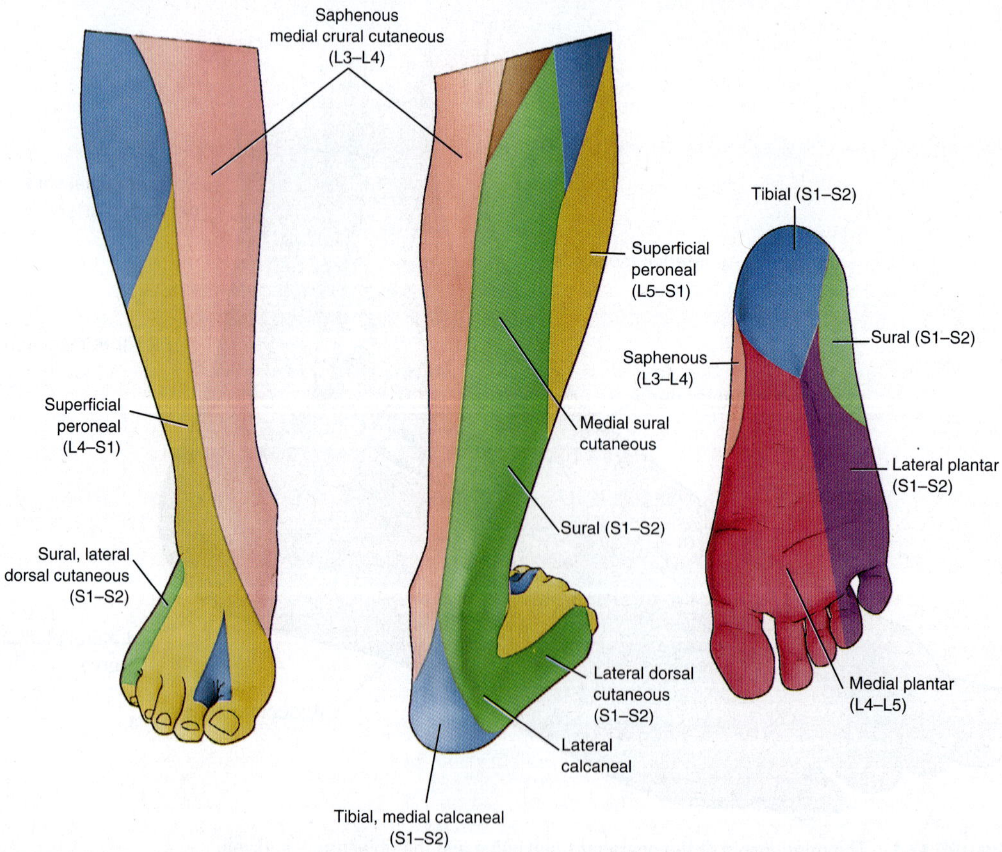

FIGURE 13.3 Sensory distribution of the distal sural nerve.

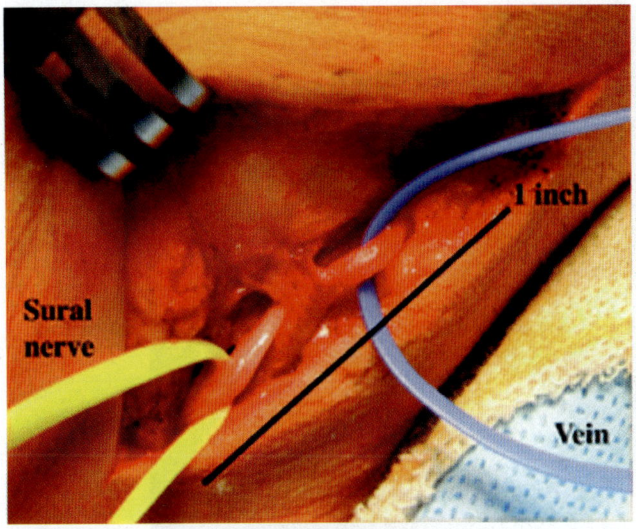

FIGURE 13.4 Ultrasound-guided sural nerve block at the ankle can also be used to localize the sural nerve when performing sural nerve biopsy. Note the anatomic relationship of the sural nerve and the small saphenous vein.

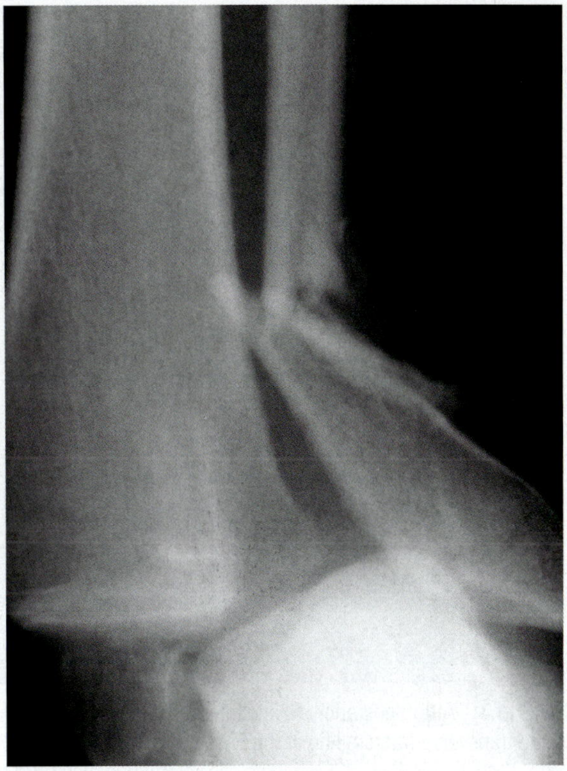

FIGURE 13.6 Radiograph demonstrating a fracture of the distal fibula and dislocation of the talus causing damage to the sural nerve. (From Bucholz RW, Heckman JD. *Rockwood & Green's Fractures in Adults.* 5th ed. Philadelphia, PA, Lippincott Williams & Wilkins; 2001.)

and crush injuries (Figs. 13.6 and 13.7). Patients suffering from compromise of the sural nerve at the ankle will complain of numbness and dysesthesias radiating into the posterior lateral aspect of the calf and the lateral surface of the foot and fifth toe and the plantar surface of the heel.

Electrodiagnostic testing should be considered in all patients who suffer from sural nerve dysfunction to provide both neuroanatomic and neurophysiologic information regarding nerve function. Magnetic resonance imaging and ultrasound imaging anywhere along the course of the sural nerve are also useful in determining the cause of sural nerve compromise (Fig. 13.8). Plain radiographs and/or computerized tomography of the ankle should be obtained in all patients who have trauma to the ankle to rule out fractures of the lateral ankle which can damage the sural nerve (Fig. 13.9).

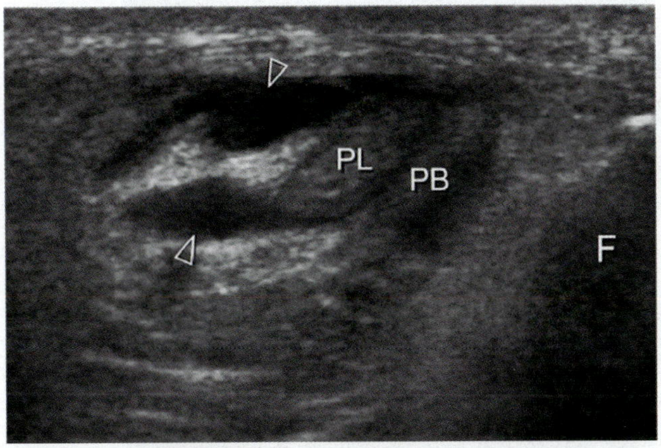

FIGURE 13.5 Peroneal tenosynovitis can compromise the sural nerve. Ultrasound transverse to the peroneus longus (PL) and peroneus brevis (PB) tendons shows anechoic fluid and isoechoic synovitis (*arrowheads*). Posterior is to the left. F, fibula. (From Femino JE, Jacobson JA, Craig CL, et al. Dynamic ultrasound of the foot and ankle: adult and pediatric applications. *Techn Foot Ankle Surg* 2007;6(1):50–61.)

ULTRASOUND TECHNIQUE

Ultrasound evaluation of the sural nerve at the ankle can be carried out by placing the patient in the lateral curled up position with the affected leg positioned up on a folded blanket. A linear high-frequency ultrasound transducer is placed in a transverse plane approximately just above and behind the lateral malleolus of the ankle and an ultrasound survey scan is taken (Fig. 13.10). The small saphenous vein is seen lying just behind the lateral malleolus, with the sural nerve lying just posterior to the vein (Fig. 13.11). Compression of the small saphenous vein with pressure on the ultrasound transducer can aid in identification of the sural nerve which lies just posterior to the vein below the tibial vein and artery (Fig. 13.12). Color Doppler can be also utilized to help identify the small saphenous vein and the adjacent sural nerve (Fig. 13.13).

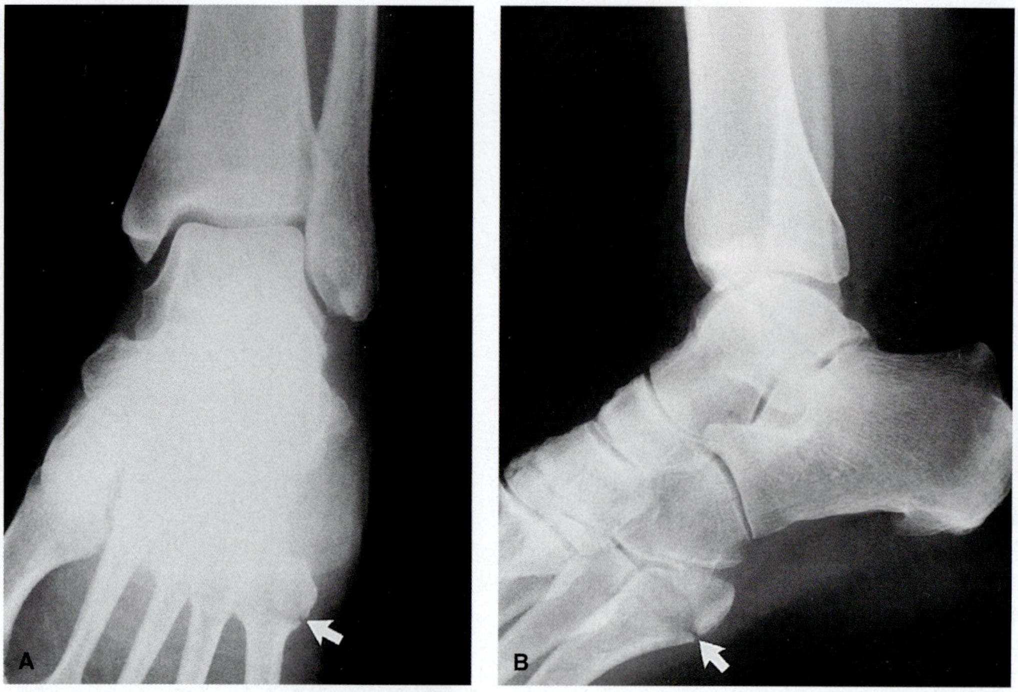

FIGURE 13.7 Anteroposterior **(A)** and lateral **(B)** ankle radiographs showing Jones fracture (dancer's fracture) at the base of the fifth metatarsal. Note the transverse fracture line at the base of the fifth metatarsal (*arrows*). (From Rowe LJ, Yochum TR, Maola CJ. Trauma. In: Rowe LJ, Yochum TR, eds. *Yochum and Rowes' Essentials of Skeletal Radiology*. 3rd ed. Vol. 1. Philadelphia, PA: Lippincott Williams & Wilkins; 2005:882.)

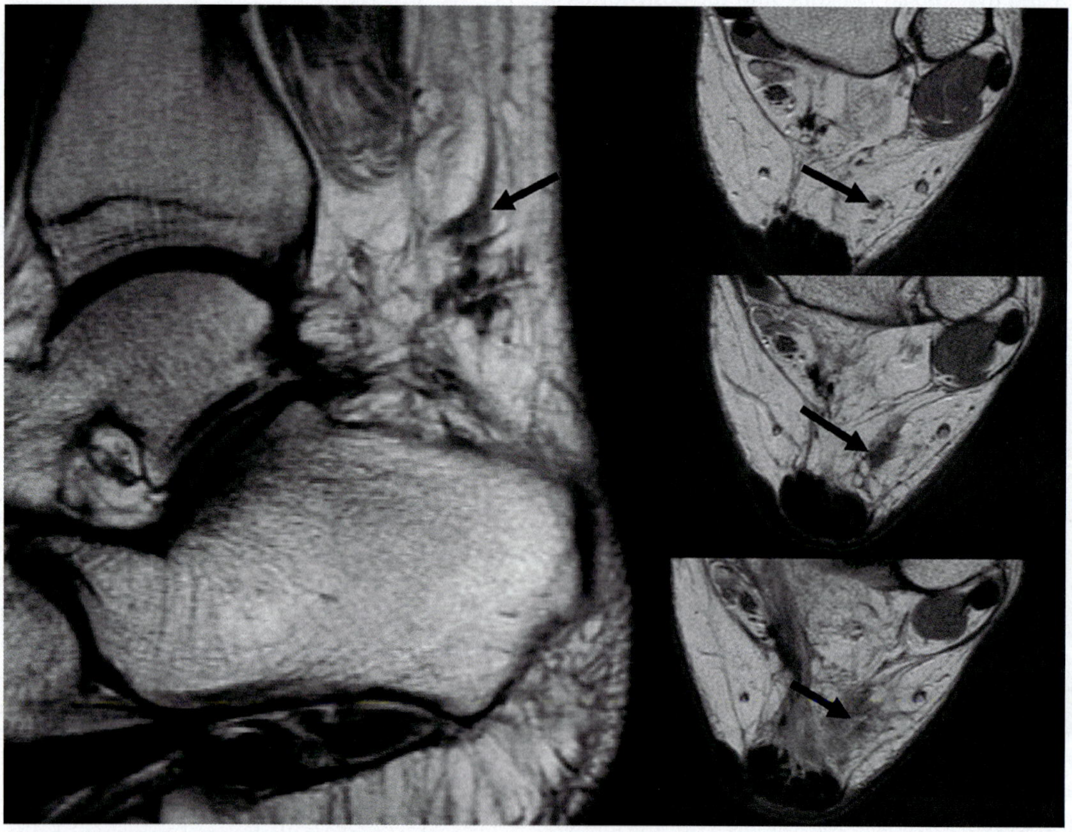

FIGURE 13.8 Posttraumatic sural neuroma. Sagittal PD and axial PD (superior to inferior) scans demonstrating focal thickening of the SN (*arrows*) just above the level of the ankle joint, with adjacent postsurgical scar, consistent with a posttraumatic neuroma. (From Simmons DN, Lisle DA, Linklater JM. Imaging of peripheral nerve lesions in the lower limb. *Top Magn Reson Imag* 2010;21(1):51–62.)

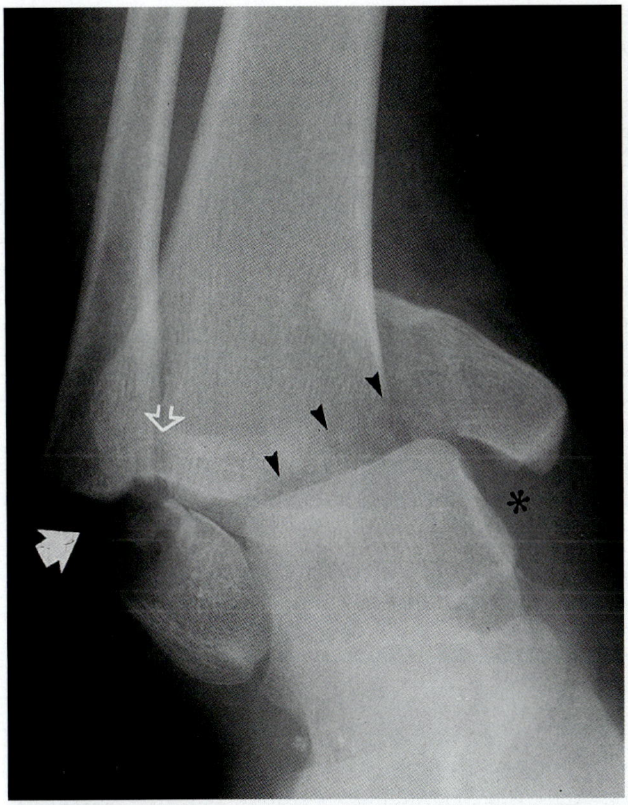

FIGURE 13.9 Bimalleolar fracture dislocation caused by an inversion injury. The impaction force of the dislocated talus striking the medial malleolus has resulted in the oblique fracture (*arrowheads*) of its base and the direction of displacement of the distal fragment. The distance between the medial malleolus and the medial surface of the talus (*asterisk*) indicates that the deltoid ligament is disrupted. The avulsion force transmitted through the intact lateral collateral ligament has caused the transverse fracture of the lateral malleolus (*solid white arrow*) at the level of the plafond. The normal relationship between the distal end of the proximal fibular fracture and the tibia (*open white arrow*) indicates that the distal tibiofibular ligaments and the interosseous membrane are intact. (From Wilson A, Harris JH Jr. Ankle. In: Pope TL Jr, Harris JH Jr, eds. *Harris & Harris' The Radiology of Emergency Medicine.* 5th ed. Philadelphia, PA: Lippincott Williams & Wilkins; 2013:938.)

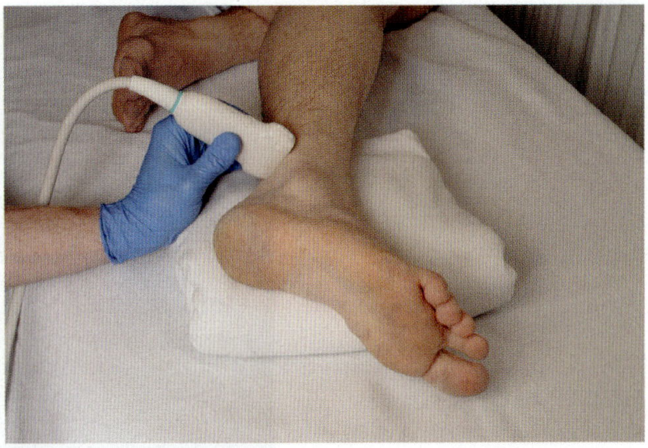

FIGURE 13.10 Proper transverse position of the ultrasound transducer for ultrasound evaluation of the sural nerve at the ankle.

When the sural nerve is identified on ultrasound imaging, the nerve is evaluated as it passes inferiorly for presence of compromise or compression by bony abnormality or soft tissue mass, cysts, neuropathy as evidence of loss of normal sonographic neurofibular architecture, and intraneural tumors (Figs. 13.14 and 13.15).

CLINICAL PEARLS

The key to performing successful ultrasound sural nerve block at the ankle is the proper identification of the sonographic anatomy and, in particular, the ability to properly identify the sural nerve. This should not be a problem if the above technique is used. Because the sural nerve is a pure sensory nerve, it is commonly sacrificed when a nerve biopsy is needed to diagnose peripheral neuropathies and, in this setting, ultrasound localization of the nerve can improve clinical outcomes (Fig. 13.16).

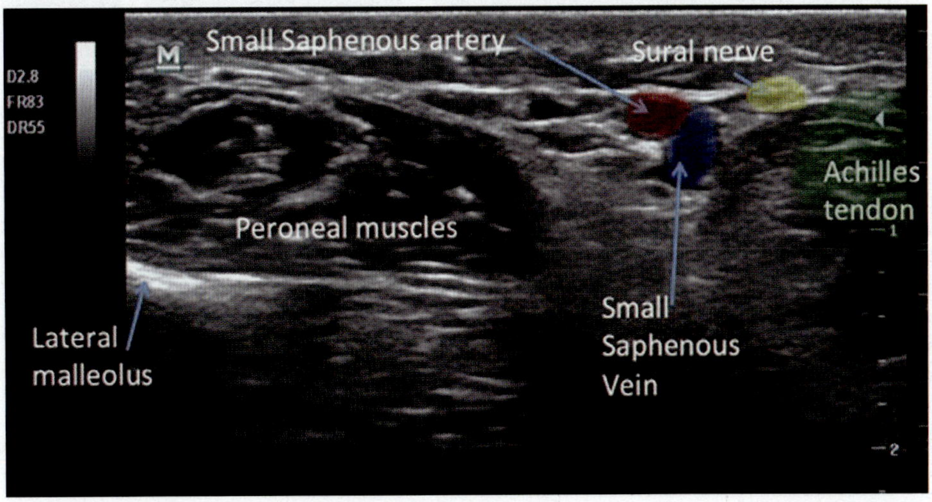

FIGURE 13.11 Transverse ultrasound image demonstrating the tibial artery and vein and the sural nerve just above and lateral to the vein.

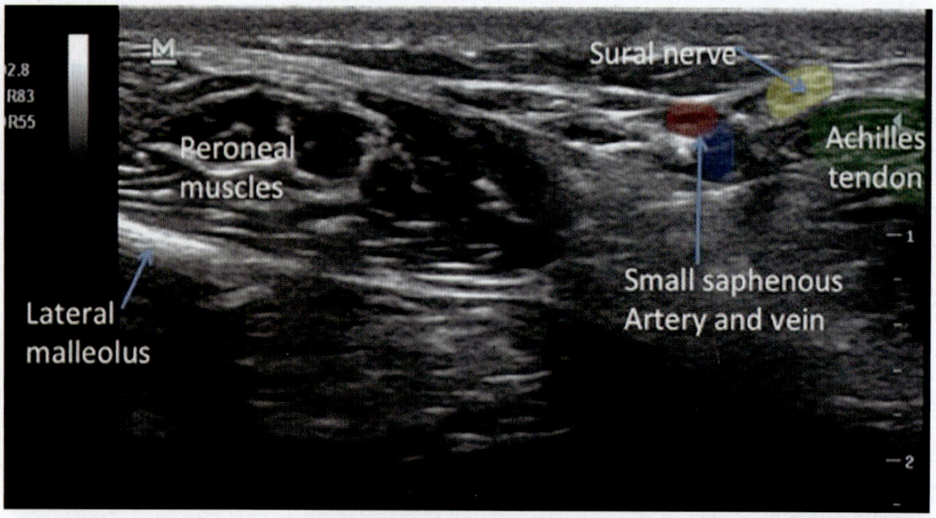

FIGURE 13.12 Compression of the small saphenous vein can aid in identification of the sural nerve which is just posterior to the vein.

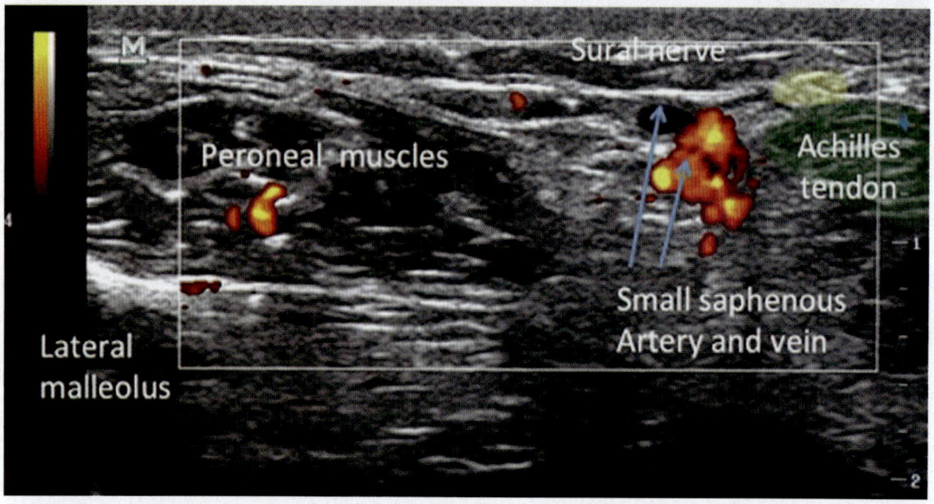

FIGURE 13.13 Transverse color Doppler image demonstrating the popliteal vein and artery and the relationship of the vein to the posterior tibial nerve.

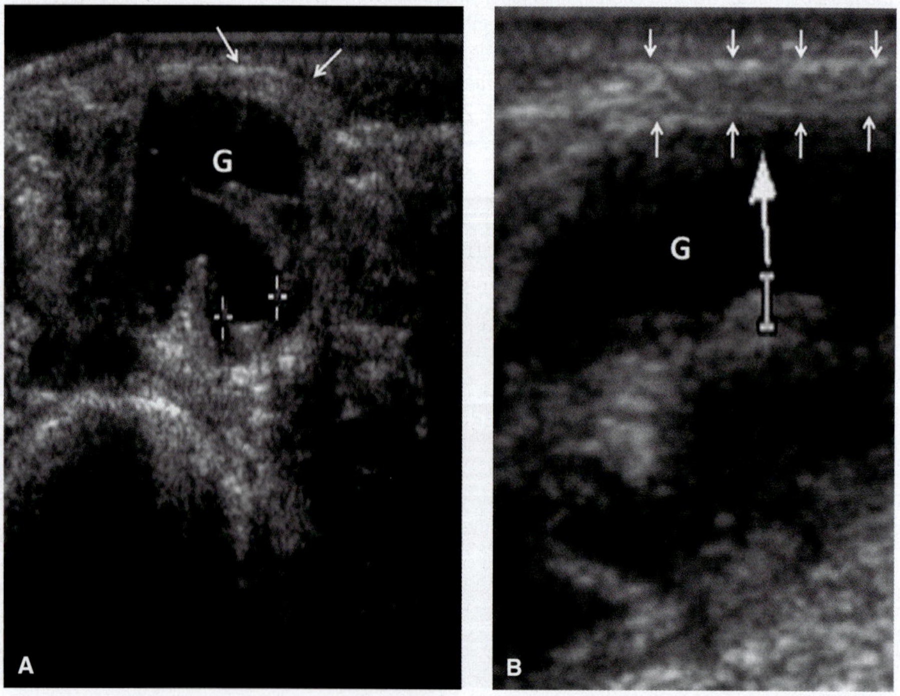

FIGURE 13.14 Longitudinal **(A)** and transverse **(B)** ultrasound images demonstrating a large ganglion (G) arising from the peroneus brevis tendon, extruding posterolaterally, displacing and compressing the sural nerve. (From Simmons DN, Lisle DA, Linklater JM. Imaging of peripheral nerve lesions in the lower limb. *Top Magn Reson Imaging* 2010;21(1):51–62.)

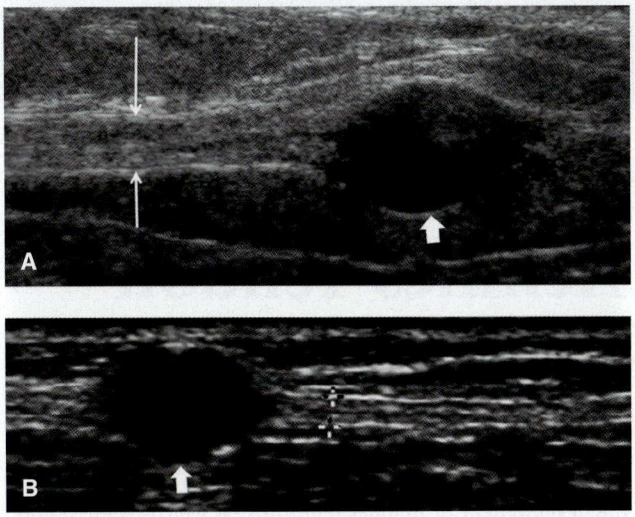

FIGURE 13.15 **A:** Longitudinal ultrasound image demonstrating a sural nerve stump neuroma (*broad arrow*), after transaction of the sural nerve at ankle reconstruction. **B:** Longitudinal ultrasound image of the sural nerve in the foot demonstrating a posttraumatic neuroma in continuity after prior surgery. (From Simmons DN, Lisle DA, Linklater JM. Imaging of peripheral nerve lesions in the lower limb. *Top Magn Reson Imaging* 2010;21(1):51–62.)

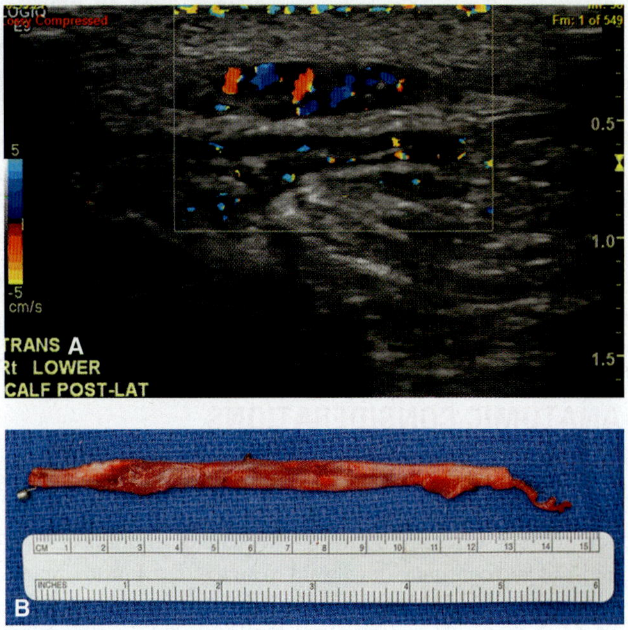

FIGURE 13.16 **A:** Preoperative color Doppler ultrasound of the lower limb showing marked thickening and increased vascularity in a long segment of the right sural nerve. **B:** At the time of resection, a 7-cm section of the right sural nerve demonstrated striking fusiform enlargement. (From Laughlin RS, Suanprasert N, Dyck P, et al. Glomangiomatosis of the sural nerve. *J Clin Pathol* 2014;67(2):190–192.)

Suggested Readings

Cho KH, Wansaicheong GKL. Ultrasound of the foot and ankle. *Ultrasound Clin* 2012;7(4):487–503.

Lopez-Ben R. Imaging of nerve entrapment in the foot and ankle. *Foot Ankle Clin* 2011;16(2):213–224.

Ricci S, Moro L, Antonelli Incalzi R. Ultrasound imaging of the sural nerve: ultrasound anatomy and rationale for investigation. *Eur J Vasc Endovasc Surg* 2010;39(5):636–641.

Waldman SD. Sural nerve block at the ankle. In: *Pain Review.* Philadelphia, PA: Saunders; 2009:579–580.

Waldman SD. Sural nerve block at the ankle. In: *Atlas of Interventional Pain Management.* 3rd ed. Philadelphia, PA: Saunders; 2009:570–574.

CHAPTER 14

Achilles Tendinitis and Other Abnormalities of the Achilles Tendon

ANATOMIC CONSIDERATIONS

The Achilles tendon is the thickest and strongest tendon in the body, yet is also very susceptible to rupture. The common tendon of the gastrocnemius muscle, the Achilles tendon, begins at mid-calf and continues downward to attach to the posterior calcaneus, where it may become inflamed (Fig. 14.1). The Achilles tendon narrows during this downward course, becoming most narrow at approximately 5 cm above its calcaneal insertion. It is at this narrowest point that tendinitis also may occur (Fig. 14.2). A bursa is located between the Achilles tendon and the base of the tibia and the upper posterior calcaneus (see Fig. 14.2). This bursa also may become inflamed as a result of coexistent Achilles tendinitis and may confuse the clinical picture.

CLINICAL CORRELATES

Achilles tendinitis is a clinical syndrome characterized by sharp, constant, and severe posterior ankle pain on plantar flexion of the ankle. Patients suffering from Achilles tendinitis will often splint the inflamed Achilles tendon by adopting a flat-footed gait to avoid plantar flexing the affected tendon. This dysfunctional gait may cause a secondary bursitis and tendinitis around the foot and ankle, which may serve to confuse the clinical picture and further increase the patient's pain and disability. Pain on palpation of the insertion of the Achilles tendon on the calcaneus or at a point approximately 5 cm above the calcaneus at the narrowest part of the Achilles tendon is a consistent finding in patients with Achilles tendinitis as is exacerbation of pain with active resisted plantar flexion. Patients suffering from Achilles tendinitis will also exhibit a positive creaking tendon test. This test is performed by having the patient sit on the edge of the examination table. The examiner then palpates the Achilles tendon while passively plantar flexing and dorsiflexing the ankle (Fig. 14.3). The test is positive if the examiner appreciates a creaking sensation. Untreated, Achilles tendinitis will result in increasing pain and functional disability, calcium deposition around the tendon occurs, making subsequent treatment more difficult (Fig. 14.4). Continued trauma to the inflamed tendon ultimately may result in tendon rupture (Fig. 14.5).

The onset of Achilles tendinitis usually is acute, occurring after overuse or misuse of the ankle joint. Inciting factors may include activities such as running and sudden stopping and starting, as when playing tennis. Improper stretching of the gastrocnemius and Achilles tendon before exercise as well as the use of quinolone antibiotics have also been implicated in the development of Achilles tendinitis, as well as acute tendon rupture.

Plain radiographs are indicated in all patients who present with posterior ankle pain (Figs. 14.6 and 14.7). Based on the patient's clinical presentation, additional testing may be indicated, including complete blood cell count, sedimentation rate, and antinuclear antibody testing. MRI and/or ultrasound imaging of the ankle is indicated if Achilles tendinitis, rupture, joint instability is suggested or the diagnosis is in question (Figs. 14.8 to 14.10). Radionuclide bone scanning is useful to identify stress fractures of the tibia not seen on plain radiographs.

ULTRASOUND TECHNIQUE

To perform ultrasound evaluation of the Achilles tendon the patient is laced in the prone position with the patient's ankle hanging off the edge of the table. With the patient in the above position, a high-frequency linear ultrasound transducer is placed in the longitudinal plane with the inferior portion of the ultrasound transducer over the insertion of the Achilles tendon on the calcaneus and an ultrasound survey scan is taken (Fig. 14.11). The linear Achilles tendon is identified as its insertion on the calcaneus (Fig. 14.12). When the insertion of the Achilles tendon is identified, the tendon is evaluated as the transducer is slowly moved in a cephalad direction while searching for fluid, extrinsic compression, tendinosis, tendinitis, tears, and rupture (Figs. 14.13 to 14.29). Ultrasound imaging of the Achilles tendon is also useful in identifying xanthomas associated with familial hypercholesterolemia. Color Doppler may aid in the identification of inflammation and the neovascularity associated with acute tears of the tendon and musculotendinous junction (Figs. 14.30 to 14.33).

CLINICAL PEARLS

Bursitis and tendinitis of the ankle and foot may coexist with Achilles tendinitis and may contribute to the patient's pain

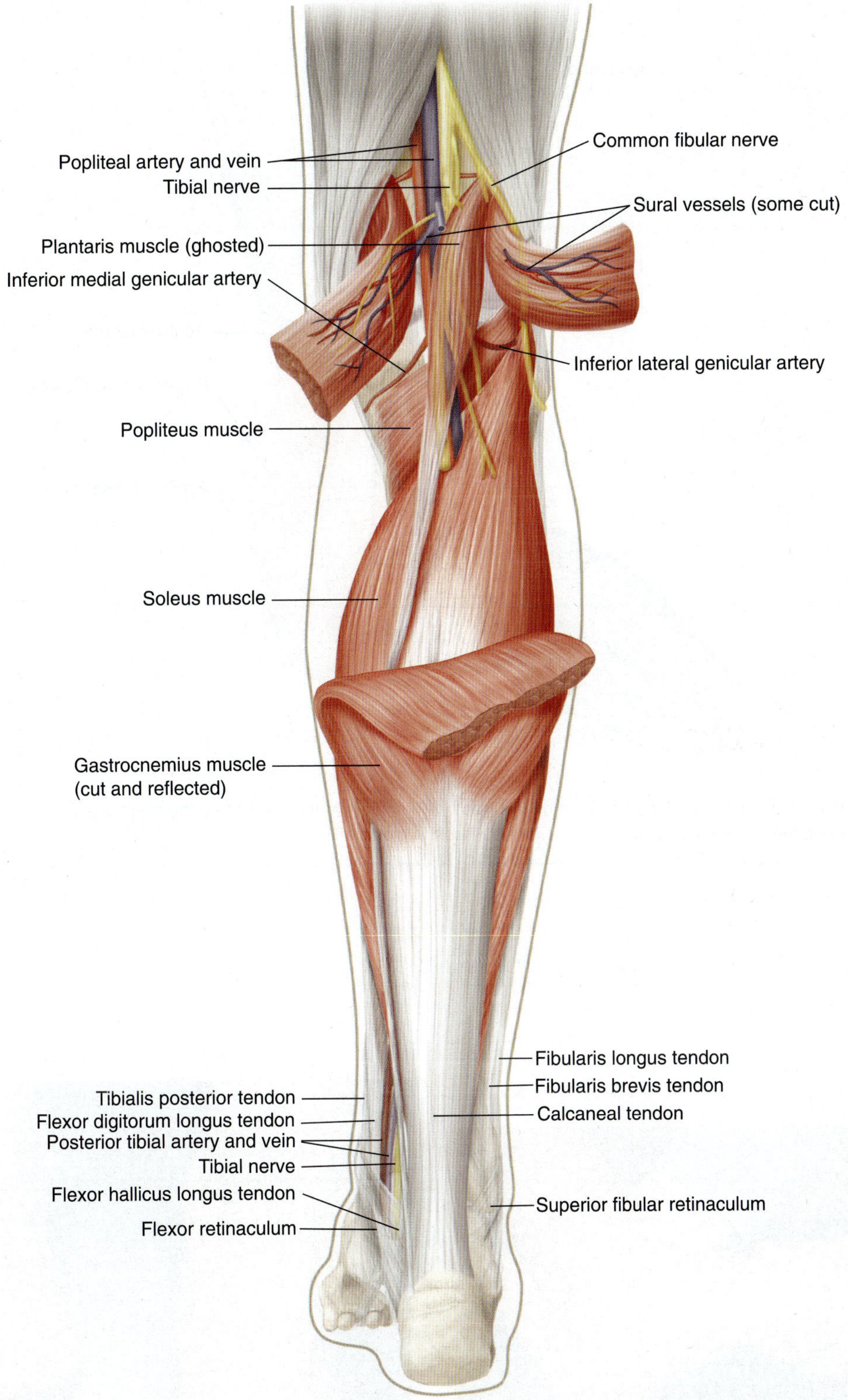

FIGURE 14.1 The common tendon of the gastrocnemius muscle, the Achilles tendon, begins at mid-calf and continues downward to attach to the posterior calcaneus, where it may become inflamed. (From Tank PW, Gest TR. The lower limb. In: *Lippincott Williams & Wilkins Atlas of Anatomy*. Philadelphia, PA: Lippincott Williams & Wilkins; 2009:117.)

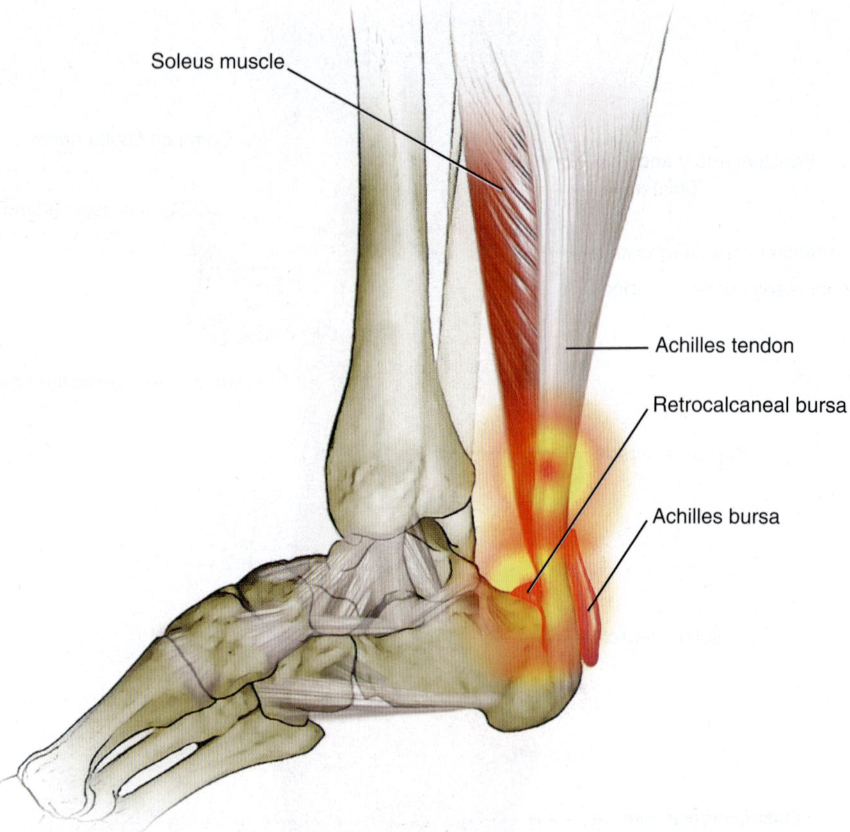

FIGURE 14.2 The Achilles tendon is susceptible to the development of tendinitis at its insertion on the calcaneus as well at its narrowest point approximately 5 cm above the calcaneal insertion.

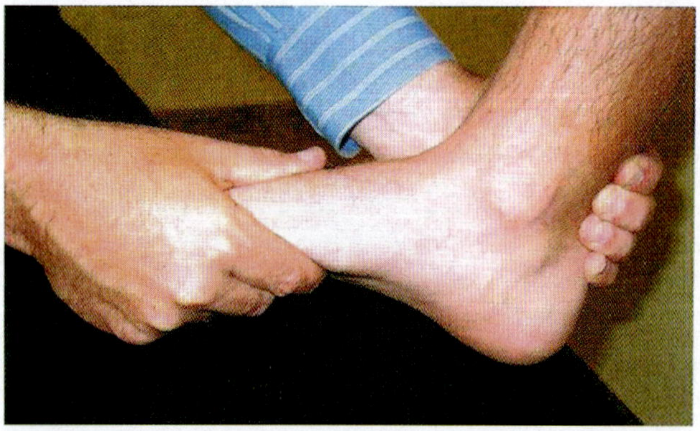

FIGURE 14.3 The creaking tendon test is performed by having the patient sit on the edge of the examination table. The examiner then palpates the Achilles tendon while passively plantar flexing and dorsiflexing the ankle. The test is positive if the examiner appreciates a creaking sensation.

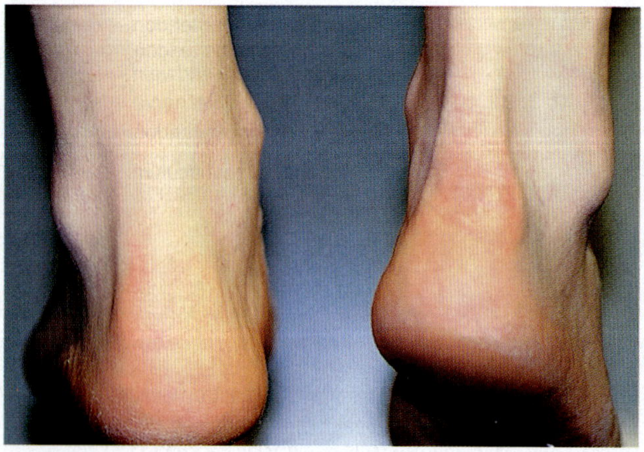

FIGURE 14.4 The patient's ruptured left Achilles tendon appears thickened and less distinct than the normal right side, and the patient is unable to plantar flex the left foot. (From Fleisher GR, Ludwig S, et al. *Atlas of pediatric Emergency medicine.* Philadelphia, PA: Lippincott Williams & Wilkins; 2004.)

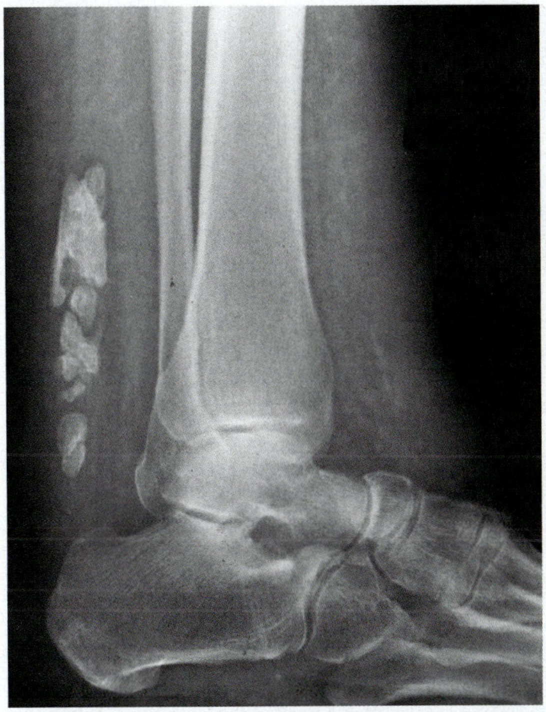

FIGURE 14.5 Lateral view of the ankle demonstrates areas of ossification in the Achilles tendon resulting from recurring injuries. (From Berquist TH. Soft tissue trauma and overuse syndromes. In: Berquist TH, ed. *MRI of the Musculoskeletal System*. 6th ed. Philadelphia, PA: Lippincott Williams & Wilkins; 2013:145.)

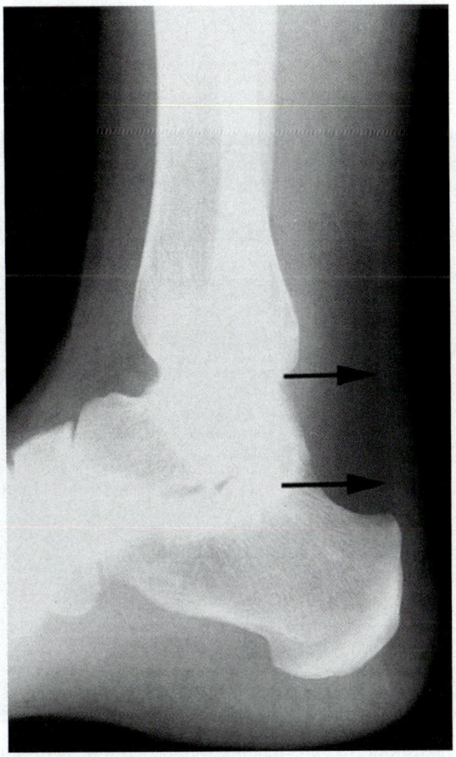

FIGURE 14.6 Lateral-view plain film demonstrating the Achilles tendon outlined by the fat in Kager's fat pad (*arrows*). (From Peduto AJ, Read JW. Imaging of ankle tendinopathy and tears. *Top Magn Reson Imaging* 2010;21(1):25–36.)

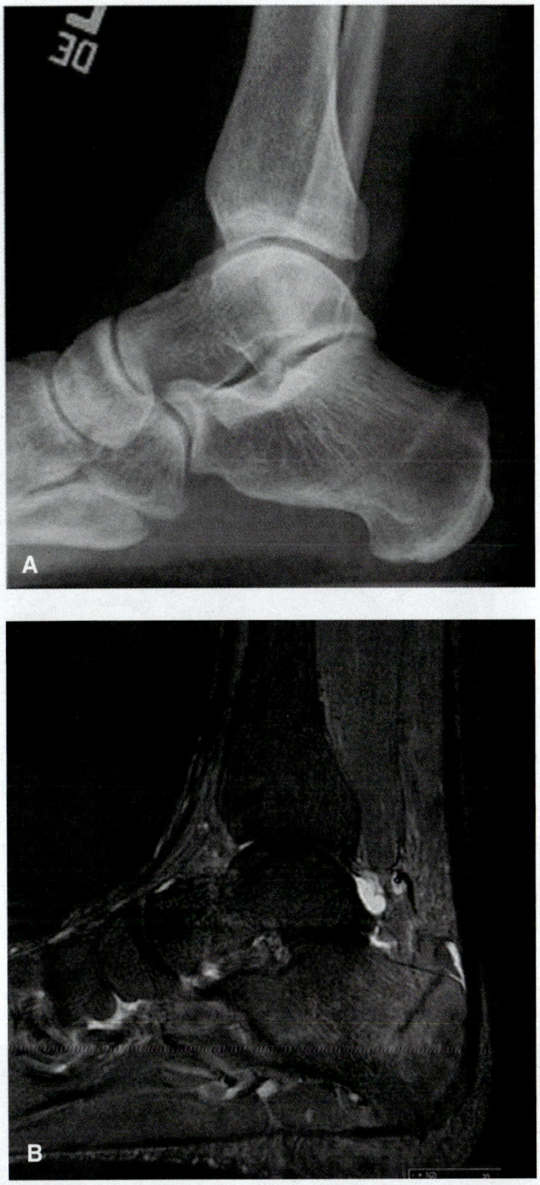

FIGURE 14.7 **A:** Standing lateral conventional radiograph of the ankle demonstrates characteristic cancellous stress fracture of the calcaneus with linear band of sclerosis oriented perpendicular to flow of trabeculae. **B:** Sagittal STIR MR image depicts calcaneal stress fracture with reactive bone marrow edema pattern surrounding the fracture. (© Hospital for Special Surgery, New York, NY. From Pavlov H, Sofka CM, Saboeiro GR, et al. Imaging of foot and ankle athletic injuries. In: Altcheck DW, DiGiovanni CW, Dines JS, et al., eds. *Foot and Ankle Sports Medicine*. Philadelphia, PA: Lippincott Williams & Wilkins; 2013:52.)

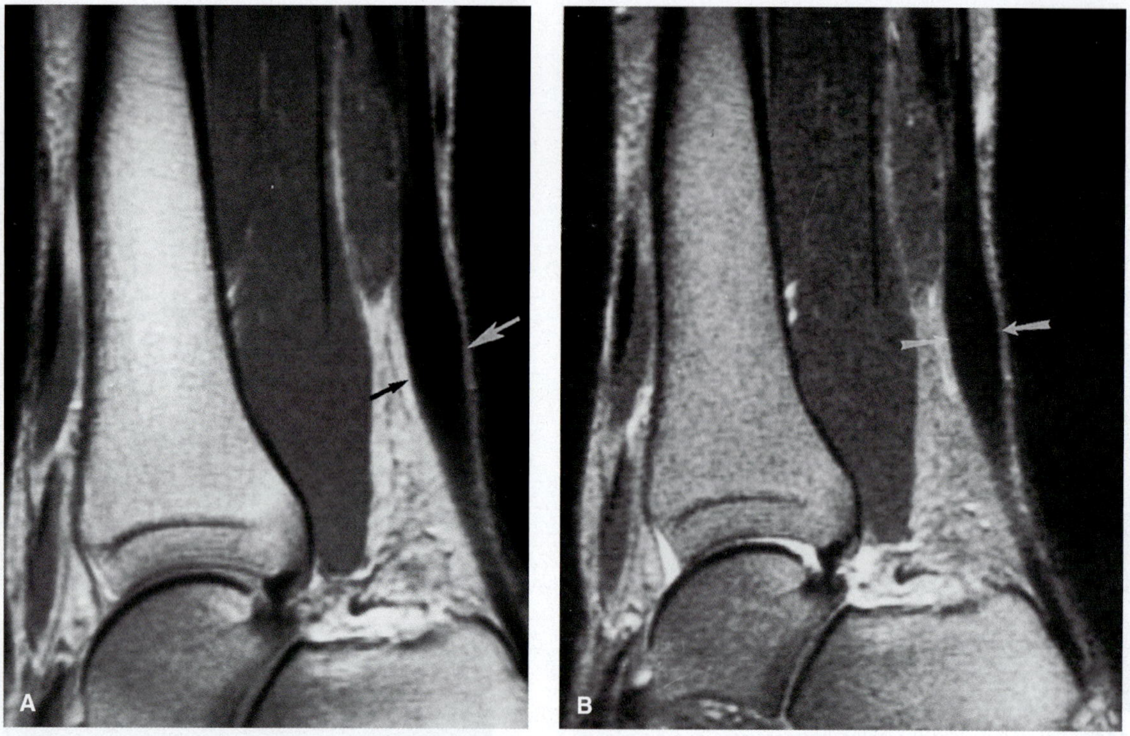

FIGURE 14.8 Sagittal proton density **(A)** and T2-weighted **(B)** images of an old low-grade tear that has filled in with scar tissue. There is tendon thickening (*arrows*) but no increased signal intensity. This has the same appearance as hypoxic tendinosis. (From Berquist TH. Soft tissue trauma and overuse syndromes. In: Berquist TH, ed. *MRI of the Musculoskeletal System*. 6th ed. Philadelphia, PA: Lippincott Williams & Wilkins; 2013:149.)

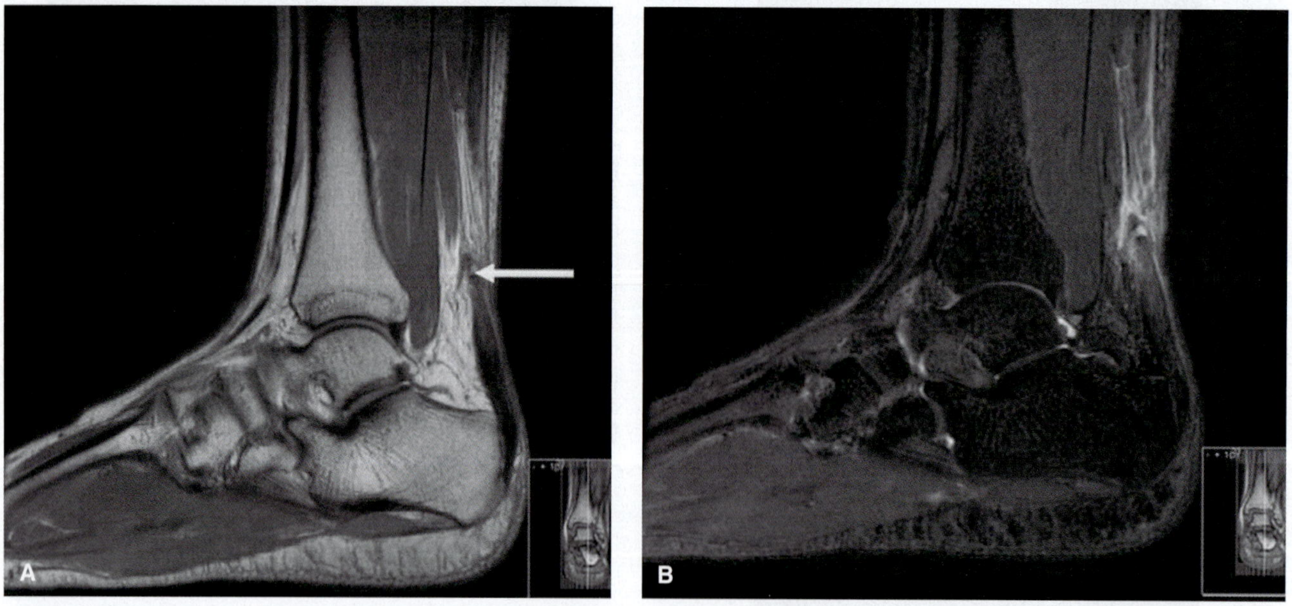

FIGURE 14.9 **A:** Sagittal FSE PD MR image of the ankle demonstrates complete disruption of the Achilles tendon with a 5-cm gap (*arrow*). **B:** Sagittal STIR MR image demonstrates that the injury is acute with hyperintensity and fluid filling the tendon gap. (© Hospital for Special Surgery, New York, NY. From Pavlov H, Sofka CM, Saboeiro GR, et al. Imaging of foot and ankle athletic injuries. In: Altcheck DW, DiGiovanni CW, Dines JS, et al., eds. *Foot and Ankle Sports Medicine*. Philadelphia, PA: Lippincott Williams & Wilkins; 2013:52.)

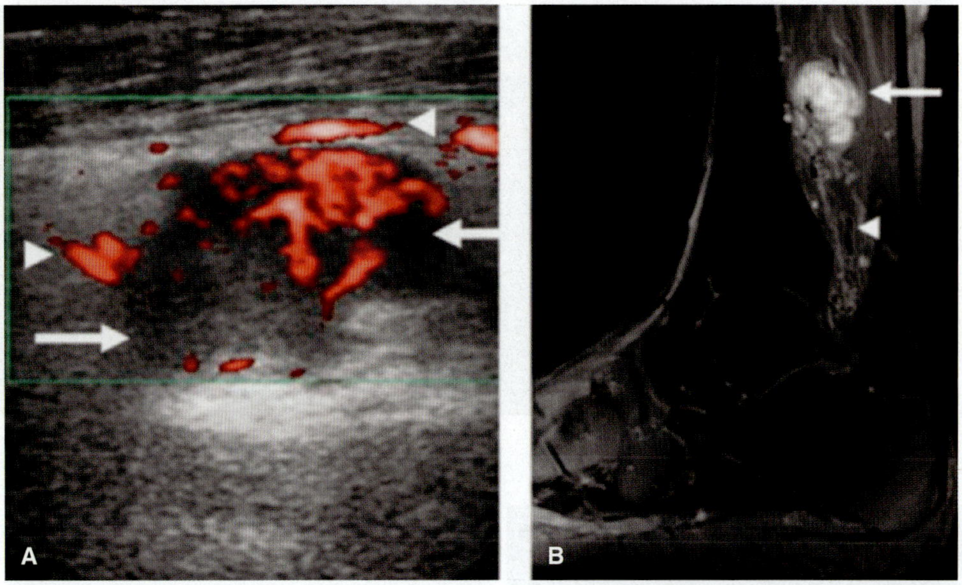

FIGURE 14.10 **A:** Ultrasound image of the lower calf shows a hypoechoic mass with marked internal vascularity (*arrows*) and surrounding vessels (*arrowheads*) seen on power Doppler interrogation in the flexor hallucis longus muscle. **B:** Sagittal T1-weighted fast spoiled gradient, fat-saturated magnetic resonance image after gadolinium administration shows homogeneous enhancement of the largest mass in the flexor hallucis longus muscle (*arrow*), with signal void seen in surrounding serpiginous vascular malformation (*arrowhead*). (From Glazebrook KN, Laundre BJ, Schiefer TK, et al. Imaging features of glomus tumors. *Skel Radiol* 2011;40:855–862.)

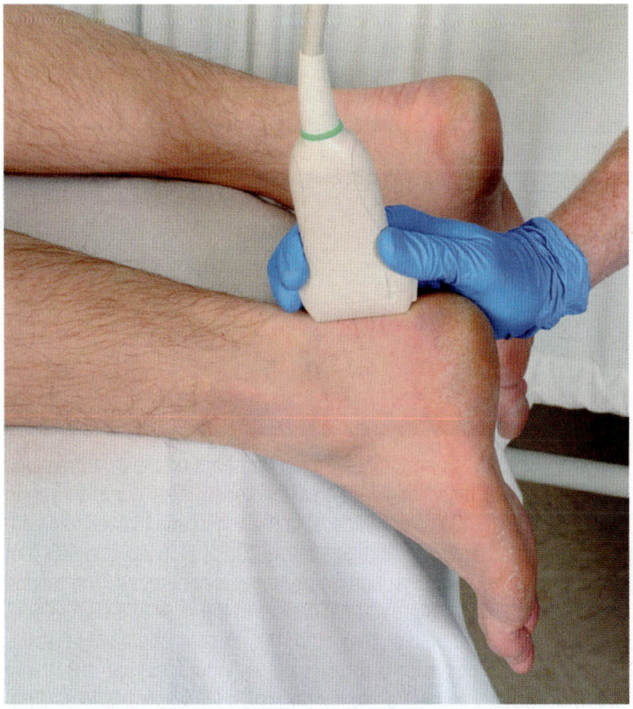

FIGURE 14.11 Proper longitudinal ultrasound transducer placement for ultrasound evaluation of the Achilles tendon.

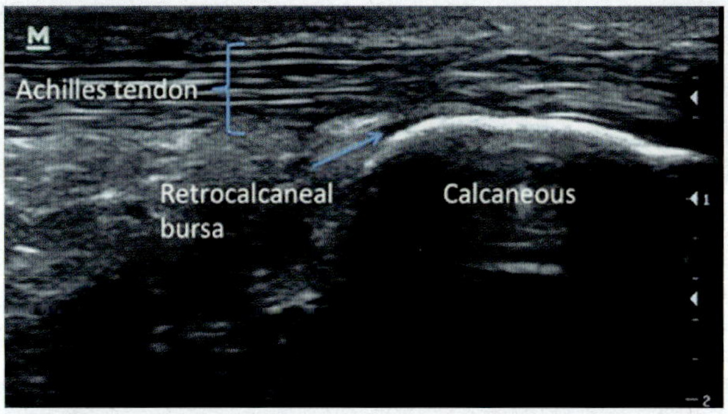

FIGURE 14.12 Longitudinal view of the Achilles tendon and its calcaneal insertion.

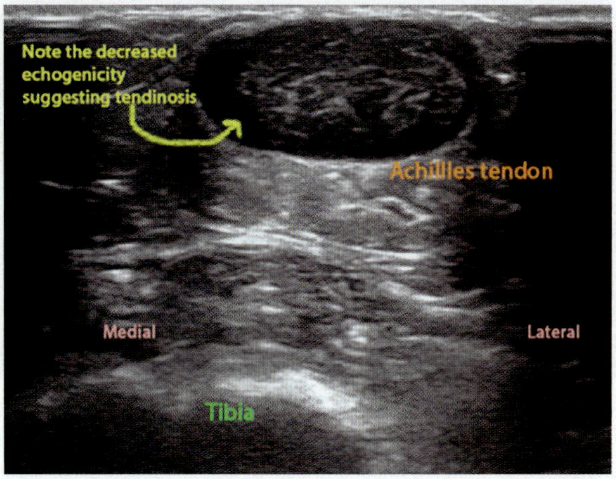

FIGURE 14.13 Achilles tendinosis. Transverse ultrasound view demonstrating thickened hypoechoic areas with inhomogeneous intratendinous architecture.

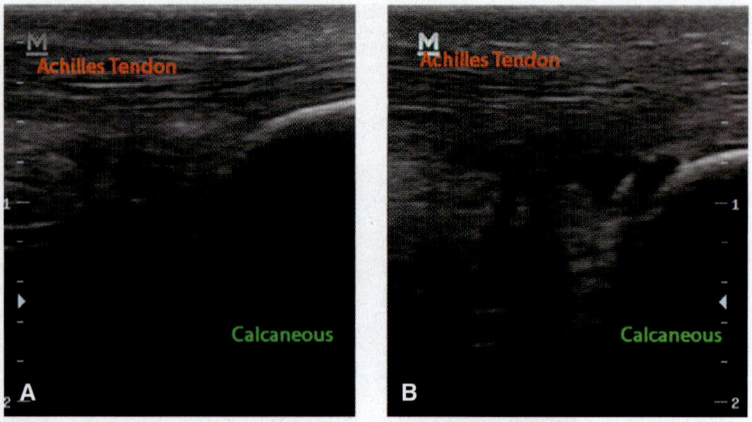

FIGURE 14.14 Longitudinal ultrasound images comparing an Achilles tendon with tendinosis **(A)** with a normal tendon **(B)**.

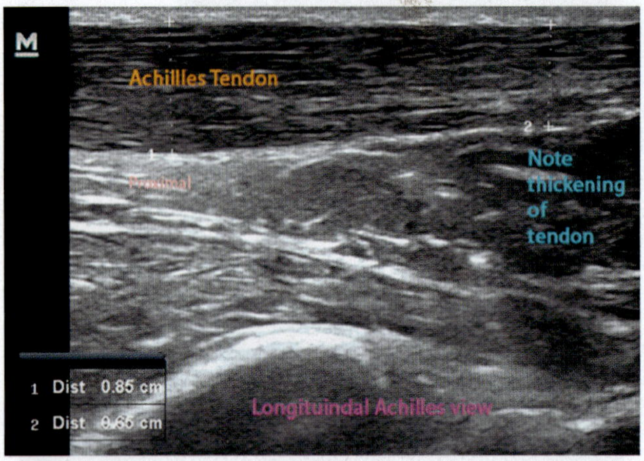

FIGURE 14.15 Longitudinal sonogram of Achilles tendinosis with fusiform thickening of the tendon and ill-defined areas of hypoechogenicity.

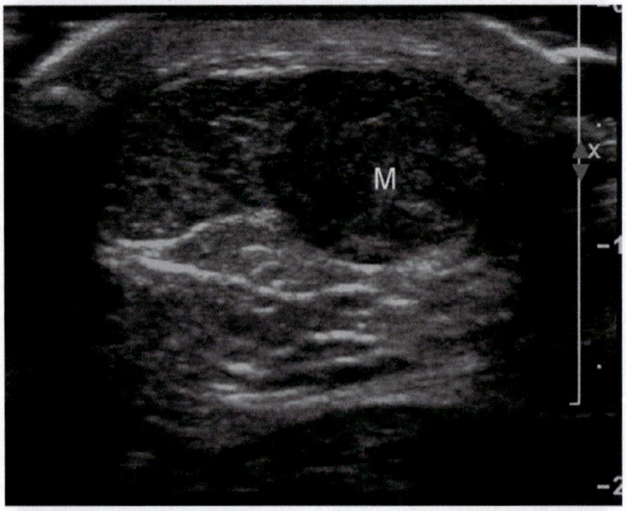

FIGURE 14.16 Medial tendinosis in the proximal Achilles. Note how the medial tendon (M) is thickened, more rounded, and heterogeneous, whereas the lateral component has a normal appearance. (From Daftary A, Adler RS. Sonographic evaluation and ultrasound-guided therapy of the Achilles tendon. *Ultrasound Q* 2009;25(3):103–110.)

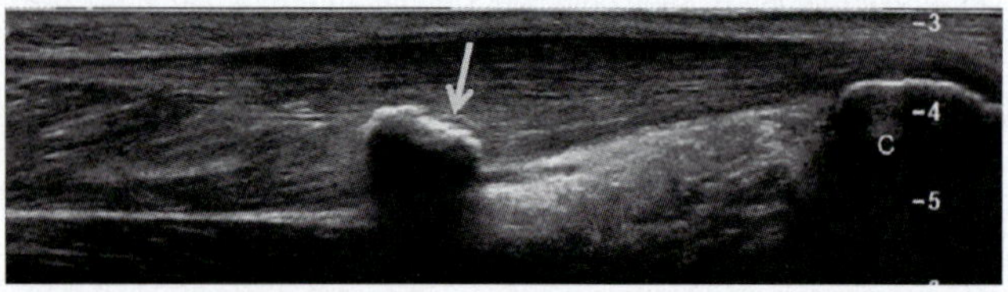

FIGURE 14.17 Calcification in the Achilles tendon (*arrow*) is seen as a well-defined area with echogenic margin and posterior shadowing in this long-axis extended-field-of-view image. C denotes the calcaneus. (From Daftary A, Adler RS. Sonographic evaluation and ultrasound-guided therapy of the achilles tendon. *Ultrasound Q* 2009;25(3):103–110.)

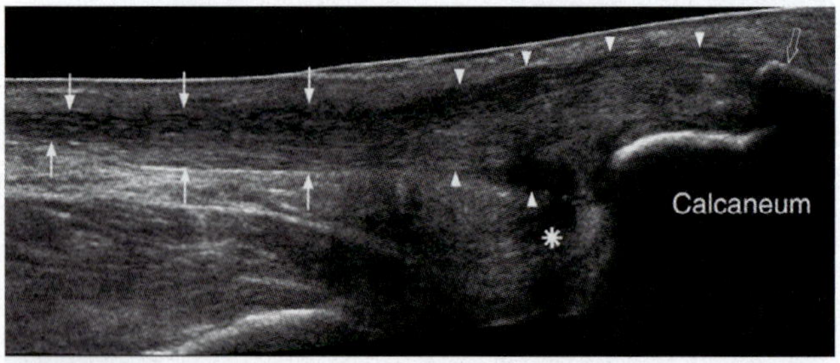

FIGURE 14.18 Longitudinal extended-field-of-view ultrasound showing severe insertional Achilles tendinosis. The distal one-third of the Achilles tendon (*arrowheads*) is thickened and hypoechoic with disruption of the normal fibrillar pattern. Color Doppler imaging (not shown) revealed mild peri- and intratendinous hyperemia. The tendon gradually tapers to a more normal caliber in the mid- to proximal one-third (*arrows*). Note mild distension of the retrocalcaneal bursa (*asterisk*) and a large posterior plantar calcaneal spur (*open arrow*). (From Lee R, Griffith J. Foot and ankle. In: Beggs I, ed. *Musculoskeletal Ultrasound*. Philadelphia, PA: Lippincott Williams & Wilkins; 2014:164.)

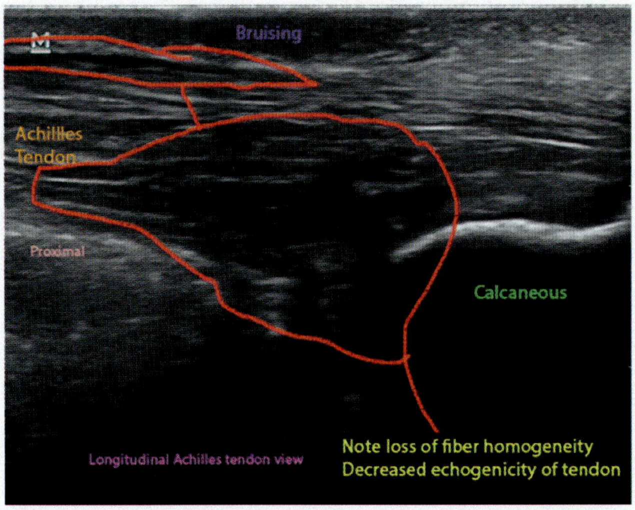

FIGURE 14.19 Longitudinal ultrasound image demonstrating bruising of the Achilles tendon from direct trauma as well as extensive tendinosis with significant tearing of the tendon substance.

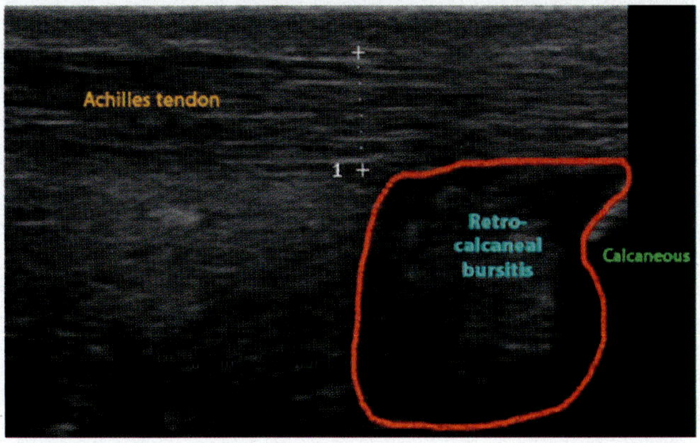

FIGURE 14.20 Longitudinal ultrasound image of the posterior leg demonstrating retrocalcaneal bursitis.

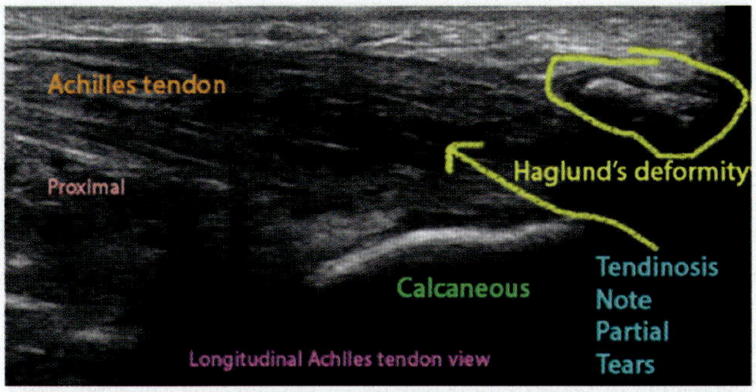

FIGURE 14.21 Haglund deformity with retrocalcaneal bursitis and insertional tendinosis. Longitudinal ultrasound image of the Achilles tendon shows it to be inhomogeneous. The posterior margin of the calcaneus is prominent, and fluid distends the retrocalcaneal. Note the partial tears of the tendon.

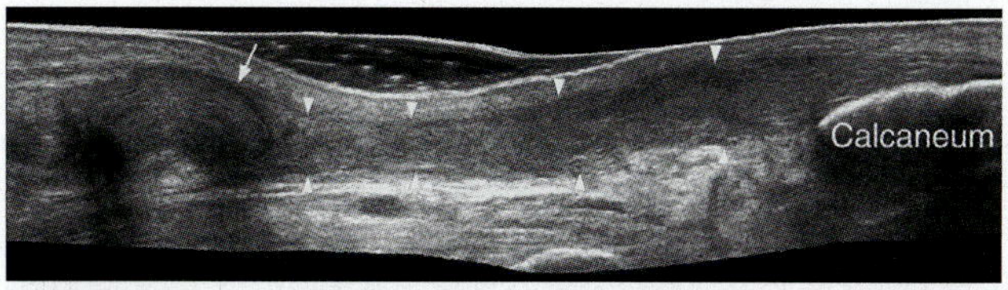

FIGURE 14.22 Longitudinal extended-field-of-view ultrasound of partial chronic Achilles tendon tear. The Achilles tendon (*arrowheads*) is elongated, although still continuous with a retracted tendon mass (*arrow*) close to the musculotendinous junction. (From Lee R, Griffith J. Foot and ankle. In: Beggs I, ed. *Musculoskeletal Ultrasound*. Philadelphia, PA: Lippincott Williams & Wilkins; 2014:165.)

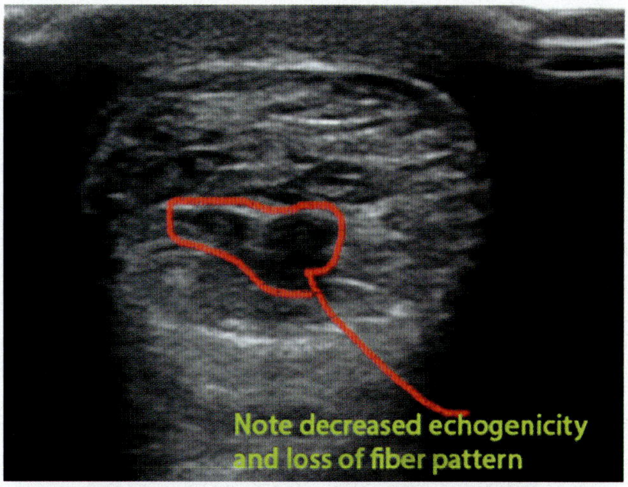

FIGURE 14.23 Transverse ultrasound image demonstrating significant tendinosis of the Achilles tendon with an intrasubstance tear.

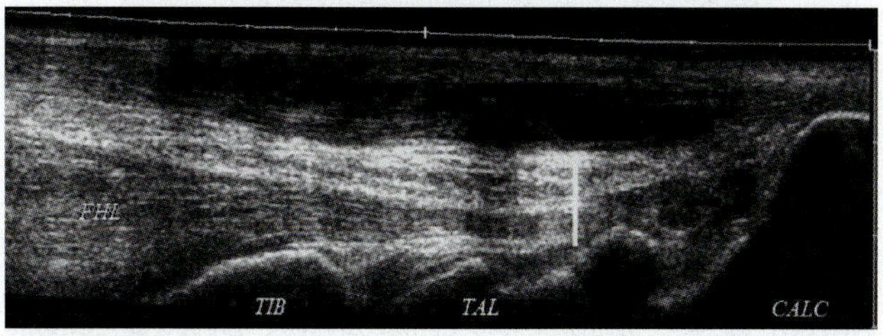

FIGURE 14.24 Longitudinal extended-field-of-view image of the Achilles tendon demonstrates advanced tendinosis with a superimposed irregular fluid-filled anechoic defect corresponding to a high-grade partial tear within the substance of tendon (*arrow*). The tibia (TIB), talus (TAL), and calcaneus (CALC) are indicated. The flexor hallucis longus (FHL) muscle belly can also be identified. (From Adler R, Sofka CM, Positano RG. *Atlas of Foot and Ankle Sonography*. Philadelphia, PA: Lippincott Williams & Wilkins; 2004:78.)

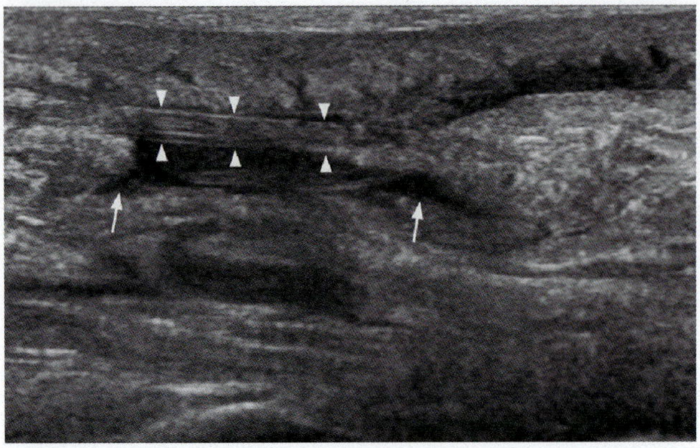

FIGURE 14.25 Longitudinal ultrasound of complete Achilles tendon tear, medial edge. The retracted ends of the tendon are shown (*arrows*) with the tendon gap filled with fluid. There is also an intact slightly swollen plantaris tendon (*arrowheads*) traversing the tendon gap. Do not confuse this with intact Achilles tendon fibers. (From Lee R, Griffith J. Foot and ankle. In: Beggs I, ed. *Musculoskeletal Ultrasound.* Philadelphia, PA: Lippincott Williams & Wilkins; 2014:164.)

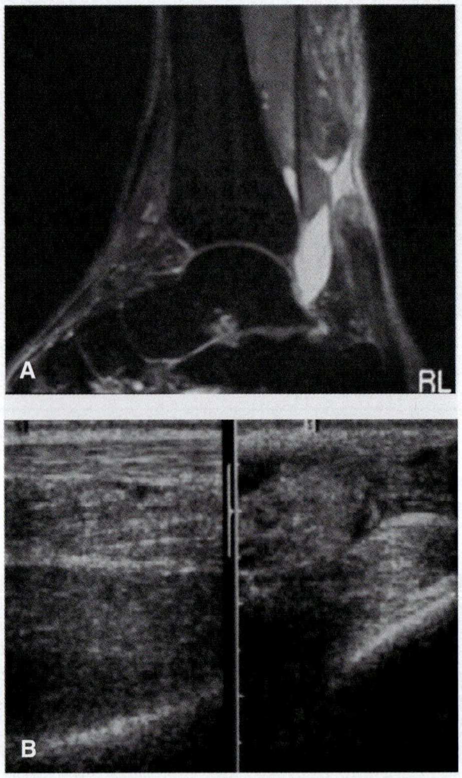

FIGURE 14.26 Complete tear of the Achilles tendon. **A:** Sagittal inversion-recovery MR image shows complete disruption and retraction of the torn edges. A fluid-filled gap and fluid within the sheet of the flexor hallucis longus tendon is seen. **B:** Longitudinal sonogram shows a normal linear fibrillar pattern in the left calf, and a full-thickness Achilles tendon tear on the right. Note that the ends of the bulged tendon are separated by the hematoma. (From Abadal JM, Fernandez JM, Rodriguez I, et al. Imaging of acute enlargement of the calf. *Radiologist* 2004;11(1):1–17.)

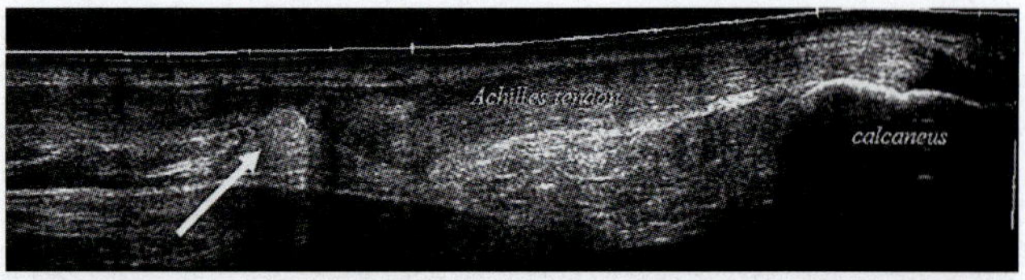

FIGURE 14.27 Longitudinal extended-field-of-view image demonstrates moderate diffuse tendinosis of the Achilles tendon with a complete muscle–tendon junction tear (*white arrow*). Note the abnormal morphology and marked attenuation of the tendon at the muscle–tendon junction. Echogenic fat herniates into the defect formed by proximally retracted tendon. (From Adler R, Sofka CM, Positano RG. *Atlas of Foot and Ankle Sonography.* Philadelphia, PA: Lippincott Williams & Wilkins; 2004:79.)

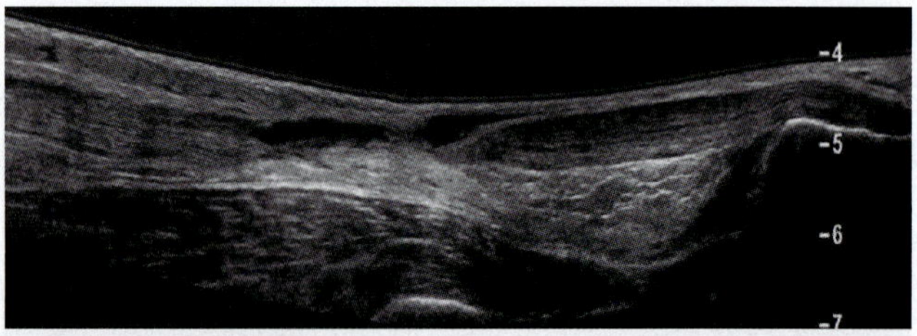

FIGURE 14.28 Typical acute Achilles tendon rupture, 4 cm from the calcaneal attachment (thinnest and possibly least vascular portion of the tendon), showing retraction and fluid in the tendon gap. Note the central herniation of fat at the site of the tear. (From Daftary A, Adler RS. Sonographic evaluation and ultrasound-guided therapy of the Achilles tendon. *Ultrasound Q* 2009;25(3):103–110.)

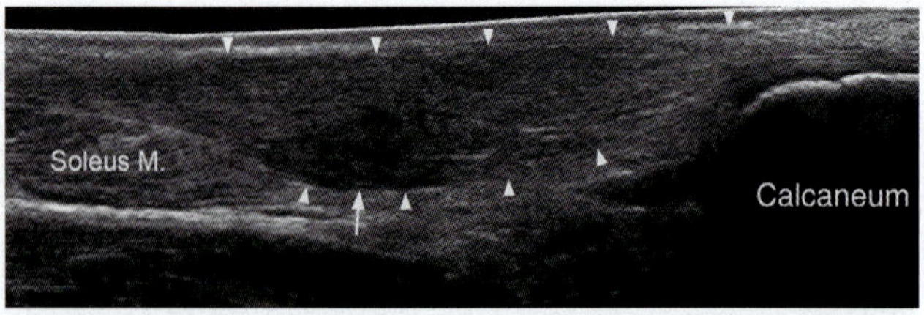

FIGURE 14.29 Longitudinal extended-field-of-view ultrasound showing diffusely thickened Achilles tendon (*arrowheads*) in a patient with familial hypercholesterolemia. The tendon thickening is due to deposition of cholesterol-rich material between the collagen fibers. There is a more discrete hypoechoic area of cholesterol deposition on the deeper aspect of the mid-tendon, which could be termed a "xanthoma" (*arrow*). (From Lee R, Griffith J. Foot and ankle. In: Beggs I, ed. *Musculoskeletal Ultrasound.* Philadelphia, PA: Lippincott Williams & Wilkins; 2014:166.)

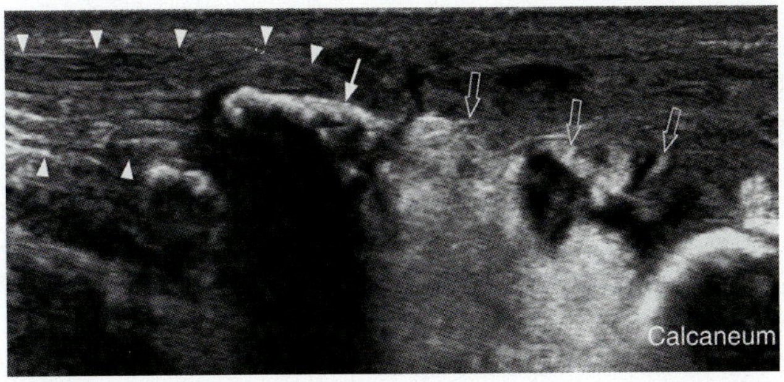

FIGURE 14.30 Longitudinal ultrasound showing Achilles fracture avulsion from calcaneal insertion. The Achilles tendon (*arrowheads*) is attached to a large fragment of bone (*closed arrow*) avulsed from the calcaneum. The intervening gap is filled with echogenic fat and hematoma (*open arrows*). (From Lee R, Griffith J. Foot and ankle. In: Beggs I, ed. *Musculoskeletal Ultrasound*. Philadelphia, PA: Lippincott Williams & Wilkins; 2014:165.)

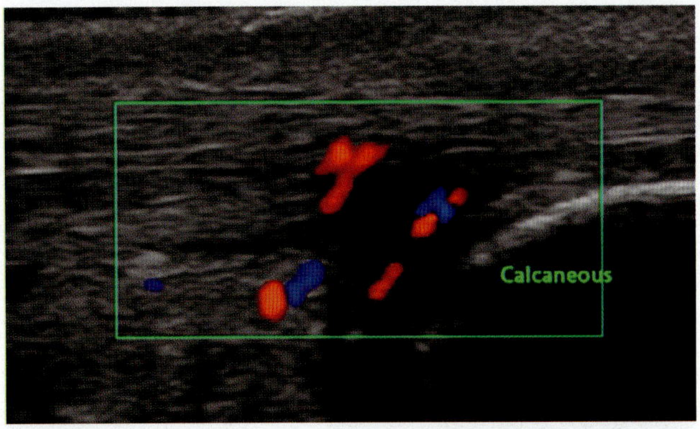

FIGURE 14.33 Longitudinal color Doppler image of the Achilles tendon. Note the neovascularity, which suggests tendinitis, not tendinosis.

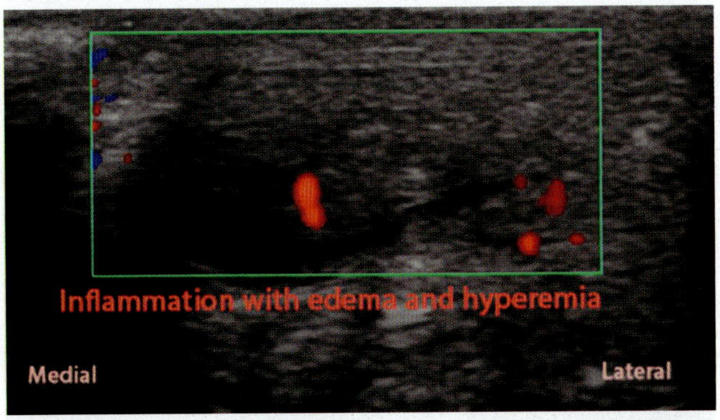

FIGURE 14.31 Transverse color Doppler image demonstrating tendinitis of the Achilles tendon.

symptoms. Early identification of pathology associated with tendinopathy of the Achilles tendon is crucial to avoid tendon rupture (Fig. 14.34). Ultrasound evaluation is also useful in assessment of healing of surgically repaired tears and ruptures of the Achilles tendon (Fig. 14.35). It is also important to identify the plantaris tendon which lies medial to the Achilles tendon and can sometimes be confused for residual Achilles tendon in the setting of complete Achilles tendon rupture (Fig. 14.36). Recent clinical experience has suggested that injection of platelet-rich plasma may be beneficial in patients with Achilles tendinosis to promote healing (Fig. 14.37).

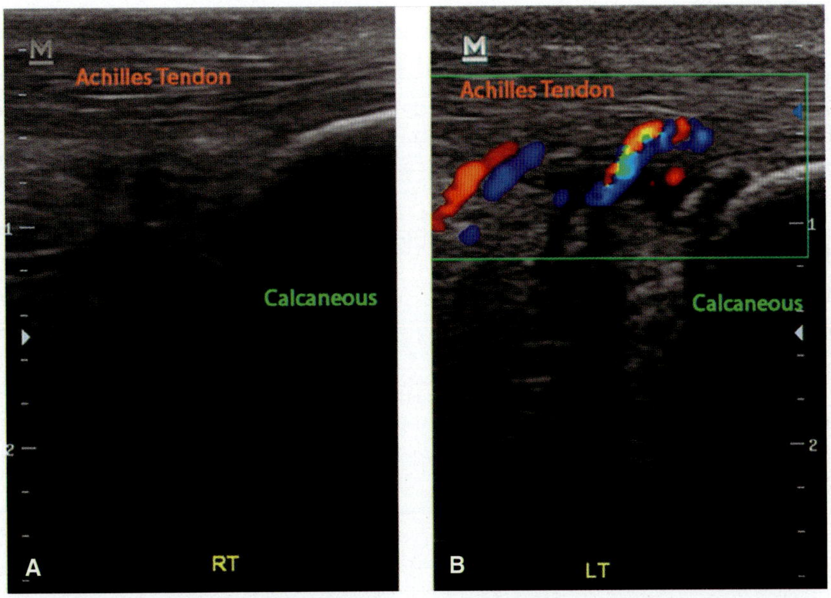

FIGURE 14.32 Longitudinal color Doppler images of right (**A**) and left (**B**) feet demonstrating tendinitis of the left foot.

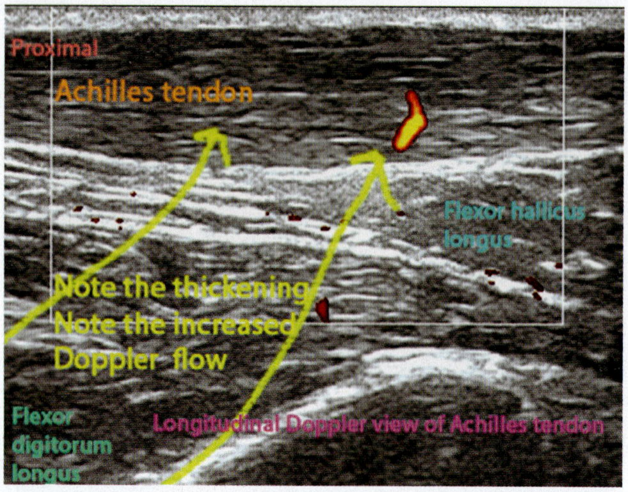

FIGURE 14.34 Partial Achilles tendon tear. A longitudinal power Doppler sonogram of the Achilles tendon showing hypoechoic flame-shaped partial tear (*arrow*) that begins interstitially and extends to the deep surface of the tendon. Normal tendon fibers are seen more proximally (*arrowhead*). A power Doppler sonogram showing proliferation of neovessels in and around the tendon. Note that the normal tendons do not show a detectable flow on the power Doppler sonography.

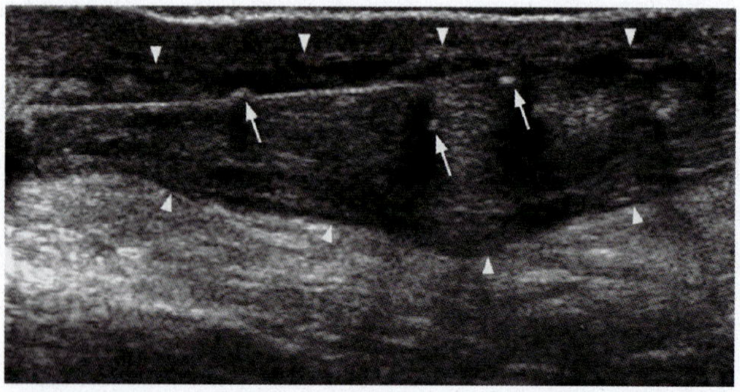

FIGURE 14.35 Postoperative appearances of Achilles tendon. The appearances vary according to the site and type of repair performed, although typically the tendon (*arrowheads*) remains thickened with clearly recognizable suture material (*arrows*). No retear is present. (From Lee R, Griffith J. Foot and ankle. In: Beggs I, ed. *Musculoskeletal Ultrasound.* Philadelphia, PA: Lippincott Williams & Wilkins; 2014:165.)

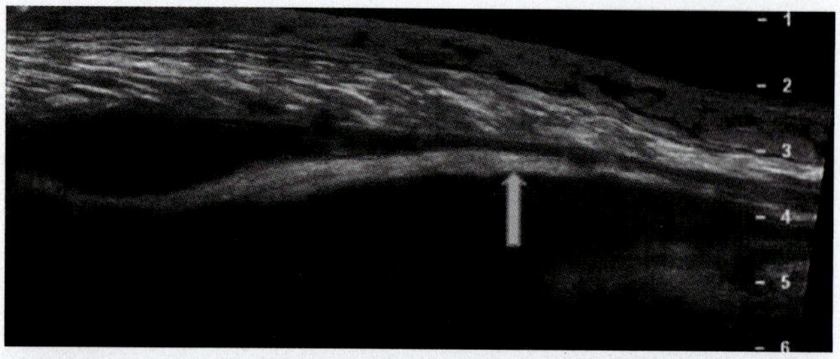

FIGURE 14.36 Plantaris tendon. The tendon is situated deep to the medial head of the gastrocnemius and medial to the Achilles tendon. It may become confluent with the Achilles tendon or have a separate insertion onto the calcaneus. In this extended-field-of-view image of the posterior calf, the tendon is apparent as a curvilinear echogenic band within a dissecting hematoma between the medial head of the gastrocnemius and soleus muscles in a patient with a complete rupture of the Achilles tendon. It is important to recognize the plantaris tendon, which can sometimes be mistaken for intact residual Achilles tendon. (From Daftary A, Adler RS. Sonographic evaluation and ultrasound-guided therapy of the Achilles tendon. *Ultrasound Q* 2009;25(3):103–110.)

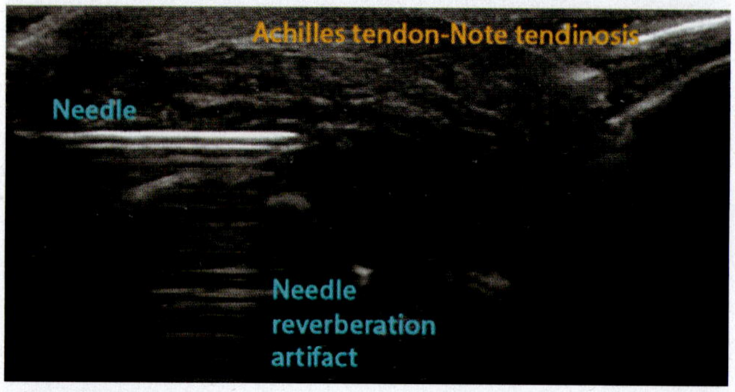

FIGURE 14.37 Transverse ultrasound image demonstrating injection of platelet-rich plasma to treat Achilles tendinosis.

Suggested Readings

Damuth E, Heidelbaugh J, Malani PN, et al. An elderly patient with fluoroquinolone-associated Achilles tendinitis. *Am J Geriatr Pharmacother* 2008;6(5):264–268.

Lesic A, Bumbasirevic M. Disorders of the Achilles tendon. *Curr Orthop* 2004;18(1):63–75.

Waldman SD. Achilles tendinitis. In: *Pain Review.* Philadelphia, PA: Saunders; 2009:325.

Waldman SD. Achilles tendinitis. In: *Atlas of Common Pain Syndromes.* 3rd ed. Philadelphia, PA: Saunders; 2011:362–364.

Waldman SD. The creaking tendon test for Achilles tendonitis. In: *Physical Diagnosis of Pain: An Atlas of Signs and Symptoms.* 2nd ed. Philadelphia, PA: Saunders; 2010:268–269.

Waldman SD. Injection technique for Achilles tendinitis. In: *Atlas of Pain Management Injection Techniques.* 3rd ed. Philadelphia, PA: Saunders; 2012:439–441.

Waldman SD, Campbell RSD. Achilles tendon rupture. In: *Imaging of Pain.* Philadelphia, PA: Saunders; 2011:431–432.

Waldman SD, Campbell RSD. Achilles tendonitis. In: *Imaging of Pain.* Philadelphia, PA: Saunders; 2011:427–428.

CHAPTER 15

Retrocalcaneal and Achilles Bursitis

ANATOMIC CONSIDERATIONS

The retrocalcaneal bursa lies between the Achilles tendon and the base of the tibia and the posterior calcaneus (Fig. 15.1). The bursa is subject to the development of inflammation after overuse, misuse, or direct trauma as is the Achilles bursa which lies posterior to the Achilles tendon at its insertion on the calcaneus. The Achilles tendon is the thickest and strongest tendon in the body, yet also very susceptible to rupture. The common tendon of the gastrocnemius muscle, the Achilles tendon, begins at mid-calf and continues downward to attach to the posterior calcaneus, where it may become inflamed. The Achilles tendon narrows during this downward course, becoming most narrow approximately 4 to 5 cm above its calcaneal insertion (Fig. 15.2). It is at this narrowmost point that tendinitis also may occur. Tendinitis, especially at the calcaneal insertion, may mimic retrocalcaneal bursitis and may make diagnosis difficult. The Achilles bursa lies between the skin and the Achilles tendon (Fig 15.1). It is an adventitious bursa which when inflamed is also known as "pump bump" due to its association with the hard back of ill-fitting pump style shoes.

CLINICAL CORRELATES

Retrocalcaneal bursitis is a common cause of posterior heel pain (Fig. 15.3). The retrocalcaneal bursa, which is also known as the subtendinous calcaneal bursa, lies between the Achilles tendon and its insertion on the calcaneus (Figs. 15.3 and 15.4). The bursa serves to cushion and facilitate sliding of the Achilles

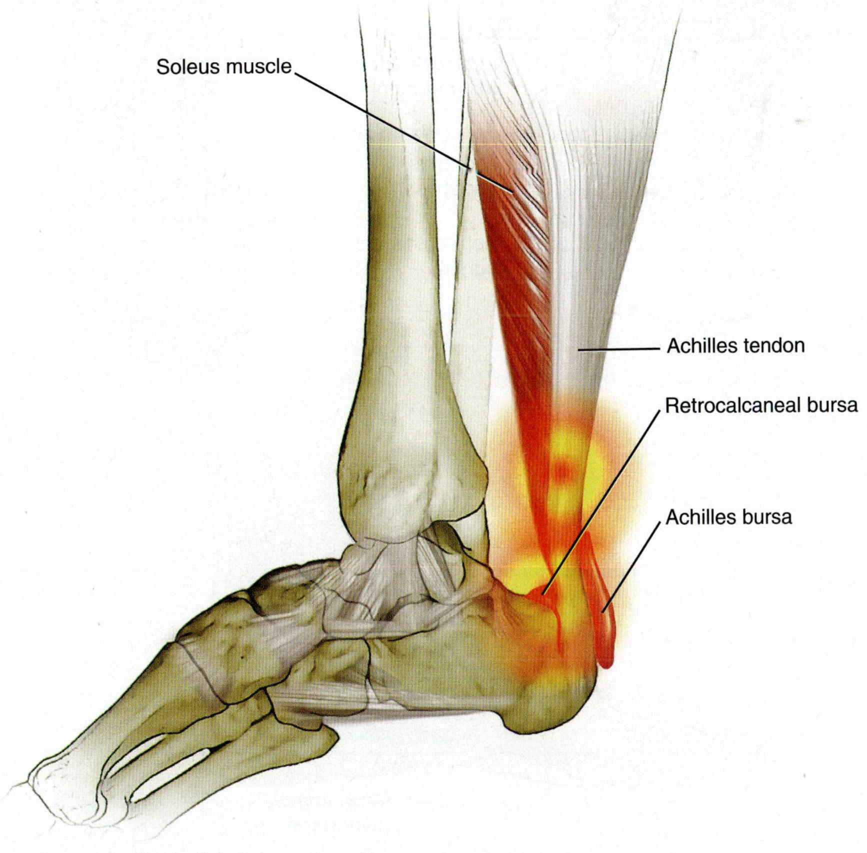

FIGURE 15.1 The bursa of the ankle.

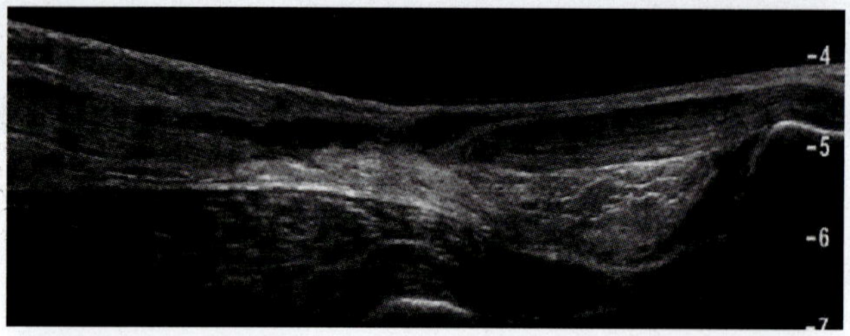

FIGURE 15.2 Achilles tendon rupture. Typical acute tendon rupture, 4 cm from the calcaneal attachment (thinnest and possibly least vascular portion of the tendon), showing retraction and fluid in the tendon gap. Note the central herniation of fat at the site of the tear. (From Daftary A, Adler RS. Sonographic evaluation and ultrasound-guided therapy of the Achilles tendon. *Ultrasound Q* 2009;25(3):103–110.)

tendon over the calcaneus. The bursa is subject to inflammation from a variety of causes with acute trauma to the knee and repetitive microtrauma being the most common. Acute injuries to the bursa can occur from direct blunt trauma to the posterior ankle such as kicks while playing sports. The bursa may also become inflammed as a result of overuse injuries, running on uneven or soft surfaces, and jobs that require repeated plantar flexion of the ankle. If the inflammation of the bursa is not treated and the condition becomes chronic, calcification of the bursa with further functional disability may occur. Gout and other crystal arthropathies may also precipitate acute retrocalcaneal bursitis as may bacterial, tubercular, or fungal infections (Fig. 15.5).

The patient suffering from retrocalcaneal bursitis most frequently present with the complaint of pain in the posterior heel which may radiate into the posterior ankle. The patient may find walking downstairs, standing on tiptoes, and kneeling increasingly difficult. Physical examination of the patient suffering from retrocalcaneal bursitis will reveal point tenderness over the heel, with the medial side affected more commonly

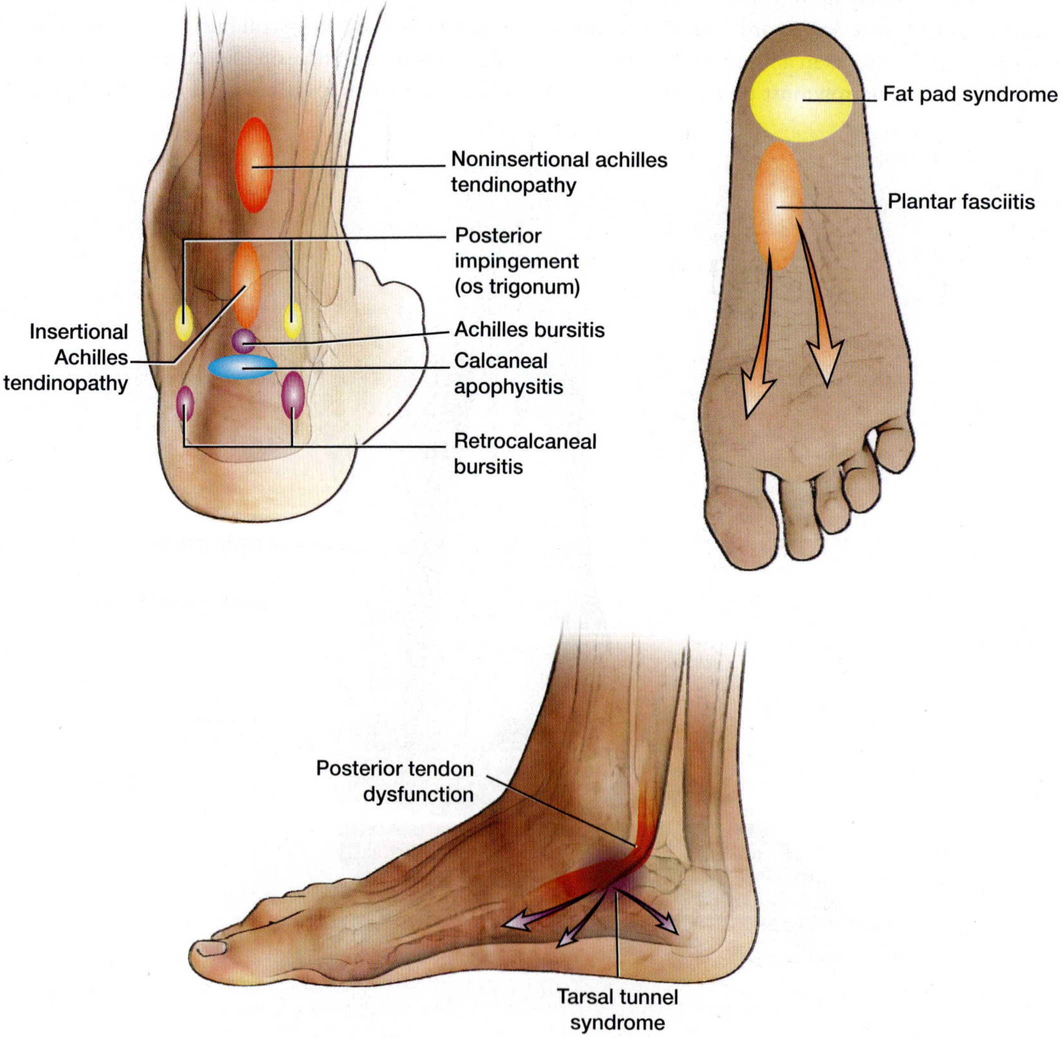

FIGURE 15.3 Common causes of heel pain.

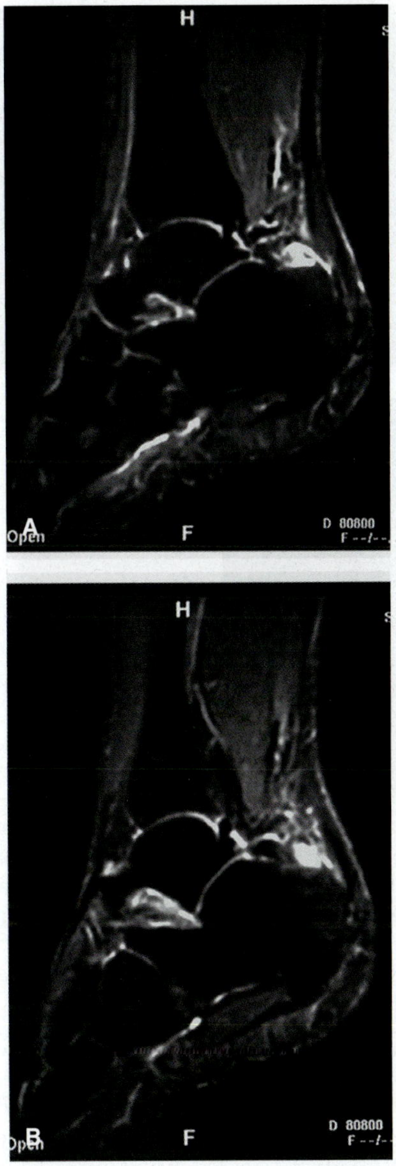

FIGURE 15.4 **A,B:** Magnetic resonance images demonstrating high signal intensity within the retrocalcaneal bursa and prominence of the posterosuperior portion of the calcaneus. (From McBryde AM, Ortmann FW. Retrocalcaneal bursoscopy. *Techn Foot Ankle Surg* 2005;4(3):174–179; Fig. 2A,B).

than the lateral. If there is significant inflammation, rubor and color may be present and the entire area may feel boggy or edematous to palpation. At times massive effusion may be present which can be quite distressing to the patient. Active plantar flexion of the affected knee will often reproduce the patient's pain. Sudden release of resistance to active plantar will markedly increase the pain. If calcification or gouty tophi or xanthomas associated with familial hypercholesterolemia of the bursa and surrounding tendons are present, the examiner may appreciate crepitus with active extension of the knee and the patient may complain of a catching sensation when moving the affected knee, especially on awaking (Fig. 15.6). Often, the

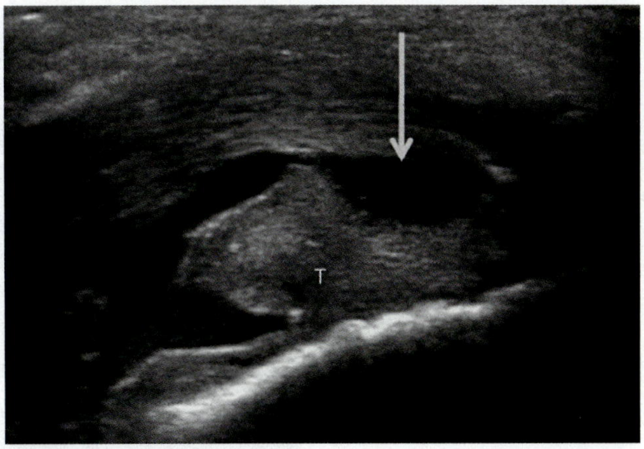

FIGURE 15.5 Longitudinal ultrasound image demonstrates deep retrocalcaneal bursitis (*long arrow*) containing tophaceous material (T) in a patient with gout. Fluid and nodular echogenic soft tissue distend the bursa. (From Daftary A, Adler RS. Sonographic evaluation and ultrasound-guided therapy of the Achilles tendon. *Ultrasound Q* 2009;25(3):103–110.)

patient will not be able to sleep on the affected side. Occasionally, the retrocalcaneal bursa may become infected, with systemic symptoms, including fever and malaise, as well as local symptoms, with rubor, color, and dolor being present.

Patients with a prominent and upturned calcaneal tuberosity are predisposed to the development of Achilles bursitis or pump bump (Fig. 15.7). When this boney abnormality is associated with Achilles bursitis, Achilles insertional tendinitis, Achilles tendinosis and tearing, and at times, retrocalcaneal bursitis, this constellation of symptoms is known as Haglund disease or deformity (Figs. 15.8 and 15.9).

Plain radiographs are indicated in all patients who present with ankle and heel pain to rule out occult ankle pathology (Fig. 15.10). Based on the patient's clinical presentation, additional testing may be indicated, including complete blood cell count, sedimentation rate, and antinuclear antibody testing. Magnetic resonance imaging or ultrasound imaging of the affected area may also confirm the diagnosis and help delineate the presence of other bursitis including coexistent Achilles bursitis, calcific tendinitis, tendinopathy, triceps tendinitis, or other ankle pathology (Figs. 15.11 and 15.12). Rarely, the inflamed bursa may become infected, and failure to diagnose and treat the acute infection can lead to dire consequences.

ULTRASOUND TECHNIQUE

To evaluate the retrocalcaneal and Achilles bursa, the patient is placed in the prone position with the patient's ankle hanging off the edge of the table. With the patient in the above position, a high-frequency linear ultrasound transducer is placed in a longitudinal plane with the inferior portion of the ultrasound transducer over the insertion of the Achilles tendon on the

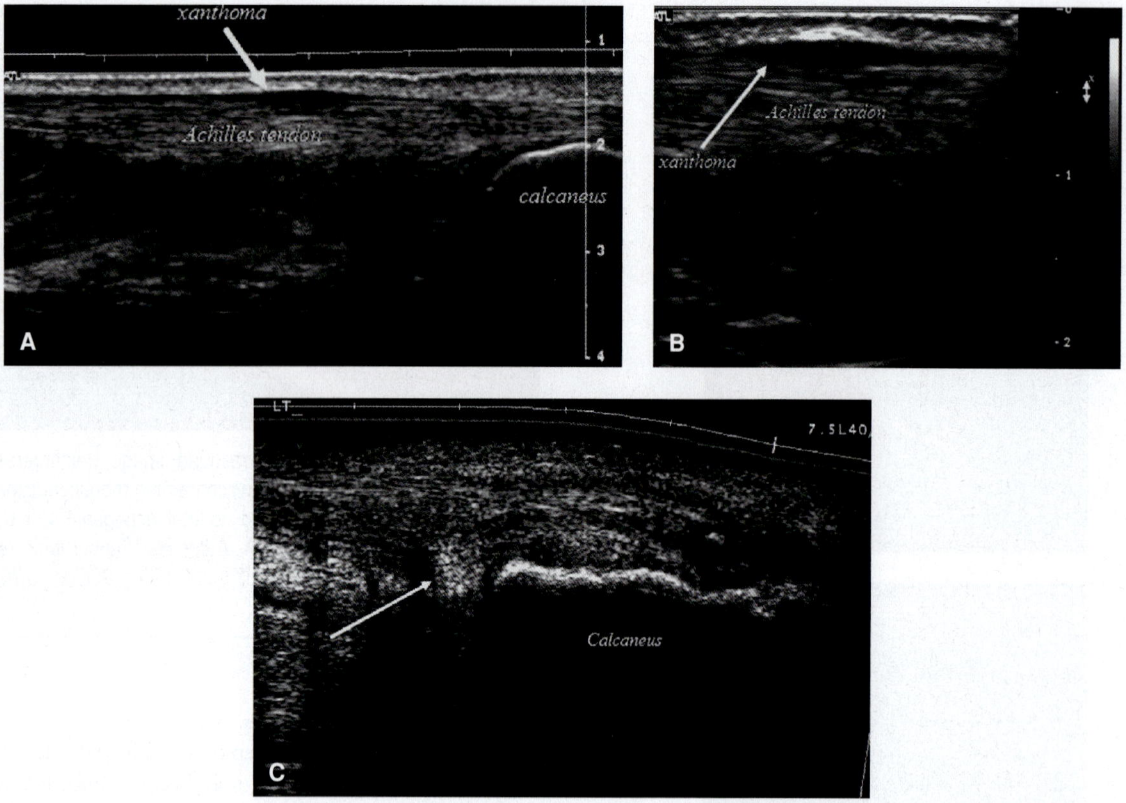

FIGURE 15.6 Ultrasound has been shown to be a sensitive technique to detect tendon xanthomas. In patients with the heterozygous form of familial hypercholesterolemia, Achilles xanthomas are an important diagnostic feature of the disease (*arrows*). **A:** This longitudinal extended-field-of-view image of the distal Achilles tendon demonstrates a hypoechoic nodule within the superficial margin of the tendon. The patient had a history of hypercholesterolemia, with a parent and sibling having died from coronary artery disease. **B:** The xanthoma is better depicted in this small field-of-view gray scale image. Typically, these are hypoechoic and oriented along the long axis of the tendon. With advanced disease, the xanthomas may become confluent and difficult to differentiate from tendinosis. **C:** Note the xanthoma just superior to the calcaneus (*arrow*). (From Adler R, Sofka CM, Positano RG. *Atlas of Foot and Ankle Sonography.* Philadelphia, PA: Lippincott Williams & Wilkins; 2004.)

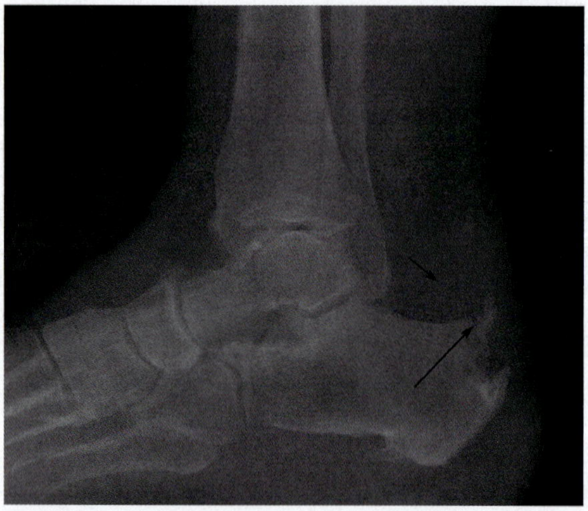

FIGURE 15.7 Haglund disease. Lateral radiograph demonstrating pre-Achilles edema (*short arrow*), prominence of the calcaneal tuberosity (*long arrow*) with calcaneal erosion, thickening of the Achilles tendon, and ossific tendinosis. (From Berquist TH. The lower limb. In: *MRI of the Musculoskeletal System.* 6th ed. Philadelphia, PA: Lippincott Williams & Wilkins; 2013:179.)

calcaneus and an ultrasound survey scan is taken (Fig. 15.13). The linear Achilles tendon is identified as its insertion on the calcaneus. Beneath the tendon lies the retrocalcaneal bursa (Fig. 15.14). When the insertion of the Achilles tendon is identified, the tendon is evaluated for the presence of insertional tendinopathy. The area above and beneath the tendon is then evaluated for the presence of retrocalcaneal and Achilles bursitis as well as for the presence of a prominent calcaneal tuberosity (Figs. 15.15 to 15.22).

CLINICAL PEARLS

Bursitis, labral tears, tedinopathy, osteoarthritis, synovitis, nerve entrapment, avascular necrosis of the knee, and impingement syndromes may coexist with other knee joint disease and may contribute to the patient's pain symptomatology. Arthroscopic treatment may be necessary to treat retrocalcaneal bursitis that is refractory to treatment with ultrasound-guided injection of local anesthetic and steroid (Fig. 15.23). The finding of bilateral retrocalcaneal bursitis is highly suggestive of coexistent inflammatory arthritis.

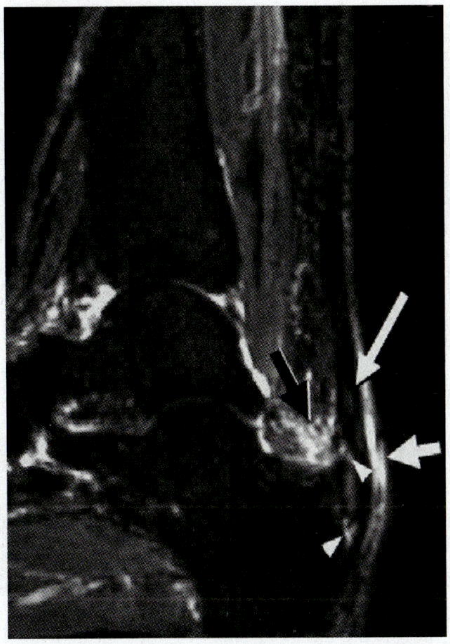

FIGURE 15.8 Sagittal STIR image shows an upturned posterior superior calcaneus ("Haglund deformity") with surrounding reactive bone marrow edema, Achilles tendinosis with mucoid degeneration (*long white arrow*), small insertional tears (*small arrowheads*), retro-Achilles bursitis (*short white arrow*), and retrocalcaneal bursitis (*black arrow*). These findings are characteristic of Haglund syndrome. (From Morrison WB. Magnetic resonance imaging of sports injuries of the ankle. *Top Magn Reson Imaging* 2003;14(2):179–197.)

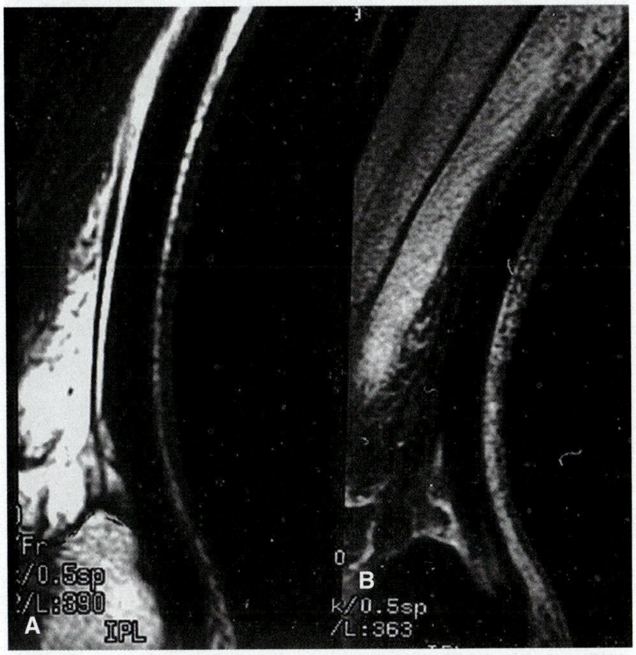

FIGURE 15.9 **A:** MRI showing the prominent Haglund's bony deformity impinging against the insertional portion of the Achilles tendon. **B:** T2 image showing the localized area of tendinosis at the site of bony impingement adjacent to the inflamed retrocalcaneal bursa. (From Sullivan M. Endoscopic resection of Haglund deformity and bursectomy. *Techn Foot Ankle Surg* 2010;9(2):48–51.)

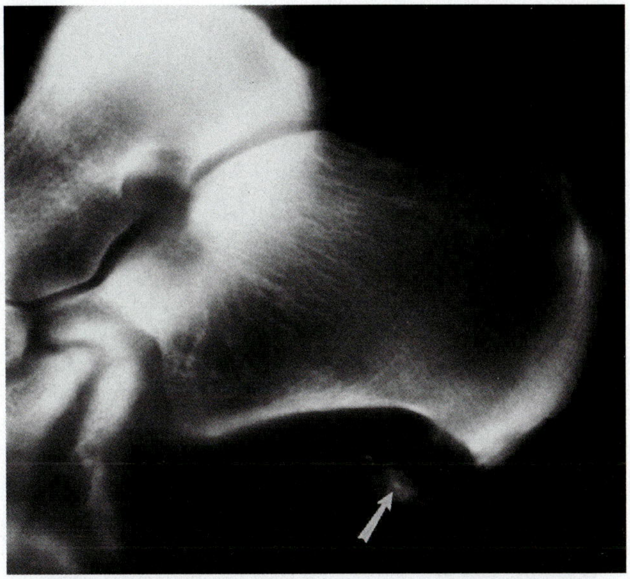

FIGURE 15.10 Lateral radiograph demonstrating an avulsed osteophyte in a patient with persistent heel pain (*arrows*). (From Berquist TH. The lower limb. In: *MRI of the Musculoskeletal System*. 6th ed. Philadelphia, PA: Lippincott Williams & Wilkins; 2013:174.)

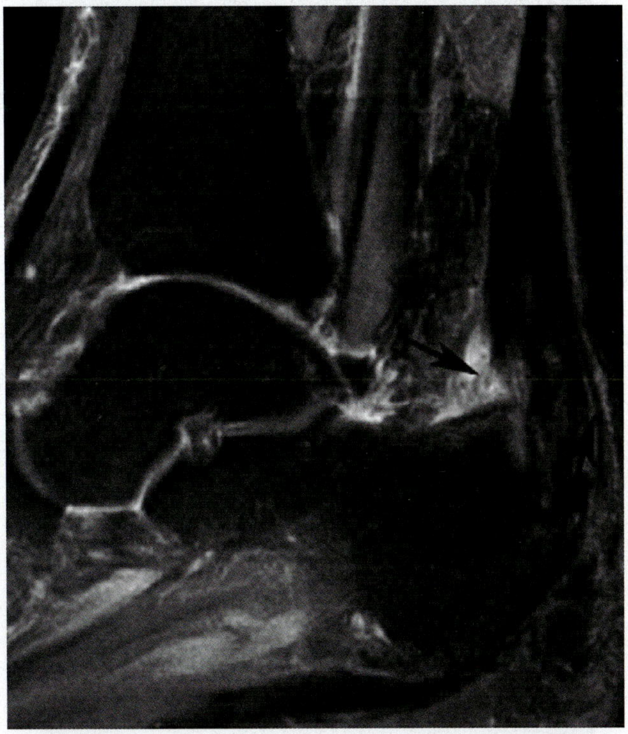

FIGURE 15.11 Sagittal fast spin-echo T2-weighted image demonstrates retro-Achilles bursitis (*short arrow*), prominence of the posterior tuberosity with marrow edema (*arrowhead*), thickening and inflammation of the Achilles tendon and fluid in the superficial bursa (*long arrow*). (From Berquist TH. The lower limb. In: *MRI of the Musculoskeletal System*. 6th ed. Philadelphia, PA: Lippincott Williams & Wilkins; 2013:180.)

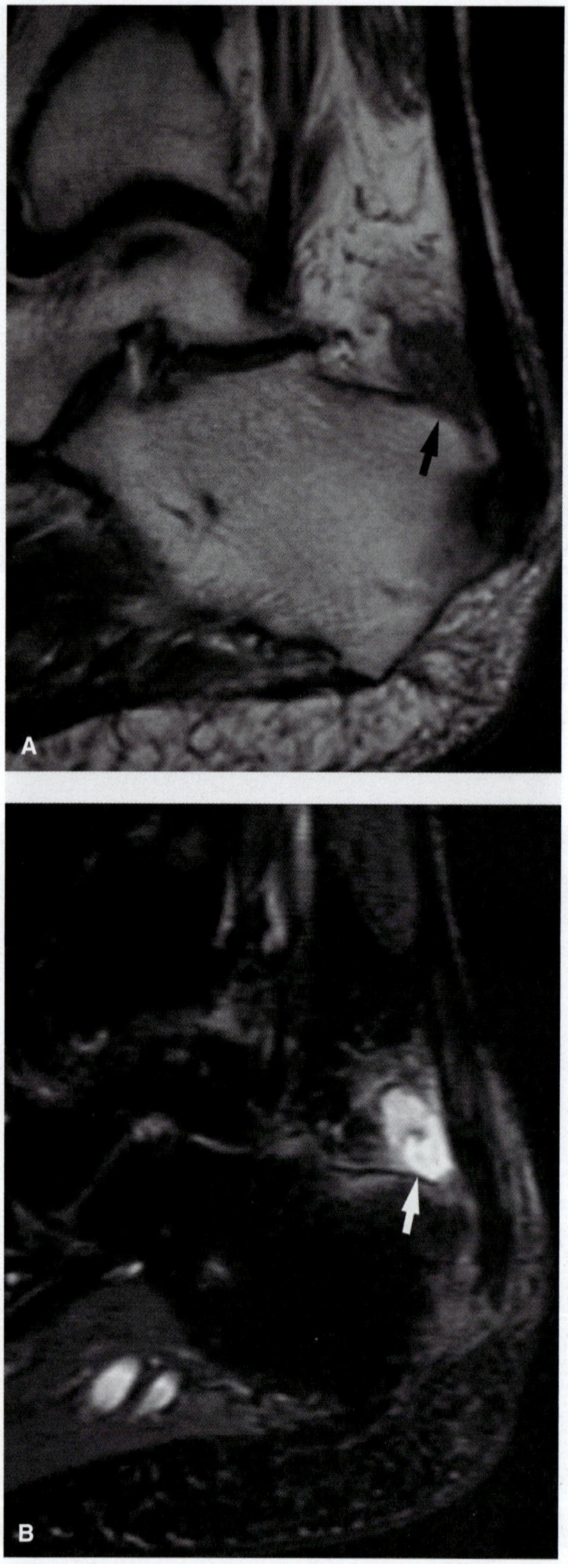

FIGURE 15.12 Retrocalcaneal bursitis. T1-weighted **(A)** and STIR **(B)** sagittal images demonstrate retrocalcaneal bursitis (*arrow*) and bone marrow edema within the posterosuperior calcaneus in this patient with persistent pain. Also note the abnormal signal within the Achilles tendon. (From Farooki S, Ashman CJ, Lee J, et al. Common bursae about the body: a review of normal anatomy and magnetic resonance imaging findings. *Radiologist* 2002;9(4):209–221.)

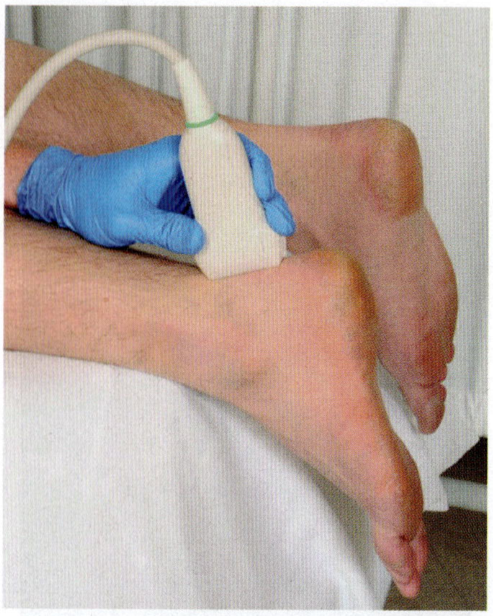

FIGURE 15.13 Proper longitudinal ultrasound transducer placement for ultrasound evaluation for retrocalcaneal and Achilles bursitis.

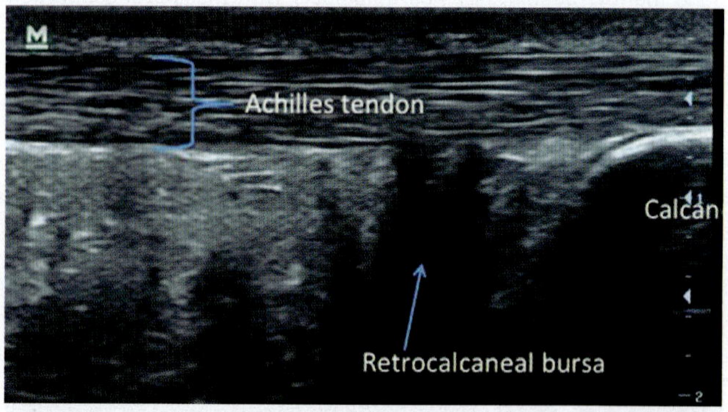

FIGURE 15.14 Longitudinal view of the Achilles tendon, its calcaneal insertion, and an enlarged retrocalcaneal bursa.

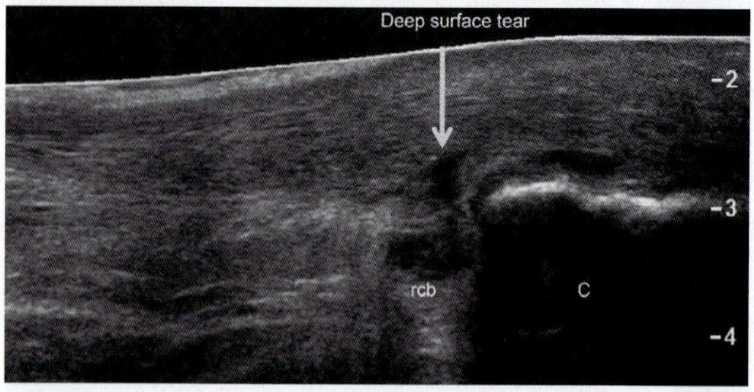

FIGURE 15.15 Haglund deformity with retrocalcaneal bursitis and insertional tendinosis. Longitudinal extended-field-of-view image of the Achilles tendon (AT) shows it to be inhomogeneous. The posterior margin of the calcaneus is prominent (C), and fluid distends the retrocalcaneal bursa, after therapeutic injection. Fluid distension of the retrocalcaneal bursa demonstrated a communication with a partially torn AT (*arrow*). As in this case, the tear appears as a well-marginated hypoechoic defect along the deep surface of the tendon. (From Daftary A, Adler RS. Sonographic evaluation and ultrasound-guided therapy of the Achilles tendon. *Ultrasound Q* 2009;25(3):103–110.)

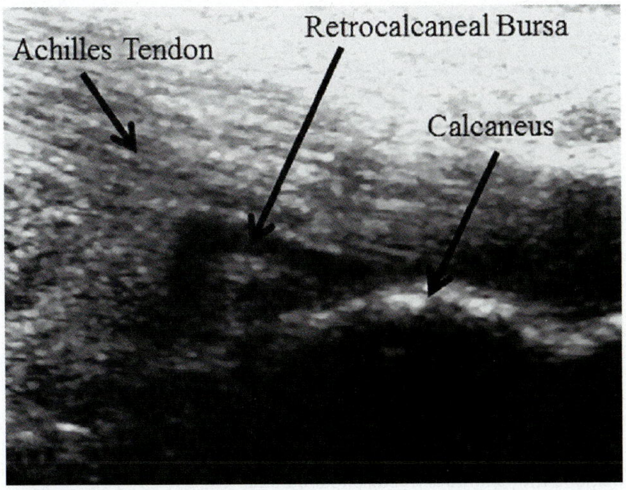

FIGURE 15.16 Longitudinal ultrasound view showing the hypoechoic triangular area of the retrocalcaneal bursa that is situated between the Achilles tendon and the calcaneus. (From Chu NK, Lew HL, Chen CP. Ultrasound-guided injection treatment of retrocalcaneal bursitis. *Am J Phys Med Rehab* 2012;91(7):635–637.)

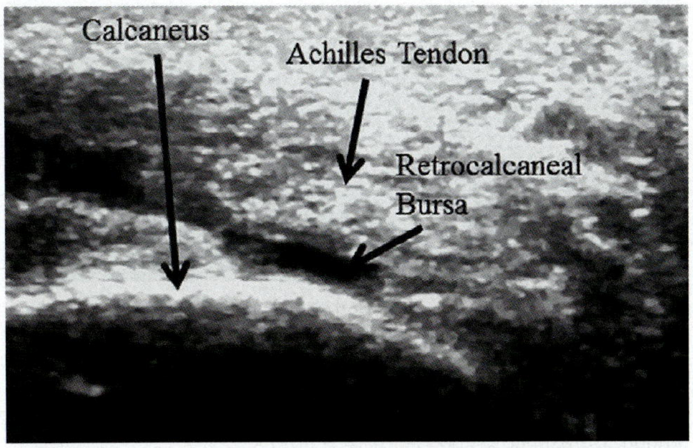

FIGURE 15.17 Transverse sonographic view showing the hypoechoic area of the retrocalcaneal bursa that is situated between the Achilles tendon and the calcaneus. (From Chu NK, Lew HL, Chen CP. Ultrasound-guided injection treatment of retrocalcaneal bursitis. *Am J Phys Med Rehab* 2012;91(7):635–637.)

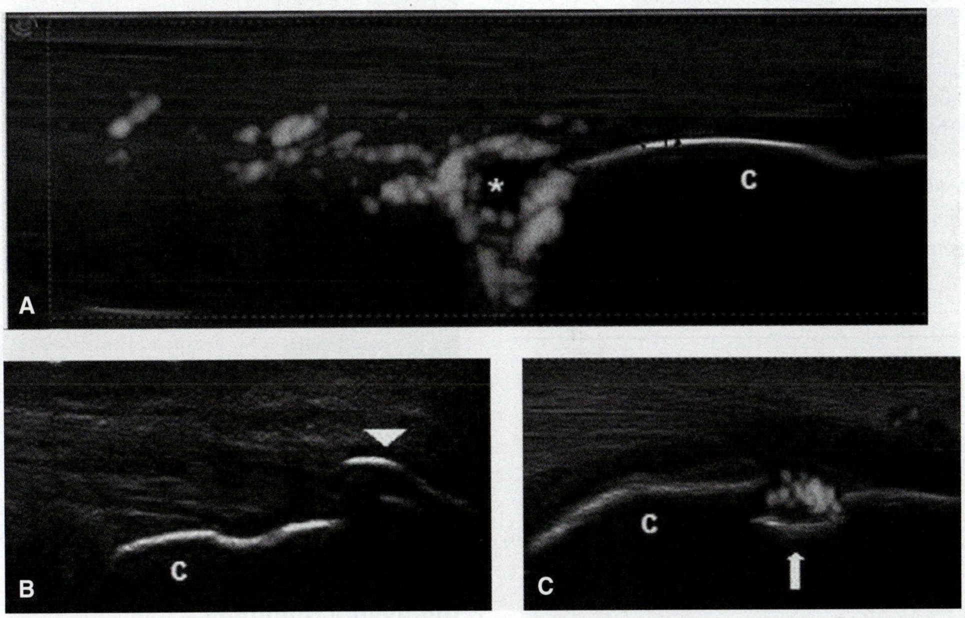

FIGURE 15.18 Longitudinal ultrasound view of patient with spondyloarthropathy. Achilles tendon insertion. **A:** Exudative retrocalcaneal bursitis (*asterisk*) with presence of intense PD signal surrounding the bursa. **B:** Loss of the typical "fibrillar" echotexture of the tendon associated with a large enthesophyte (*arrowhead*) generating acoustic shadow. **C:** Presence of large calcaneal erosion with presence of PD signal (*arrow*). c, calcaneus bone. (From Daftary A, Adler RS. Sonographic evaluation and ultrasound-guided therapy of the Achilles tendon. *Ultrasound Q* 2009;25(3):103–110.)

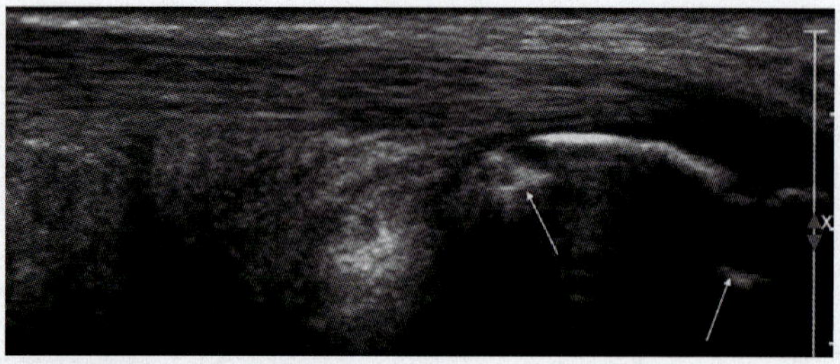

FIGURE 15.19 Inflammatory enthesitis. Longitudinal sonographic image demonstrates insertional erosions (*arrows*) in a male patient with suspected seronegative arthritis. (From Daftary A, Adler RS. Sonographic evaluation and ultrasound-guided therapy of the Achilles tendon. *Ultrasound Q* 2009;25(3):103–110.)

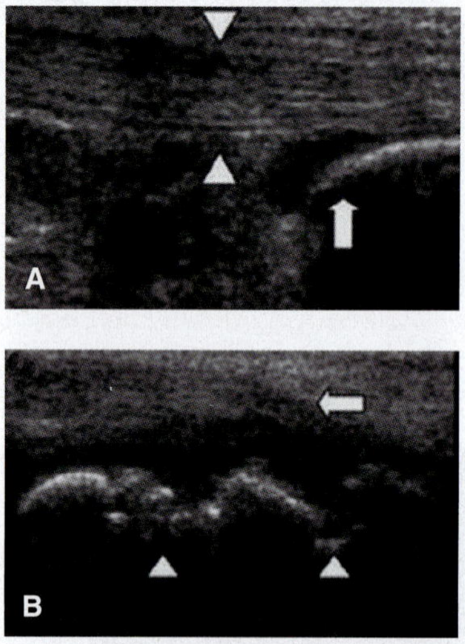

FIGURE 15.20 **A:** Mild retrocalcaneal bursitis (*arrow*) near the insertion of the Achilles tendon (*arrowheads*). **B:** Enthesopathy (*arrowheads*) at the distal insertion of the Achilles tendon (*arrow*). (From Demirkaya E, Ozcakar L, Turker T, et al. Musculoskeletal sonography in juvenile systemic lupus erythematosus. *Arthr Rheum* 2009;61(1):58–60.)

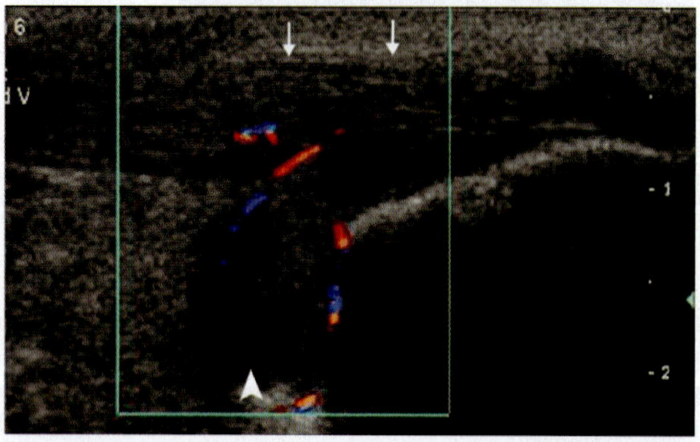

FIGURE 15.21 Longitudinal ultrasound image showing distended retrocalcaneal bursa (*arrowhead*) filled with pannus. Increased flow on color Doppler sonography is present both in the bursa and in the adjacent Achilles tendon (*arrows*). Differential diagnosis includes retrocalcaneal bursitis secondary to gout and insertional Achilles tendinosis. (From Ahmed R, Nazarian LN. Overview of musculoskeletal sonography. *Ultrasound Q* 2010;26(1):27–35.)

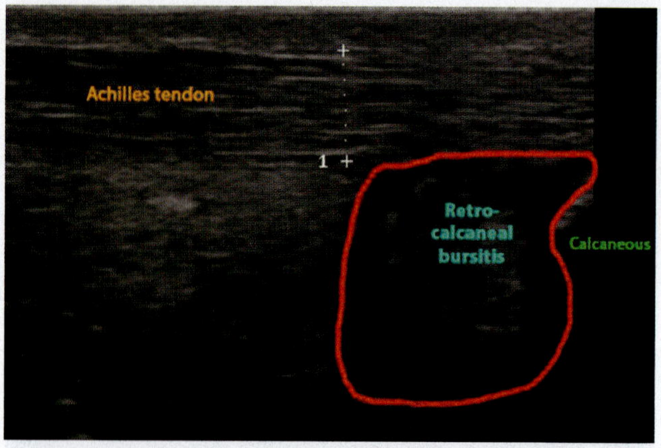

FIGURE 15.22 Longitudinal ultrasound view of the posterior leg demonstrating large retrocalcaneal bursitis.

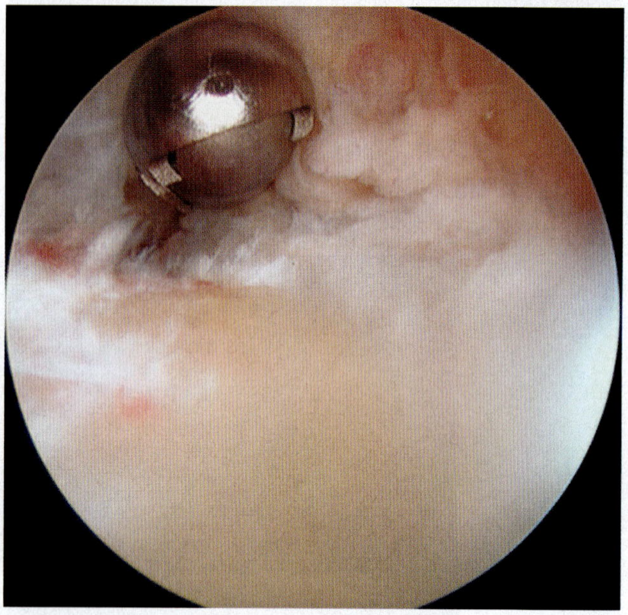

FIGURE 15.23 The shaver is seen in the retrocalcaneal bursa on the superior aspect of the calcaneus. (From Sullivan M. Endoscopic resection of Haglund deformity and bursectomy. *Techn Foot Ankle Surg* 2010;9(2):48–51.)

Suggested Readings

Aronow MS. Posterior heel pain (retrocalcaneal bursitis, insertional and noninsertional Achilles tendinopathy). *Clin Podiatr Med Surg* 2005;22(1):19–43.

Hochman MG, Ramappa AJ, Newman JS, et al. Imaging of tendons and bursae. *Imag Arthritis Metab Bone Dis* 2009:196–238.

Lesic A, Bumbasirevic M. Disorders of the Achilles tendon. *Curr Orthop* 2004;18(1):63–75.

Van der Wall H, Lee A, Magee M, et al. Radionuclide bone scintigraphy in sports injuries. *Semin Nucl Med* 2010;40(1):16–30.

Vyce SD, Addis-Thomas E, Mathews EE, et al. Painful prominences of the heel. *Clin Podiatr Med Surg* 2010;27(3):443–462.

Waldman SD. Achilles bursitis. In: *Atlas of Uncommon Pain Syndromes.* 3rd ed. Philadelphia, PA: Saunders; 2011:302–306.

Waldman SD. Achilles bursa injection. In: *Atlas of Pain Management Injection Techniques.* 3rd ed. Philadelphia, PA: Saunders; 2012:443–445.

CHAPTER 16

Plantar Fasciitis and Other Abnormalities of the Plantar Fascia

ANATOMIC CONSIDERATIONS

The plantar fascia is made up of thick, longitudinally oriented connective tissue that is tightly attached to the plantar skin (Fig. 16.1). It attaches to the medial calcaneal tuberosity and then runs forward, dividing into five bands, one going to each toe (Fig. 16.2). The plantar fascia provides dynamic support to the arch of the foot, tightening as the foot bears weight.

CLINICAL CORRELATES

Plantar fasciitis is a clinical syndrome characterized by pain and tenderness over the plantar surface of the calcaneus made immediately worse by dorsiflexion of the toes. Occurring twice as often in women, plantar fasciitis is thought to be caused by an inflammation of the plantar fascia. Inflammation of the plantar fascia can occur alone or be part of a systemic inflammatory condition, such as rheumatoid arthritis, Reiter syndrome, or gout. Obesity also seems to predispose to the development of plantar fasciitis, as does going barefoot or wearing house slippers for prolonged periods. High-impact aerobic exercise also has been implicated.

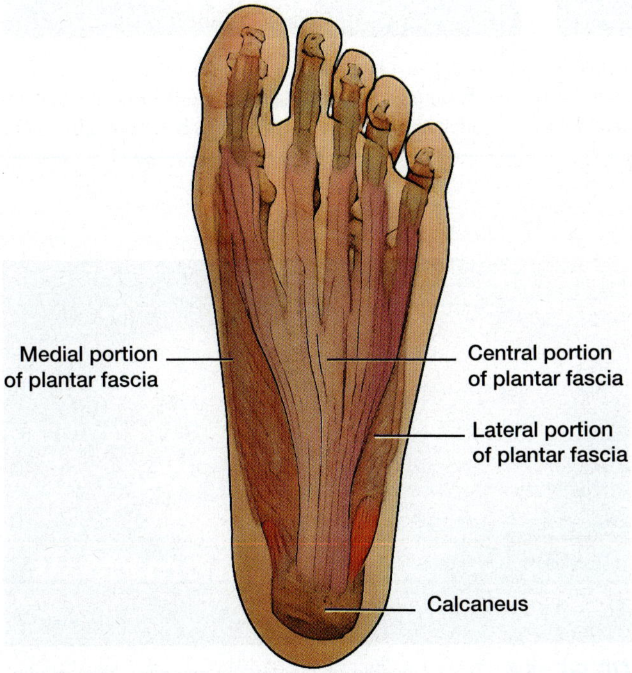

FIGURE 16.1 The anatomy of the plantar fascia.

Pain on palpation of the insertion of the plantar fascia on the plantar medial calcaneal tuberosity is a consistent finding in patients with plantar fasciitis as is exacerbation of pain with active resisted dorsiflexion of the toes. Patients suffering from plantar fasciitis will also exhibit pain on deep palpation of the plantar fascia, especially when the toes are dorsiflexed pulling the plantar fascia taunt. The pain of plantar fasciitis is most severe on taking the first few steps after having not borne weight and is made worse by prolonged standing or walking.

Plantar fibromatosis, which is also known as Ledderhose disease, is a common cause of heel and foot pain and functional disability (Fig. 16.3). It is caused by a progressive fibrosis of the plantar fascia and was first described by Dr. George Ledderhose in 1894. Early symptoms of plantar fibrosis are tender fibrotic nodules along the course of the plantar fascia with the initial nodules first appearing at the medial aspect of the arch of the foot (Figs. 16.4 and 16.5). Frequently, the painful, fibrotic nodules of the plantar surface that are seen early in the course of the disease are misdiagnosed as plantar warts, corns, or ganglion cysts (Fig 16.6).

As the disease progresses, these isolated nodules begin to coalesce. Untreated, flexion contractures of the toes in a manner analogous to Dupuytrens contraction will develop. The pain of plantar fibrosis tends to burn itself as the disease progresses.

The exact cause of Dupuytren contracture remains unknown although the disease seems to have a genetic basis with an autosomal dominant inheritance pattern with variable penetrance. A biochemical pathogenesis has been hypothesized which suggests that excess deposition of Type I collagen combined with abnormal myofibroblast formation and increased levels of beta-catenin are responsible for the disease. Dupytren contraction occurs with increased frequency in individuals of European descent with a gender predilection approaching ten males for every female affected. The disease rarely occurs before the fourth decade. Diabetes, smoking, cirrhosis of the liver, chronic barbiturate use, trauma to the palmar fascia, and alcoholism are risk factors.

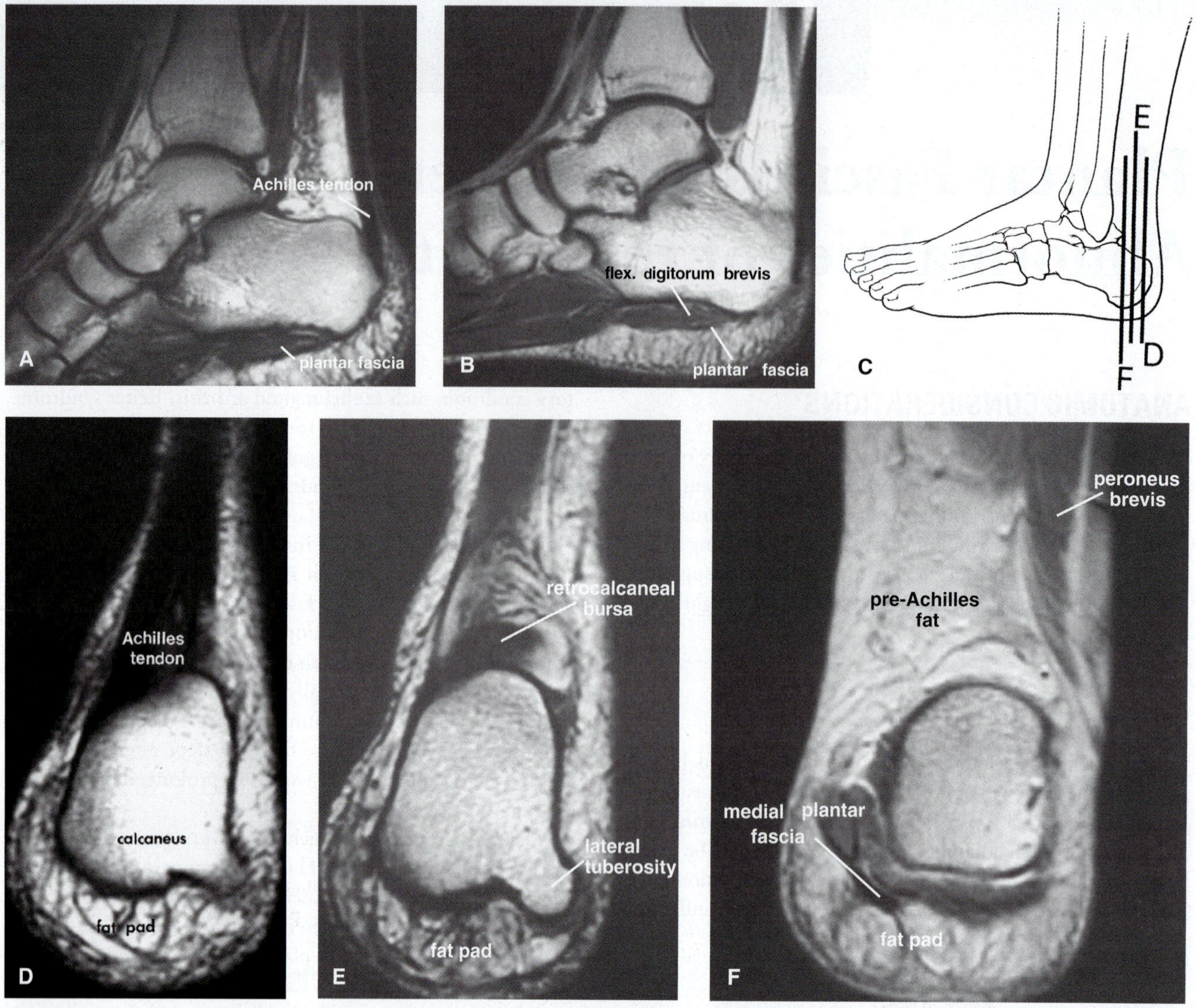

FIGURE 16.2 Normal MR images of the heel. **A,B:** Sagittal MR images demonstrating the heel pad, plantar fascia, and Achilles tendon insertion. **C:** Coronal illustration localizing coronal images. **D:** Coronal image at the Achilles insertion. **E:** Coronal image just anterior to the Achilles tendon. **F:** Coronal image through the calcaneus. (From Berquist TH. *Imaging of the Foot and Ankle*. Philadelphia, PA: Lippincott Williams & Wilkins; 2011:171.)

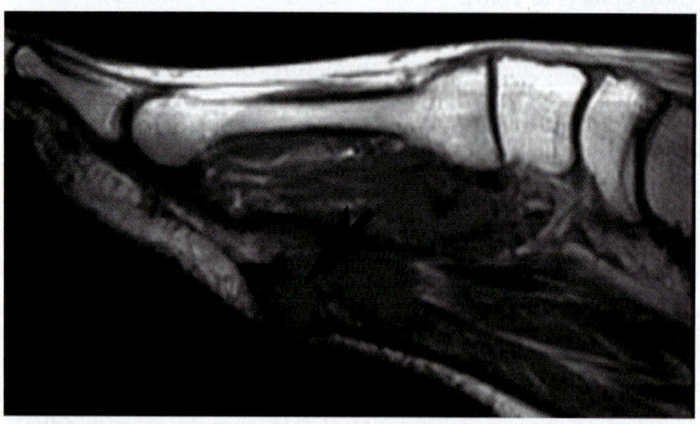

FIGURE 16.3 Plantar fibromatosis. Sagittal T1-weighted image demonstrating a focal nodule (*arrow*) of muscle density in the plantar fascia at the level of the junction of the first metatarsal shaft and neck. (From Berquist TH. *Imaging of the Foot and Ankle*. Philadelphia, PA: Lippincott Williams & Wilkins; 2011:177.)

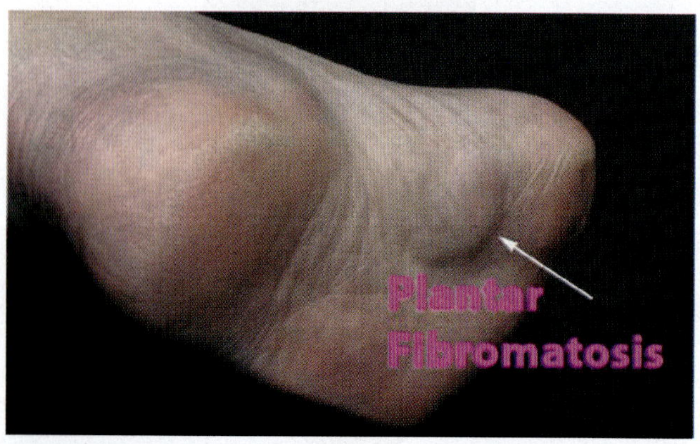

FIGURE 16.4 Typical nodule of plantar fibromatosis. Note medial location.

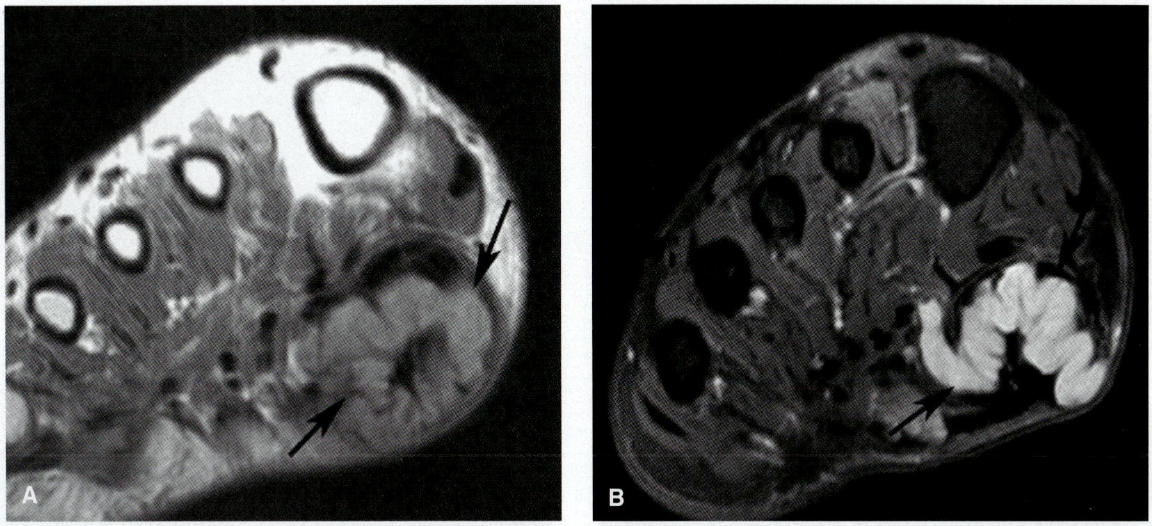

FIGURE 16.5 Plantar fibromatosis. Axial T1-weighted **(A)** and postcontrast fat-suppressed T1-weighted **(B)** images demonstrate a large enhancing mass with displacement of the flexor tendons located beneath the first metatarsal. (From Berquist TH. *Imaging of the Foot and Ankle*. Philadelphia, PA: Lippincott Williams & Wilkins; 2011:177.)

Plain radiographs are indicated in all patients who present with heel and foot pain (Fig. 16.7). Based on the patient's clinical presentation, additional testing may be indicated, including complete blood cell count, sedimentation rate, and antinuclear antibody testing. MRI and/or ultrasound imaging of the ankle is indicated if plantar fasciitis, rupture, or joint instability is suggested or the diagnosis is in question (Figs. 16.8 to 16.15). Radionuclide scanning is useful to identify stress fractures of the calcaneus and foot not seen on plain radiographs and may aid in the diagnosis of plantar fasciitis as there may be increased uptake of radionucleotide at the insertion of the plantar fascia at the calcaneus (Fig. 16.16).

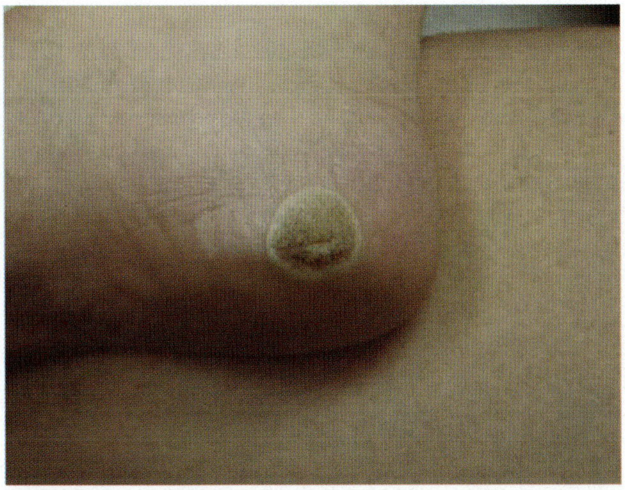

FIGURE 16.6 Frequently, the painful, fibrotic nodules of the plantar surface that are seen early in the course of the disease are misdiagnosed as plantar warts, corns, or ganglion cysts. (From Sanders MJ, De Ybarrondo LE. Foot rashes and lumps. In: Chung EK, ed. *Visual Diagnosis and Treatment in Pediatrics*. 3rd ed. Philadelphia, PA: Lippincott Williams & Wilkins; 2015:410. Courtesy of Denise W. Metry, MD.)

ULTRASOUND TECHNIQUE

To perform ultrasound evaluation of the plantar fascia, the patient is placed in the prone position with the patient's ankle hanging off the edge of the table. With the patient in the above position, a high-frequency linear ultrasound transducer is placed in a longitudinal plane with the inferior portion of the

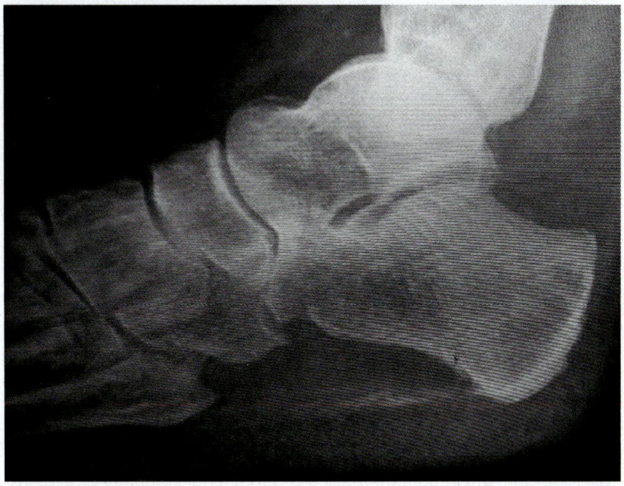

FIGURE 16.7 Stippled calcifications in the plantar fascia seen on a lateral radiograph. (From Monto RR. Platelet-rich plasma and plantar fasciitis. *Sports Med Arthrosc* 2013;21(4):220–224.)

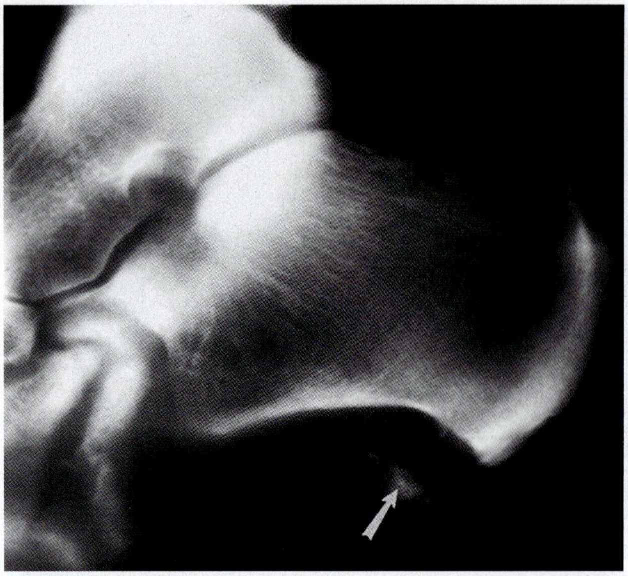

FIGURE 16.8 Lateral radiograph of the calcaneus demonstrates an avulsed osteophyte (*arrow*) in a patient with chronic heel pain with a recent acute exacerbation. (From Berquist TH. *Imaging of the Foot and Ankle*. Philadelphia, PA: Lippincott Williams & Wilkins; 2011:174.)

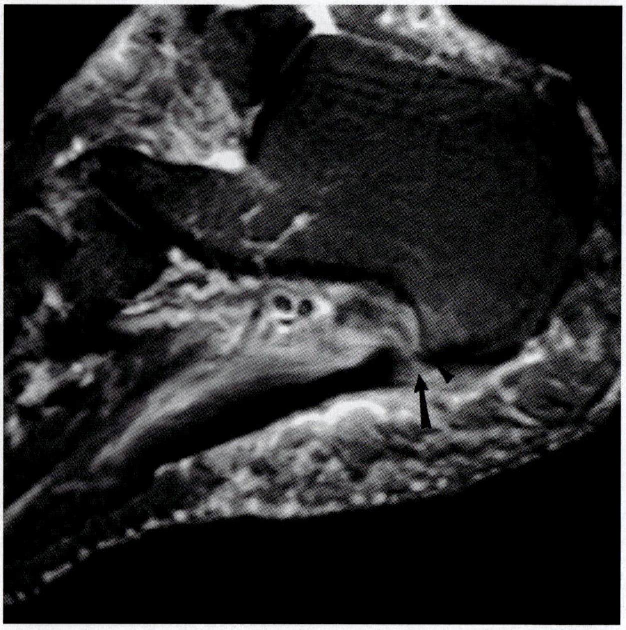

FIGURE 16.10 Sagittal T2-weighted MR image demonstrates thickening of the plantar fascia distal to the complete tear (*arrow*) with high-signal intensity due to complete disruption near the calcaneal attachment. The proximal remnant is partially visualized (*arrowhead*). (From Berquist TH. *Imaging of the Foot and Ankle*. Philadelphia, PA: Lippincott Williams & Wilkins; 2011:177.)

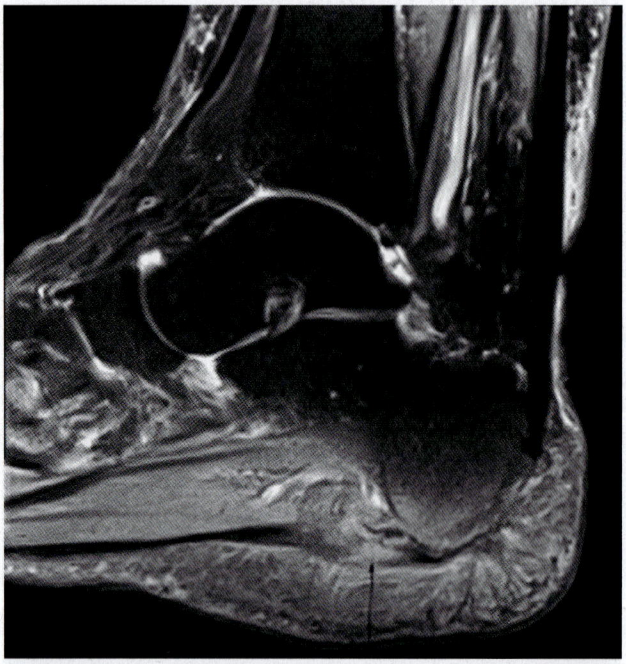

FIGURE 16.9 Partial tear of the plantar fascia near the calcaneal attachment. Sagittal T2-weighted MR image demonstrates thickening of the fascia with a partial tear (*arrow*). (From Berquist TH. *Imaging of the Foot and Ankle*. Philadelphia, PA: Lippincott Williams & Wilkins; 2011:176.)

ultrasound transducer over plantar surface of the foot with the superior end of the transducer centered on the anterior portion of the calcaneus. An ultrasound survey scan is then taken (Fig. 16.17). The calcaneus and linear plantar fascia is identified at its insertion on the calcaneus (Fig. 16.18). When the insertion of the plantar fascia is identified, the insertion is evaluated for tendinopathy and then the plantar fascia is evaluated along its length for tears, rupture, and fibromatosis, and tumors that may produce symptoms that may mimic plantar fasciitis (Figs. 16.19 to 16.34). Recent reports suggest that ultrasound elastography may improve the diagnostic accuracy of plantar fasciitis (Figs. 16.35 and 16.36).

CLINICAL PEARLS

Bursitis and tendinitis of the ankle and foot may coexist with plantar fasciitis and may contribute to the patient's pain symptoms. It should be remembered that there are many diseases that may mimic the symptoms of plantar fasciitis and plantar fibromatosis and the use of multiple imaging modalities will improve the accuracy of diagnosis (Figs. 16.37 to 16.40).

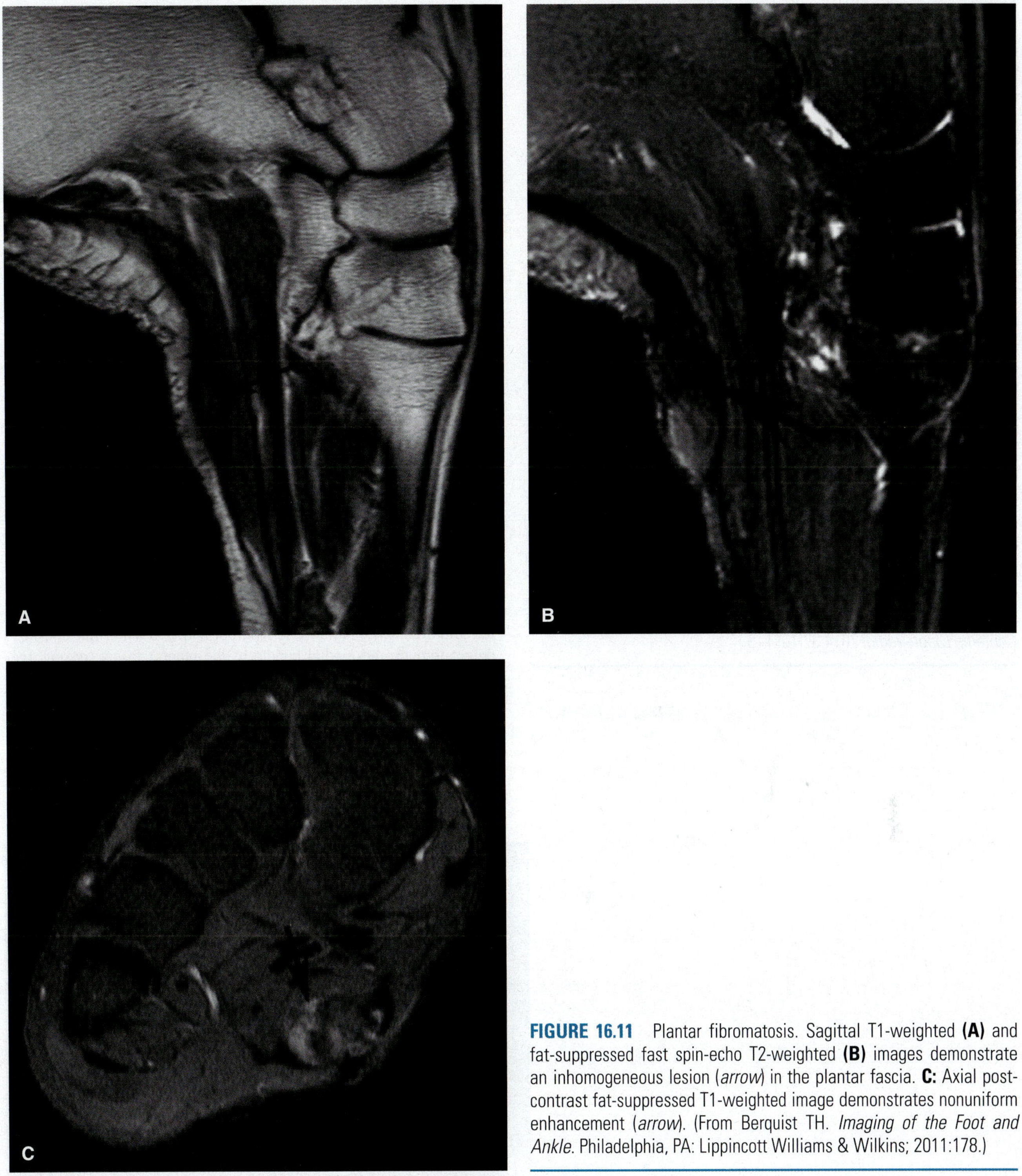

FIGURE 16.11 Plantar fibromatosis. Sagittal T1-weighted **(A)** and fat-suppressed fast spin-echo T2-weighted **(B)** images demonstrate an inhomogeneous lesion (*arrow*) in the plantar fascia. **C:** Axial post-contrast fat-suppressed T1-weighted image demonstrates nonuniform enhancement (*arrow*). (From Berquist TH. *Imaging of the Foot and Ankle*. Philadelphia, PA: Lippincott Williams & Wilkins; 2011:178.)

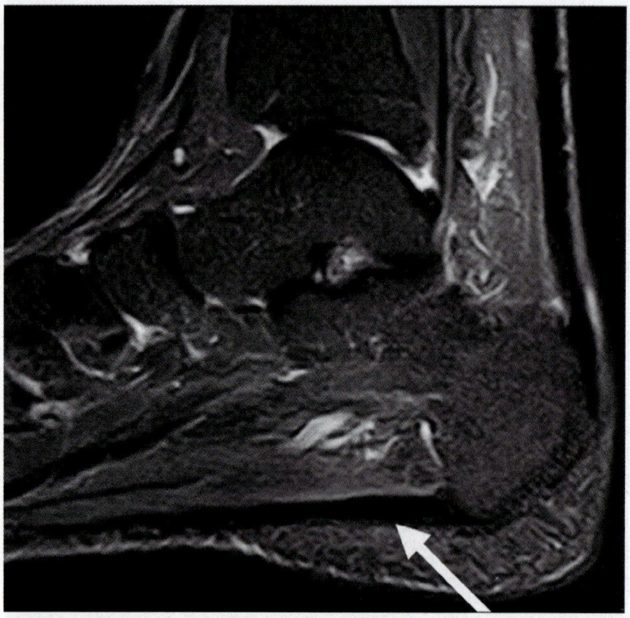

FIGURE 16.12 Plantar fasciitis. A 28-year-old runner presented with localized tenderness over the anteromedial aspect of the calcaneus, which was worse in the morning after arising from sleep. This sagittal STIR MR image shows thickening of the plantar fascia, measuring up to 7 mm proximally (*arrow*), representing plantar fasciitis. (From Verma S, Feldman J, Mohsen N. MR imaging for evaluation of plantar pain. *Contemp Diagn Radiol* 2014;37(10):1–5.)

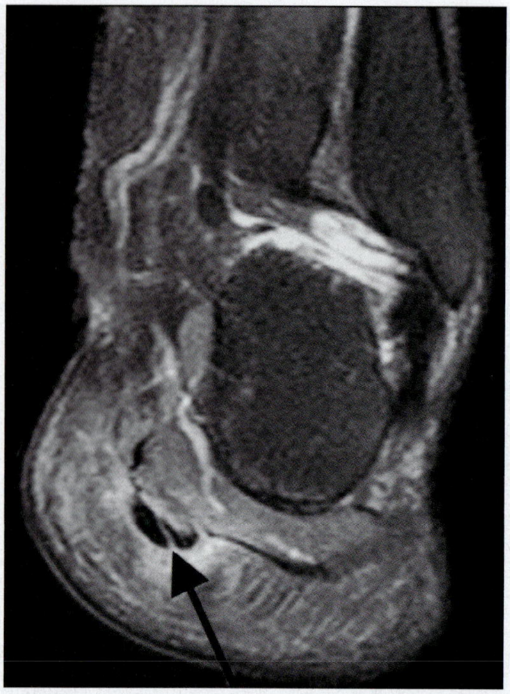

FIGURE 16.13 Plantar fascial rupture. A 22-year-old male professional basketball player presented with severe medial plantar heel pain after rebounding. This coronal, proton density, T2-weighted, fat-saturated MR image of the hindfoot shows a linear full-thickness defect through the medial bundle of the plantar fascia (*arrow*), representing a fascial rupture with associated soft tissue edema. (From Verma S, Feldman J, Mohsen N. MR imaging for evaluation of plantar pain. *Contemp Diagn Radiol* 2014;37(10):1–5.)

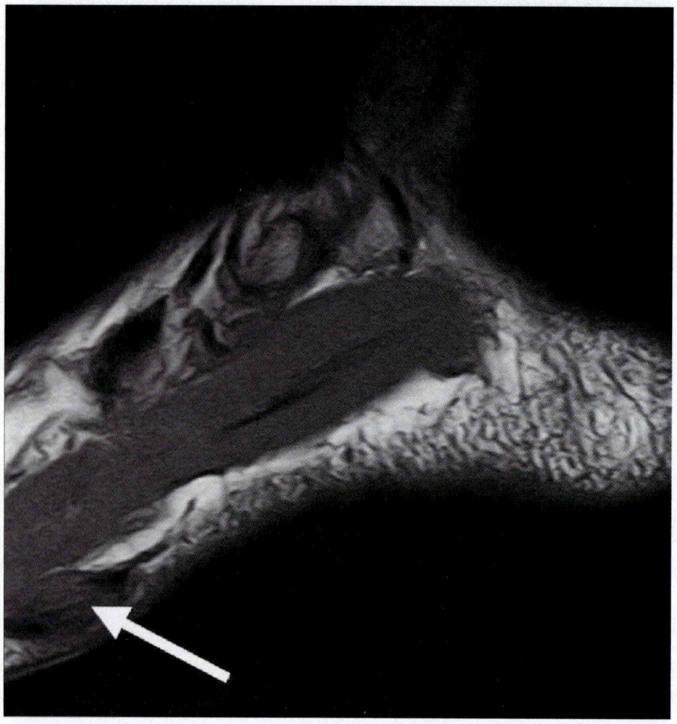

FIGURE 16.14 Plantar fibromatosis. A 19-year-old man presented with a mildly painful soft tissue mass along the plantar aspect of his midfoot medially. This sagittal, T1-weighted MR image of the midfoot shows an ovoid, soft tissue mass within the plantar fascia along the base of the first metatarsal (*arrow*), which is isointense to muscle, representing a fibrous nodule of plantar fibromatosis. (From Verma S, Feldman J, Mohsen N. MR imaging for evaluation of plantar pain. *Contemp Diagn Radiol* 2014;37(10):1–5.)

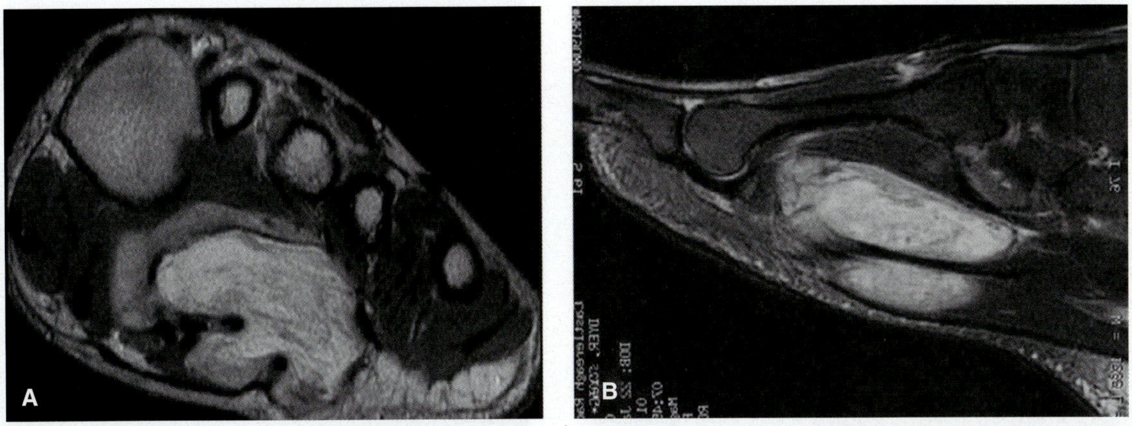

FIGURE 16.15 Synovial sarcoma. Coronal PD **(A)** and sagittal fat-suppressed T2 MR images **(B)** showing a large, deep, soft tissue mass in the plantar aspect of the foot in a 26-year-old man. It involves the flexor digitorum brevis and longus muscles and wraps around and between the tendons, penetrating into subcutaneous fat. It is T2-bright but heterogeneous. (From Schatz J, Soper J, McCormack S, et al. Imaging of tumors in the ankle and foot. *Top Magn Reson Imaging* 2010;21(1):37–50.)

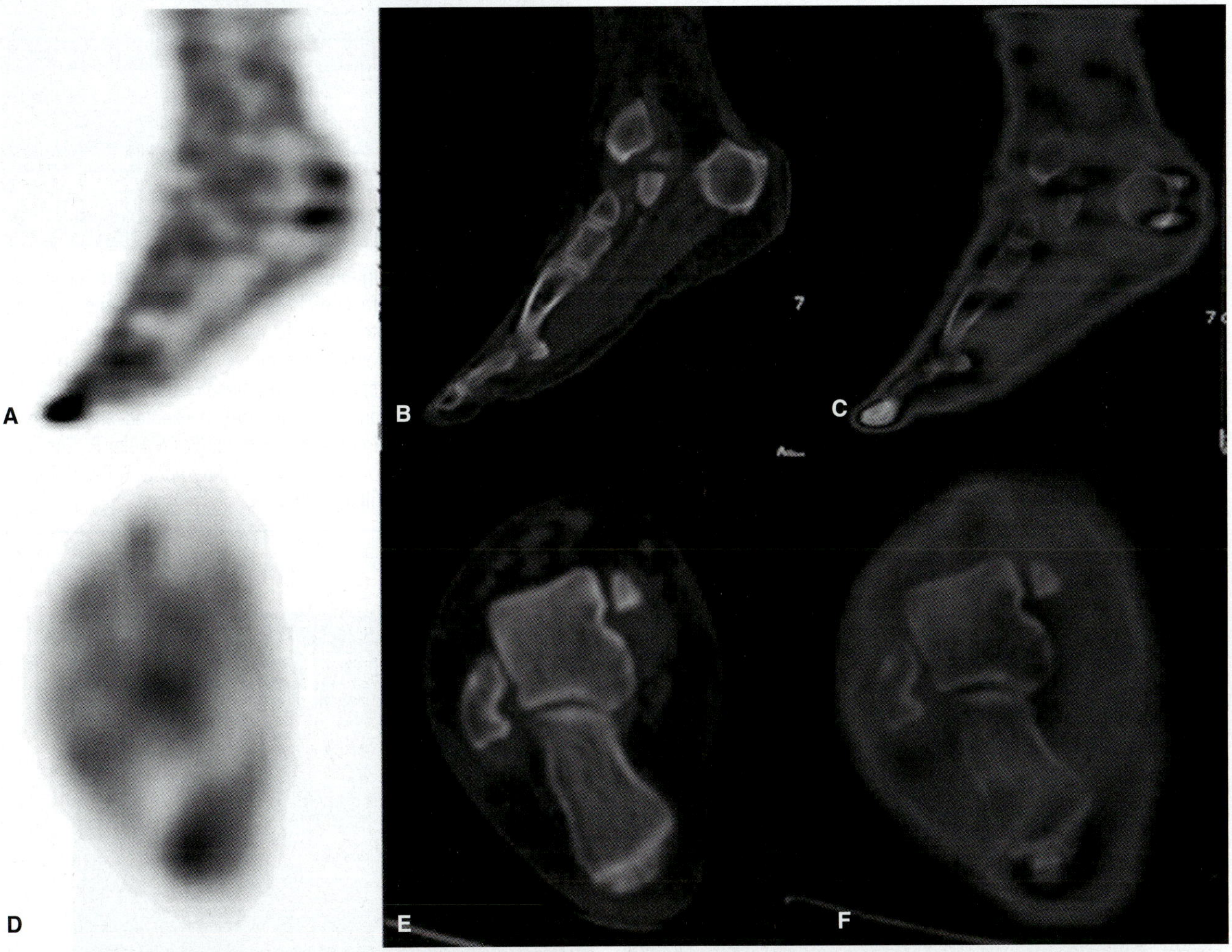

FIGURE 16.16 Sagittal SPECT **(A)**, CT **(B)**, and fused SPECT/CT **(C)** images showing moderate uptake associated with both the posterosuperior and plantar aspects of the calcaneus with associated structural changes. Axial SPECT **(D)**, CT **(E)**, and fused SPECT/CT **(F)** images showing enthesopathic changes at the posterosuperior aspect of the calcaneus, suggestive of Achilles tendinitis. Uptake at the inferior aspect of the calcaneus is suggestive of plantar fasciitis. SPECT/CT, single-photon emission computed tomography/computed tomography. (From Nathan M, Mohan H, Vijayanathan S, et al. The role of 99mTc-diphosphonate bone SPECT/CT in the ankle and foot. *Nuclear Med Comm* 2012;33(8):799–807.)

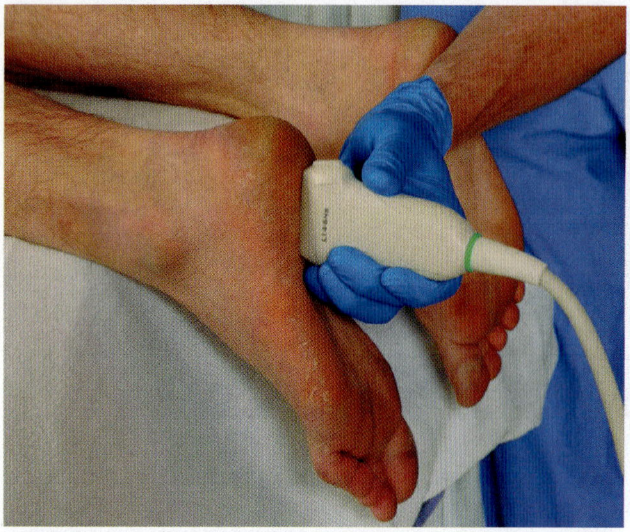

FIGURE 16.17 Proper longitudinal ultrasound transducer placement for ultrasound evaluation of the plantar fascia.

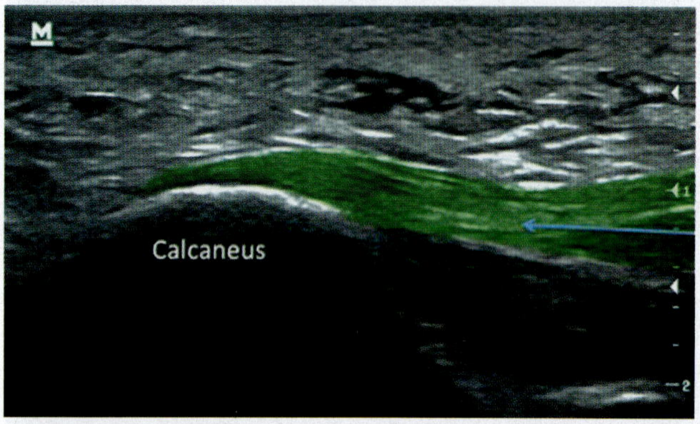

FIGURE 16.18 Longitudinal view of the plantar fascia (*green band*) and its calcaneal insertion.

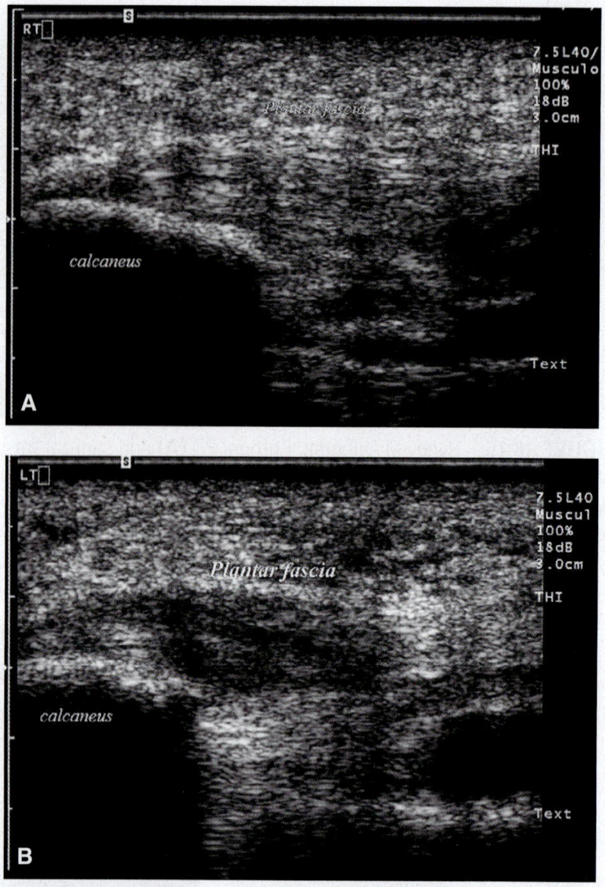

FIGURE 16.20 **A:** Longitudinal image of the plantar fascia demonstrates mild plantar fasciitis. There is thickening and decreased echogenicity of the plantar fascia at calcaneus. Normally, the plantar fascia should measure less than 4 mm at the calcaneal origin. Note the presence of a small spur along the base of the calcaneus. **B:** Longitudinal ultrasound image demonstrates thickening and decreased echogenicity of the proximal plantar fascia. (From Adler R, Sofka CM, Positano RG. *Atlas of Foot and Ankle Sonography.* Philadelphia, PA: Lippincott Williams & Wilkins; 2004:88.)

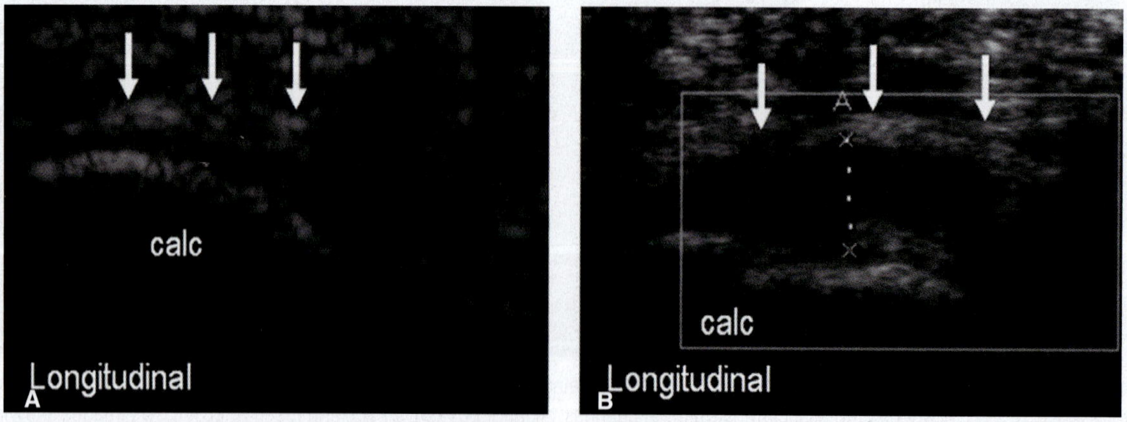

FIGURE 16.19 Longitudinal ultrasound image of normal plantar fascia (*arrows* in **A**) and plantar fasciitis **(B)**, demonstrating a thickened hypoechoic plantar fascia (*arrows*) inserting into the calcaneus (*calc*). (From Chew K, Stevens KJ, Wang T-G, et al. Introduction to diagnostic musculoskeletal ultrasound: part 2: examination of the lower limb. *Am J Phys Med Rehabil* 2008;87(3):238–248.)

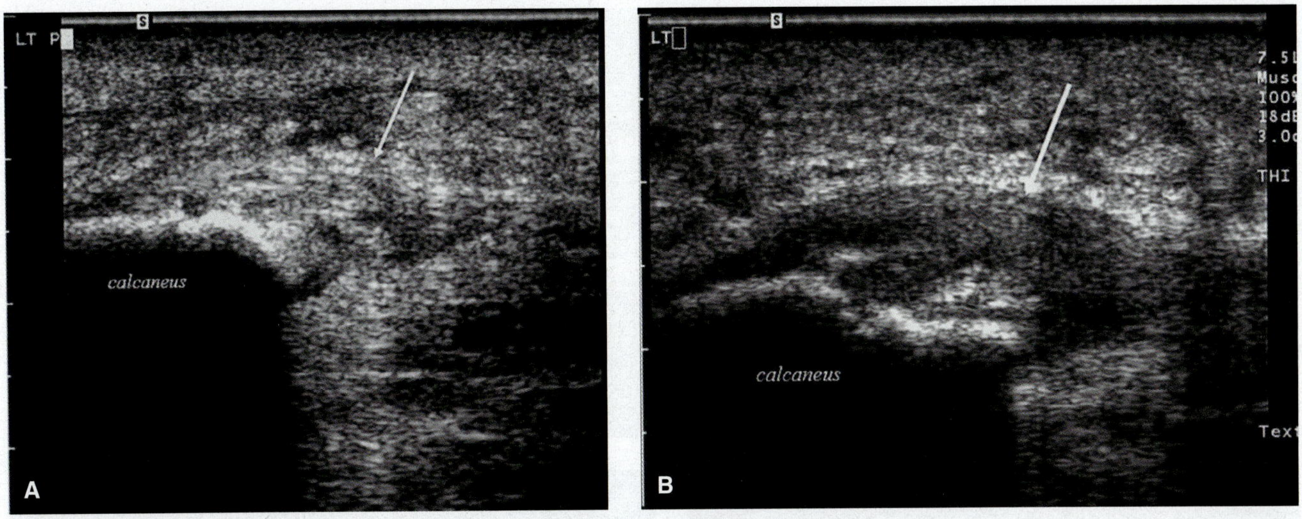

FIGURE 16.21 **A:** Longitudinal ultrasound image demonstrates thickening and deep surface fissures (*arrow*). Note the presence of mild reactive edema in the overlying fat pad. **B:** In this case the plantar fascia is markedly enlarged and diffusely hypoechoic with remodeling of the calcaneus (*arrow*). (From Adler R, Sofka CM, Positano RG. *Atlas of Foot and Ankle Sonography*. Philadelphia, PA: Lippincott Williams & Wilkins; 2004:89.)

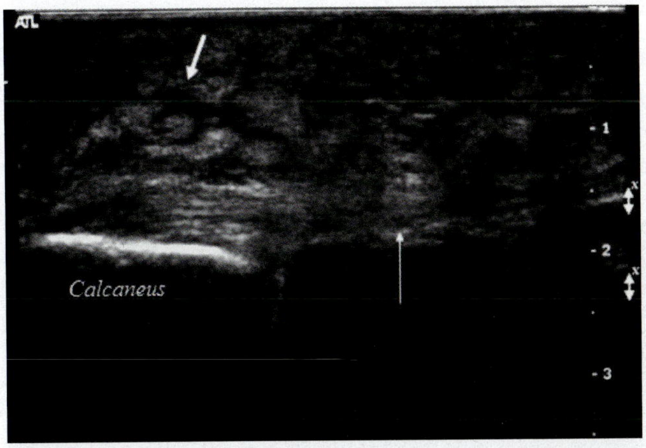

FIGURE 16.22 Edema in the fat pad overlying the plantar fascia often presents as a concomitant finding seen in association with plantar fasciitis. In this case, there is striking edema (*thick arrow*) in the fat pad overlying the abnormal plantar fascia (*thin arrow*). (From Adler R, Sofka CM, Positano RG. *Atlas of Foot and Ankle Sonography*. Philadelphia, PA: Lippincott Williams & Wilkins; 2004:90.)

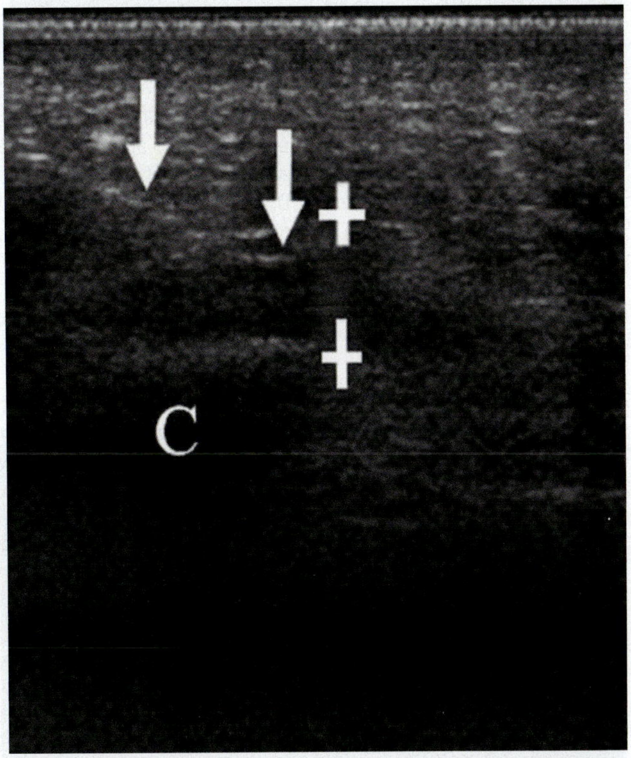

FIGURE 16.23 Longitudinal ultrasound image of the proximal plantar fascia. The target lies on the line of comet-tail effect passing through the inflamed proximal plantar fascia (between the two *crosses*). *C* indicates the calcaneus. *Arrows* indicate needle entry. (From Chen CM, Chen JS, Tsai WC, et al. Effectiveness of device-assisted ultrasound-guided steroid injection for treating plantar fasciitis. *Am J Phys Med Rehabil* 2013;92(7):597–605.)

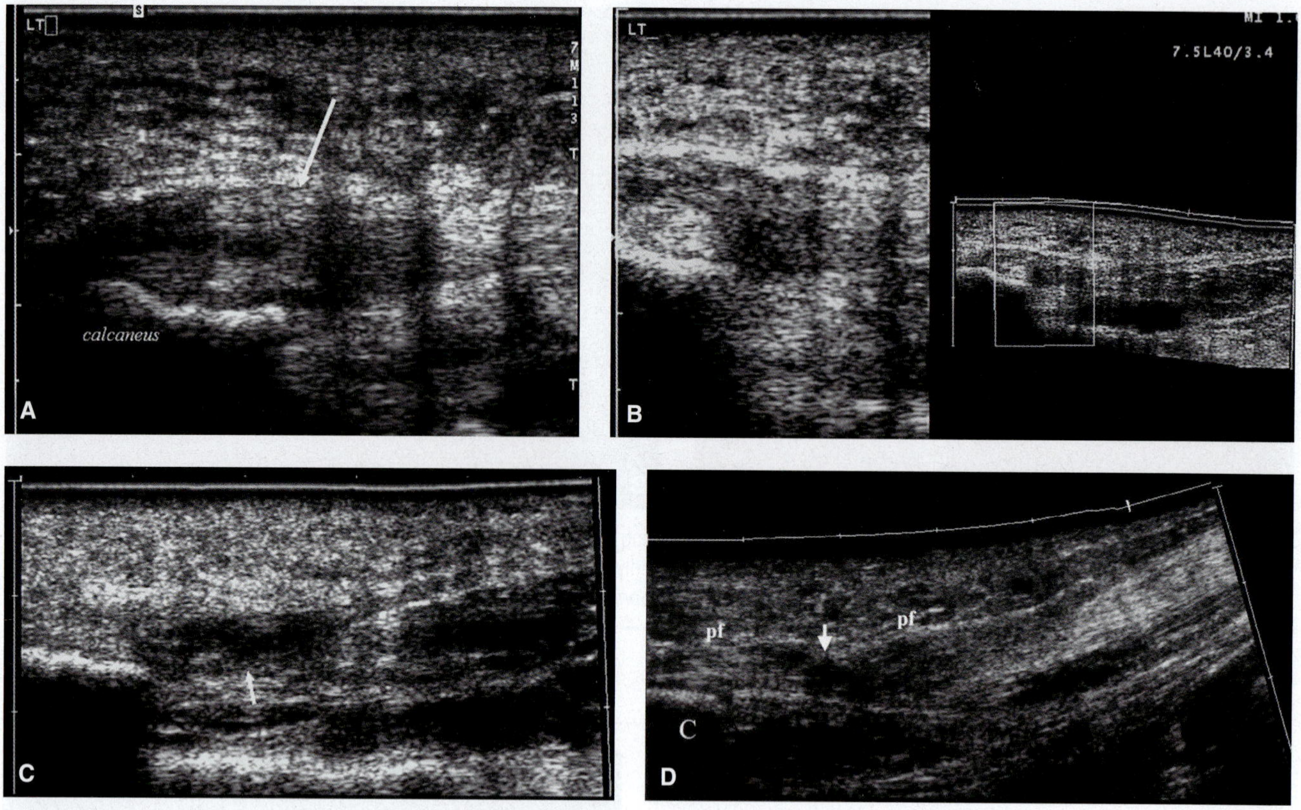

FIGURE 16.24 Tears of the plantar fascia. These may occur in association with plantar fasciitis, as a result of trauma or iatrogenically, through a misplaced cortisone injection. **A:** In this patient with plantar fasciitis, a well-marginated hypoechoic split is seen within the fascia, representing an intrasubstance tear. **B:** More commonly, tears appear as discretely marginated defects along the deep surface of the plantar fascia, near the calcaneal margin. **C:** This patient is a professional dancer who experienced sudden onset of plantar pain during rehearsal. A partial-thickness deep surface tear is present (*arrow*). **D:** Longitudinal extended-field-of-view image in a patient with heel pain and difficulty walking following a blind cortisone injection. There is complete rupture of the plantar fascia (*arrow*). Blind cortisone injections can result in intrafascial deposition and have been associated with plantar fascia rupture. C, calcaneus. (From Adler R, Sofka CM, Positano RG. *Atlas of Foot and Ankle Sonography*. Philadelphia, PA: Lippincott Williams & Wilkins; 2004:91–92.)

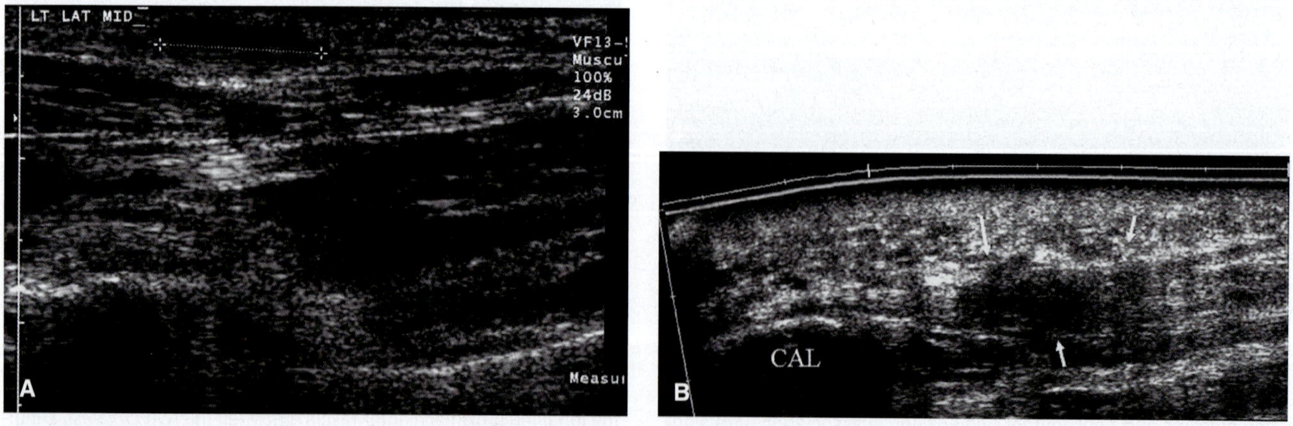

FIGURE 16.25 **A:** Plantar fibromas present as hard palpable nodules along the plantar aspect of the foot and distal to the origin of the plantar fascia (usually >2 to 3 cm). Sonographically, these appear as hypoechoic nodules oriented along the fascial axis and often arising from the superficial margin. **B:** This longitudinal extended-field-of-view image at the level of the midfoot demonstrates fusiform dilation of the plantar fascia, with replacement of the normally thin hyperechoic plantar fascia fibers with a hypoechoic heterogeneous mass, consistent with a plantar fibroma. Note that the origin of the plantar fascia is normal. (From Adler R, Sofka CM, Positano RG. *Atlas of Foot and Ankle Sonography*. Philadelphia, PA: Lippincott Williams & Wilkins; 2004:93.)

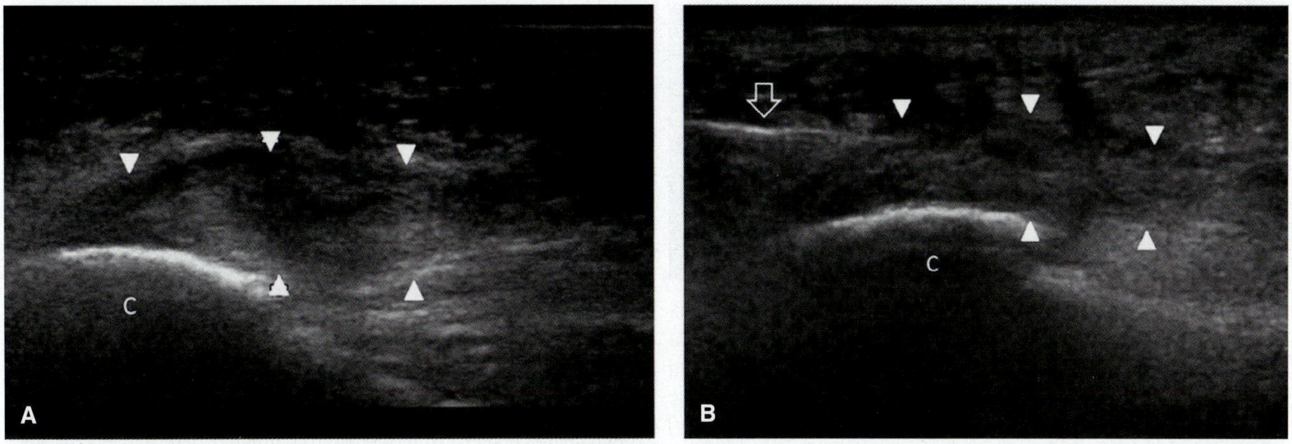

FIGURE 16.26 Ultrasound-guided corticosteroid injection of the proximal plantar fasciitis by posterior approach in the long-axis view. **A:** Thickening of the plantar fascia greater than 4 to 5 mm with decreased echogenicity at its insertion to the calcaneal tuberosity is the typical feature of the proximal plantar fasciitis. **B:** Administration of corticosteroid by posterior approach. *Solid arrowheads,* plantar fascia; *blank arrow,* injection needle; *c,* calcaneus. (From Chen CK, Lew HL, Chu NC. Ultrasound-guided diagnosis and treatment of plantar fasciitis. *Am J Phys Med Rehabil* 2012;91(2):182–184.)

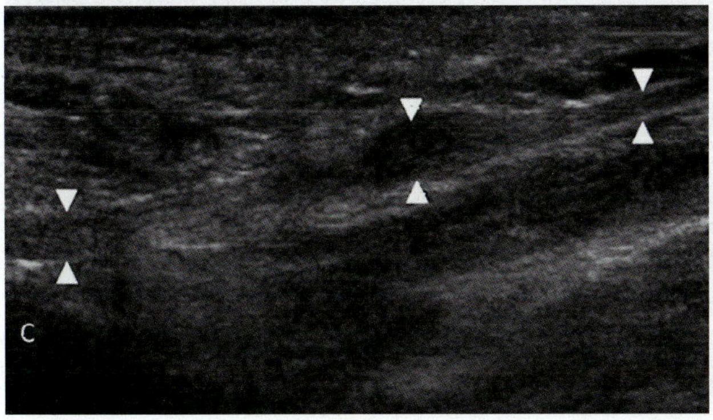

FIGURE 16.27 In the long-axis ultrasound view, the plantar fasciitis is observed far anterior to the calcaneus. (From Chen CK, Lew HL, Chu NC. Ultrasound-guided diagnosis and treatment of plantar fasciitis. *Am J Phys Med Rehabil* 2012;91(2):182–184.)

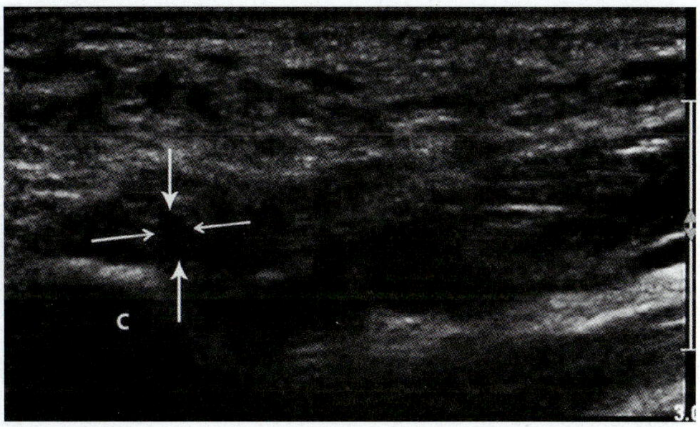

FIGURE 16.29 Left plantar fascia. The darker, or more hypoechoic, focus represents a small insertional plantar fascia tear. *c,* calcaneus. (From Louwers MJ, Sabb B, Pangilinan PH. Ultrasound evaluation of a spontaneous plantar fascia rupture. *Am J Phys Med Rehabil* 2010;89(11):941–944.)

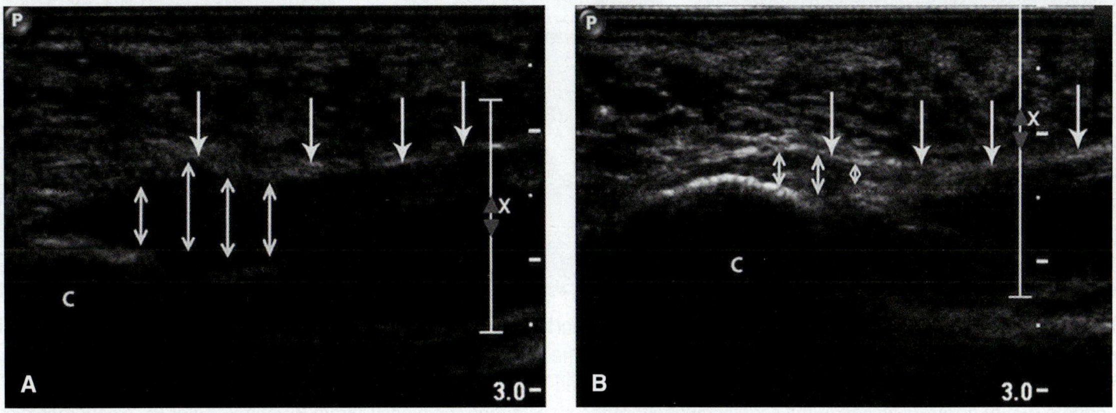

FIGURE 16.28 **A:** Left plantar fascia. Note the thickening (more than 4 mm) and hypoechogenicity of the plantar fascia. **B:** Right plantar fascia. Note the normal thin and homogeneous plantar fascia. *c,* calcaneus. (From Louwers MJ, Sabb B, Pangilinan PH. Ultrasound evaluation of a spontaneous plantar fascia rupture. *Am J Phys Med Rehabil* 2010;89(11):941–944; Fig. 1A,B.)

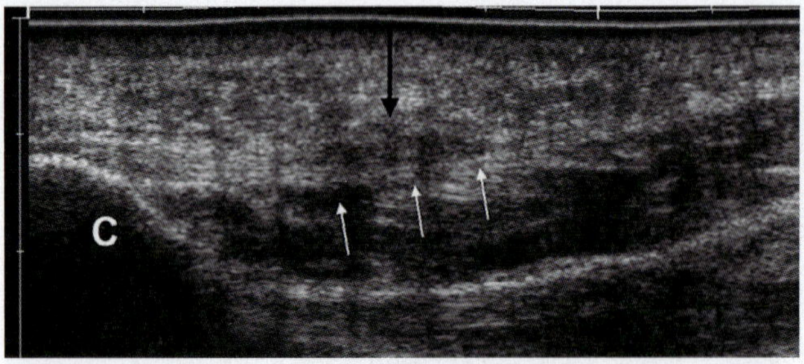

FIGURE 16.30 Superficial fibromatosis. A longitudinal gray scale image of the plantar foot shows a subcutaneous hypoechoic nodule (*black arrow*) within the plantar fascia (*white arrows*), separate from the calcaneal insertion (c). (From Hwang S, Adler RS. Sonographic evaluation of the musculoskeletal soft tissue masses. *Ultrasound Q* 2005;21(4):259–270.)

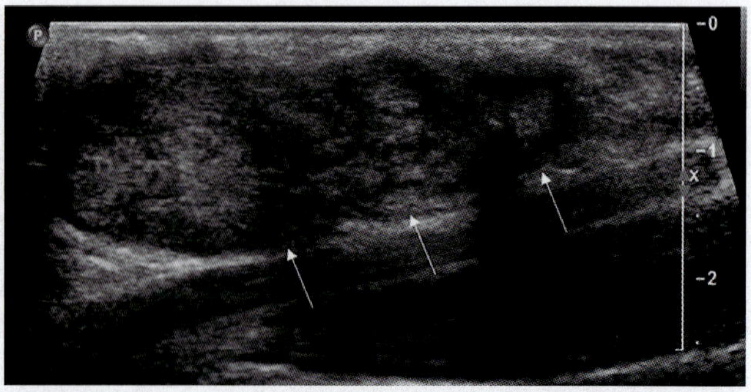

FIGURE 16.31 Superficial fibromatosis. A longitudinal gray scale image of a foot demonstrates multiple plantar nodules (*white arrows*) becoming confluent along plantar aspect. The patient had both plantar and palmar nodules with Dupuytren contracture. (From Hwang S, Adler RS. Sonographic evaluation of the musculoskeletal soft tissue masses. *Ultrasound Q* 2005;21(4):259–270.)

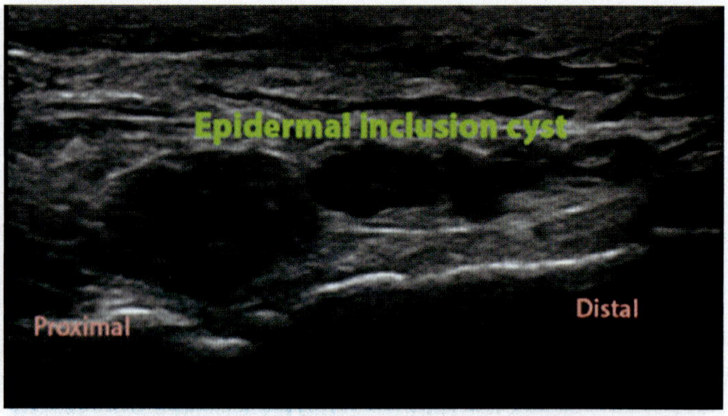

FIGURE 16.32 Longitudinal ultrasound image of the plantar surface demonstrating an epidermoid inclusion cyst.

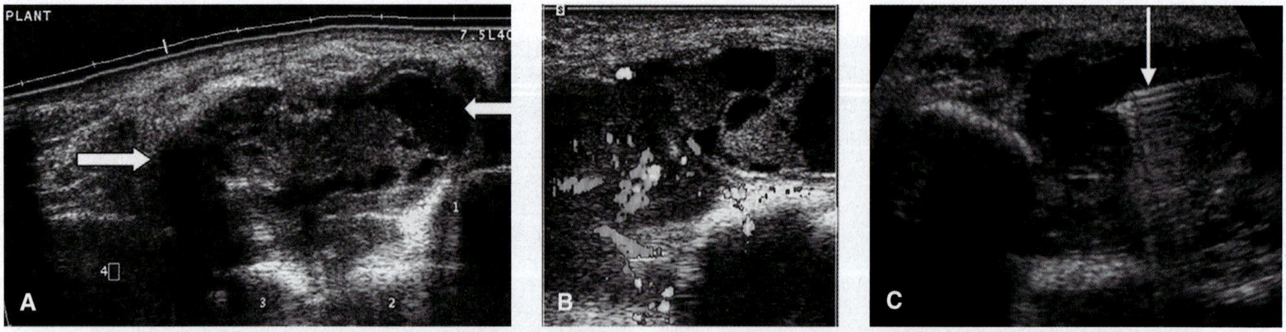

FIGURE 16.33 Synovial sarcoma. Patient with a history of excised Morton neuroma, underwent a sonographically guided biopsy of a recurrent mass in a plantar aspect of the foot. **A:** A coronal gray scale image of the plantar aspect of the foot demonstrates a complex solid mass (*arrows*) with mixed echogenicity with cystic areas. The metatarsals are numbered 1 to 4. **B:** On power Doppler, the mass demonstrates increased vascular flow. **C:** A needle (*white arrow*) is placed in the solid component of the mass during the biopsy. (From Hwang S, Adler RS. Sonographic evaluation of the musculoskeletal soft tissue masses. *Ultrasound Q* 2005;21(4):259–270.)

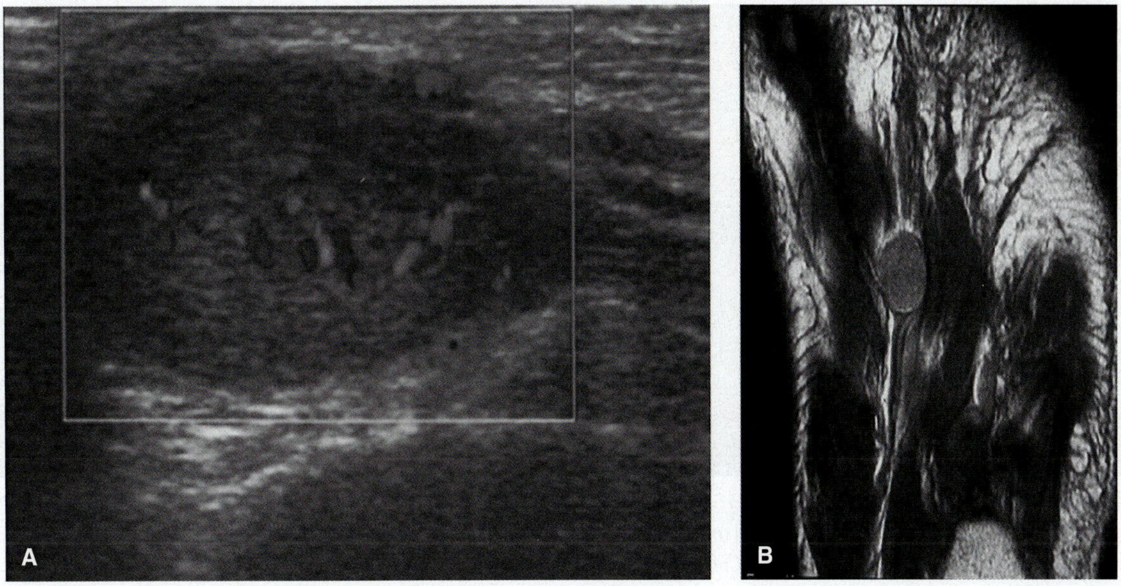

FIGURE 16.34 Schwannoma. **A:** Ultrasound image showing a circumscribed ovoid mass, long axis parallel to the skin surface, vascular on a color Doppler echocardiographic image V features typical but not diagnostic of a schwannoma. **B:** Coronal PD MR image demonstrating the medial plantar nerve passing directly into and exiting from the mass. (From Schatz J, Soper J, McCormack S, et al. Imaging of tumors in the ankle and foot. *Top Magn Reson Imaging* 2010;21(1):37–50.)

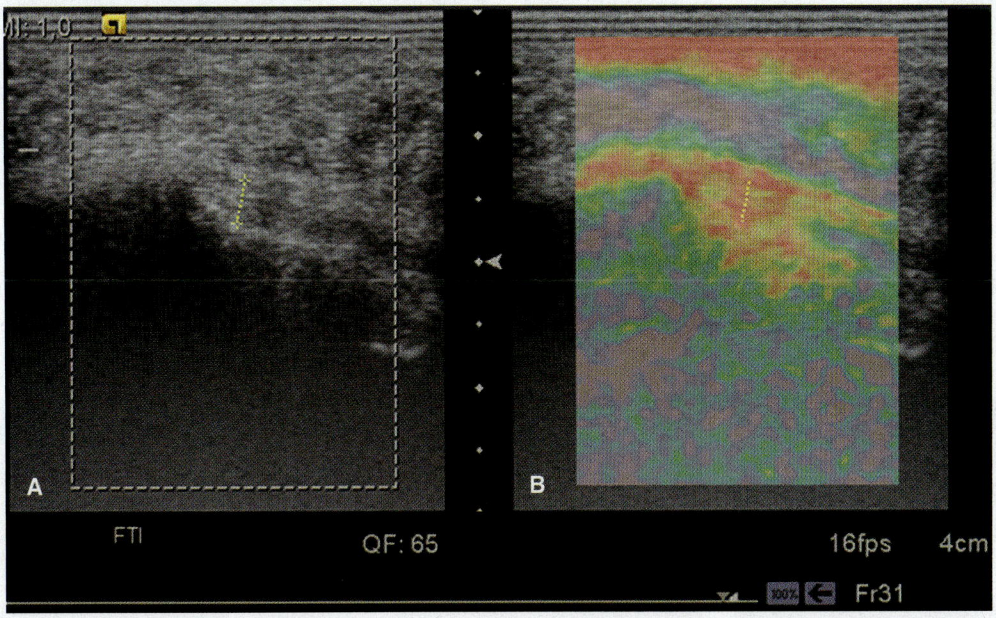

FIGURE 16.35 Ultrasound **(A)** and elastography **(B)** of the normal plantar fascia showing normal homogeneous (*red*) stiffness of plantar fascia. (From Kapoor A, Sandhu HS, Sandhu PS, et al. Realtime elastography in plantar fasciitis comparison with ultrasonography and MRI. *Curr Orthopaed Pract* 2010;21(6):600–608.)

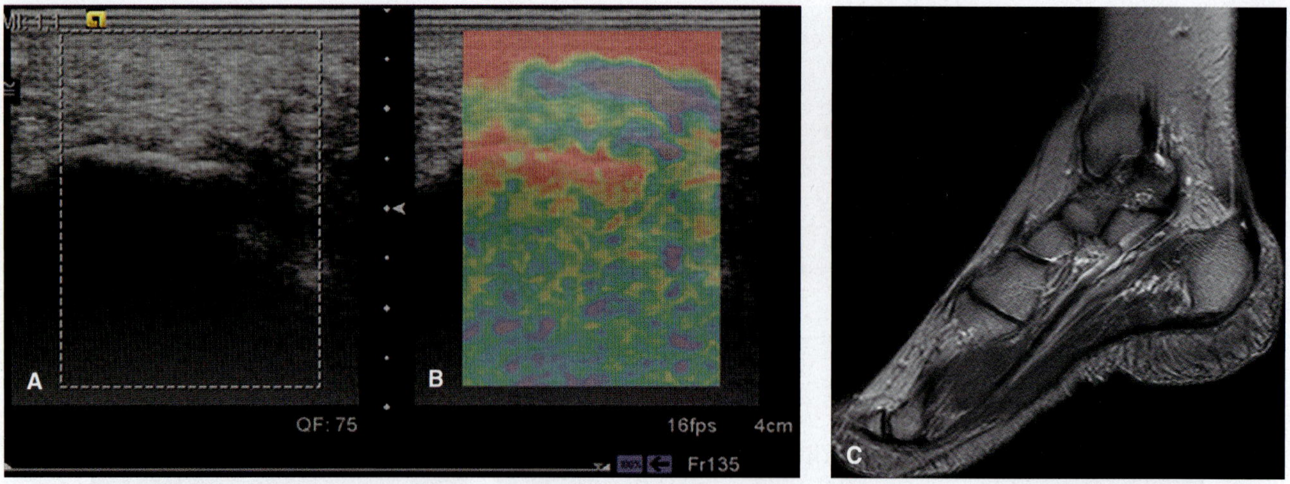

FIGURE 16.36 Ultrasound **(A)** shows normal fascia, while elastography **(B)** shows abnormal changes seen as *blue* in the fascia. **C:** Plain MRI showing abnormal signal change at the calcaneal end of the fascia. (From Kapoor A, Sandhu HS, Sandhu PS, et al. Realtime elastography in plantar fasciitis comparison with ultrasonography and MRI. *Curr Orthopaed Pract* 2010;21(6):600–608.)

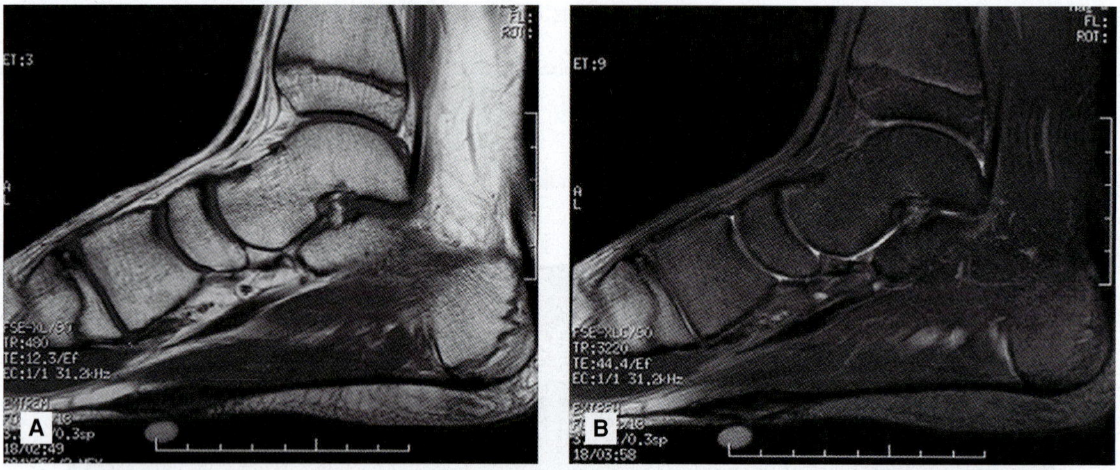

FIGURE 16.37 Plantar fibromatosis. Sagittal T1-weighted **(A)** and fat-suppressed T2-weighted **(B)** MR images showing a fusiform mass in the plantar aponeurosis and extending into subcutaneous fat. It is predominantly low signal, but there is a small area of higher signal deep into its plantar surface. (From Schatz J, Soper J, McCormack S, et al. Imaging of tumors in the ankle and foot. *Topics Magn Reson Imaging* 2010;21(1):37–50.)

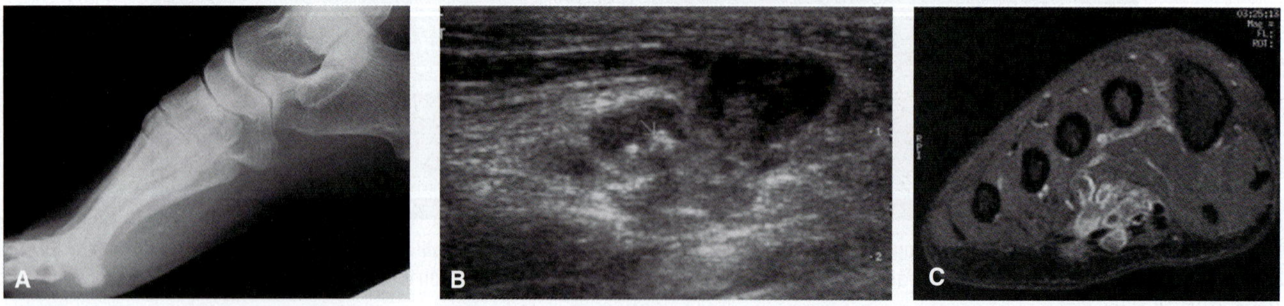

FIGURE 16.38 Hemangioma. **A:** Lateral radiograph showing increased density and soft tissue swelling in the plantar aspect of the foot, containing several round smooth calcifications indicating phleboliths, which are virtually diagnostic of a vascular malformation/tumor. **B:** Ultrasound image revealing a poorly defined mass of mixed echotexture; the phleboliths are distinct echogenic foci causing posterior acoustic shadowing. **C:** Coronal postcontrast fat-suppressed T1 MR image showing a poorly defined mass consisting of enhancing vascular spaces associated with a feeding artery. (From Schatz J, Soper J, McCormack S, et al. Imaging of tumors in the ankle and foot. *Top Magn Reson Imaging* 2010;21(1):37–50.)

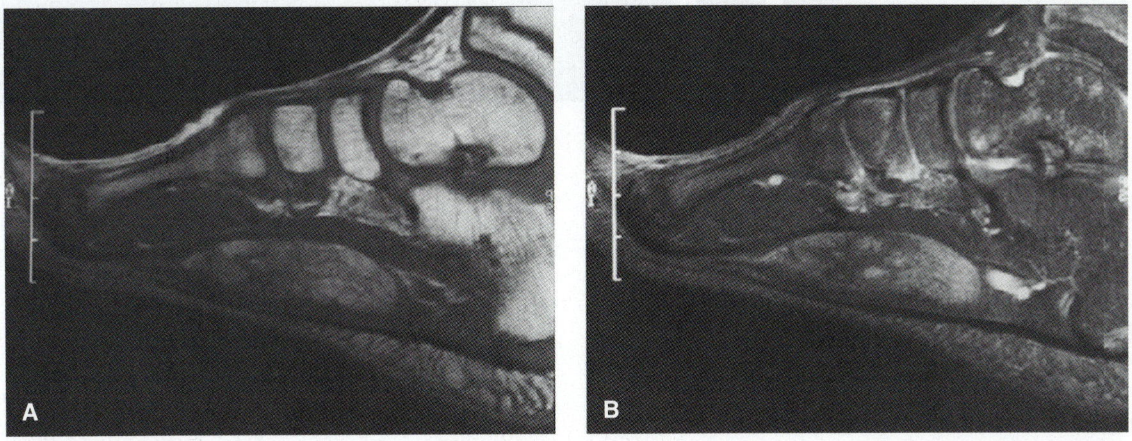

FIGURE 16.39 Spindle cell lipoma. **A:** Sagittal T1-weighted MR image showing a well-defined mass in the deep plantar midfoot of a 10-year-old boy. It contains tissue of fat signal intensity, but also septations and strands of lower signal. **B:** T2-weighted image showing signal hyperintensity consistent with edema in much of the lesion, which is not typical of a simple lipoma and raises concerns of liposarcoma. It was excised and found to be a spindle cell lipoma, which is a benign variant, uncommon in children and in the extremities. (From Schatz J, Soper J, McCormack S, et al. Imaging of tumors in the ankle and foot. *Top Magn Reson Imaging* 2010;21(1):37–50.)

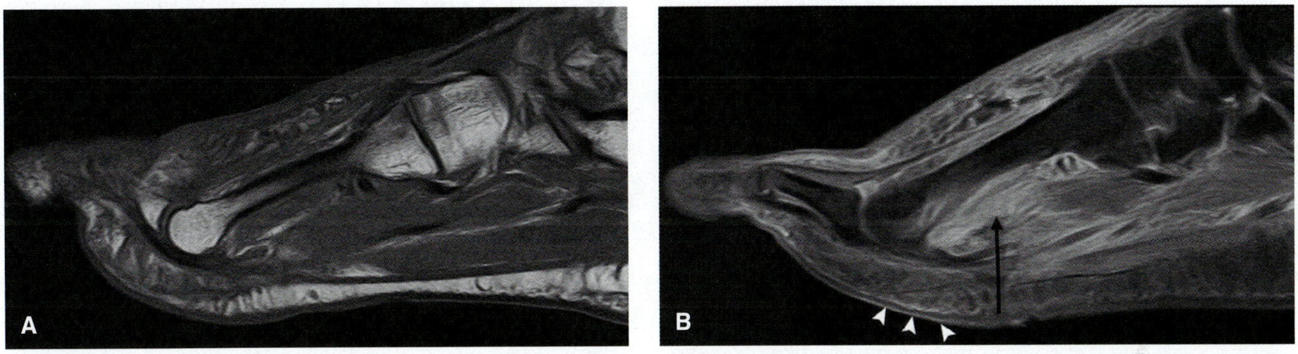

FIGURE 16.40 Cellulitis and myositis. Precontrast, sagittal, T1-weighted **(A)** and postcontrast, sagittal, fat-saturated **(B)** MR images of the forefoot show enhancement of the skin (*arrowheads*) and muscle (*arrow*), consistent with cellulitis and myositis. (From Verma S, Feldman J, Mohsen N. MR imaging for evaluation of plantar pain. *Contemp Diagn Radiol* 2014;37(10):1–5.)

Suggested Readings

Buccilli TA Jr, Hall HR, Solmen JD. Sterile abscess formation following a corticosteroid injection for the treatment of plantar fasciitis. *J Foot Ankle Surg* 2005;44(6):466–468.

Puttaswamaiah R, Chandran P. Degenerative plantar fasciitis: a review of current concepts. *Foot* 2007;17(1):3–9.

Rajput B, Abboud RJ. Common ignorance, major problem: the role of footwear in plantar fasciitis. *Foot* 2004;14(4):214–218.

Toomey EP. Plantar heel pain. *Foot Ankle Clin* 2009;14(2):229–245.

Waldman SD. Plantar fasciitis. In: *Pain Review.* Philadelphia, PA: Saunders; 2009:327.

Waldman SD. Injection technique for plantar fasciitis. In: *Atlas of Pain Management Injection Techniques.* 3rd ed. Philadelphia, PA: Saunders; 2012:453–455.

Waldman SD, Campbell RSD. Plantar fasciitis. In: *Atlas of Common Pain Syndromes.* 3rd ed. Philadelphia, PA: Saunders; 2012:377–379.

Waldman SD, Campbell RSD. Plantar fasciitis. In: *Imaging of Pain.* Philadelphia, PA: Saunders; 2011:457–459.

CHAPTER 17

Calcaneal Spurs

ANATOMIC CONSIDERATIONS

The calcaneus is the largest of the tarsal bones (Fig. 17.1). The main function of the calcaneus is to transfer the weight of the body to the ground, as well as to serve as a lever for the muscles of the calf. The plantar surface of the calcaneus is elevated posteriorly to form the calcaneal tuberosity. The calcaneal tuberosity is depressed centrally, with lateral and medial processes. It is at the medial process that symptomatic calcaneal spurs most commonly occur. The plantar fascia is made up of thick, longitudinally oriented connective tissue that is tightly attached to the plantar skin. It attaches to the medial calcaneal tuberosity and then runs forward, dividing into five bands, one going to each toe (Fig. 17.2). The plantar fascia provides dynamic support to the arch of the foot, tightening as the foot bears weight.

CLINICAL CORRELATES

Calcaneal spurs are a common cause of heel pain (Fig. 17.3). Calcaneal spurs may be asymptomatic or symptomatic. When symptomatic, calcaneal spurs are usually seen in conjunction with plantar fasciitis. The clinical syndrome associated with symptomatic calcaneal spurs is characterized by pain and tenderness over the plantar surface of the calcaneus made immediately worse by dorsiflexion of the toes. Calcaneal spurs are thought to be caused by an inflammation of the insertional fibers of plantar fascia onto the medial tuberosity of the calcaneus (Fig. 17.4). Inflammation of these insertional fibers of the plantar fascia can occur alone or can be part of a systemic inflammatory condition, such as rheumatoid arthritis, plantar fasciitis, Reiter syndrome, or gout (Figs. 17.5 and 17.6). In some patients, suffering from symptomatic heel spurs, there does not appear to be an inflammatory basis for the patient's pain symptomatology and the etiology of the pain appears to be entirely mechanical as is seen with patients with gait abnormalities that include an excessive heel strike. High-impact aerobic exercise also has been implicated.

Pain on palpation of the insertion of the plantar fascia on the plantar medial calcaneal tuberosity is a consistent finding in patients with calcaneal spurs as is exacerbation of pain with active resisted dorsiflexion of the toes. Patients suffering from calcaneal spurs will also exhibit pain on deep palpation of the plantar fascia, especially when the toes are dorsiflexed pulling the plantar fascia taunt. The pain of calcaneal spurs is most severe on taking the first few steps after having not borne weight and is made worse by prolonged standing or walking. The pain of symptomatic heel spurs is made worse by standing for long periods or by weight bearing and is often relieved by padding of the affected heel.

Compromise of the inferior calcaneal nerve, which is known as Baxter neuropathy produces medial heel pain similar to that of plantar fasciitis and calcaneal spurs. Causes of Baxter neuropathy, may occur because of plantar fasciitis, calcaneal spur, or secondary to internal foot derangement. Baxter neuropathy is diagnosed on MRI of the calcaneus which will demonstrate a distinctive sign of selective fatty atrophy of the abductor digiti minimi muscle (Fig. 17.7).

Plain radiographs are indicated in all patients who present with heel and foot pain (Figs. 17.8 and 17.9). Based on the patient's clinical presentation, additional testing may be indicated, including complete blood cell count, sedimentation rate, and antinuclear antibody testing. MRI and/or ultrasound imaging of the ankle is indicated if calcaneal spurs, rupture of the plantar fascia, or joint instability is suggested (Figs. 17.10 to 17.13). Radionuclide bone scanning is useful to identify stress fractures of the calcaneus and foot, not seen on plain radiographs, and may aid in the diagnosis as there may be increased uptake of radionucleotide at the insertion of the plantar fascia at the calcaneus (Figs. 17.14 and 17.15).

ULTRASOUND TECHNIQUE

To perform ultrasound evaluation of the calcaneus, the patient is placed in the prone position with the patient's ankle hanging off the edge of the table. With the patient in the above position, a high-frequency linear ultrasound transducer is placed in a longitudinal plane with the inferior portion of the ultrasound transducer over plantar surface of the foot with the superior end of the transducer on the anterior portion of the calcaneus, and an ultrasound survey scan is taken (Fig. 17.16). The calcaneus, calcaneal spur, and linear plantar fascia are identified at its insertion on the calcaneus (Fig. 17.17). When the insertion of the plantar fascia is identified, it is evaluated for evidence of calcaneal spurs, insertional tendinopathy, and plantar fasciitis (Figs. 17.18 to 17.20).

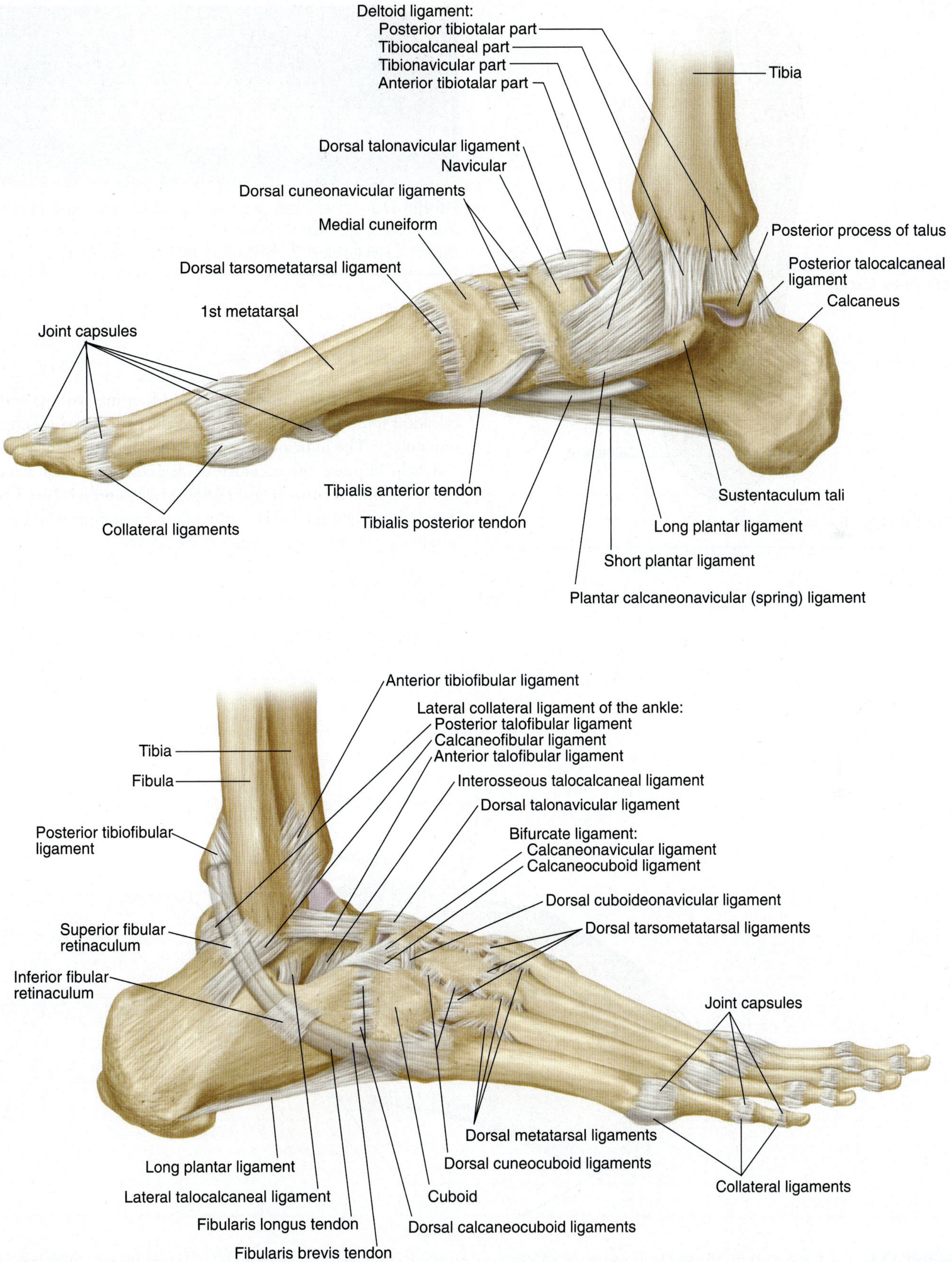

FIGURE 17.1 The calcaneus is the largest of the tarsal bones. The main function of the calcaneus is to transfer the weight of the body to the ground, as well as to serve as a lever for the muscles of the calf. (From Tank PW, Gest TR. The lower limb. In: *Lippincott Williams & Wilkins Atlas of Anatomy*. Philadelphia, PA: Lippincott Williams & Wilkins; 2009:146.)

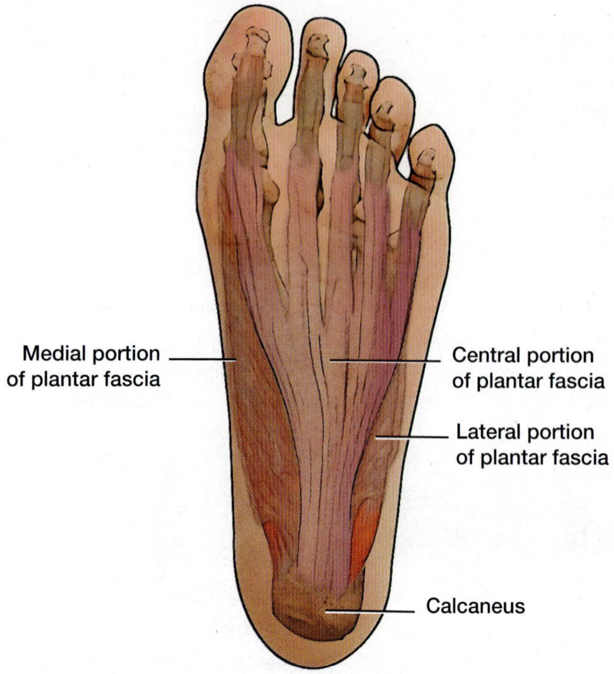

FIGURE 17.2 The anatomy of the plantar fascia.

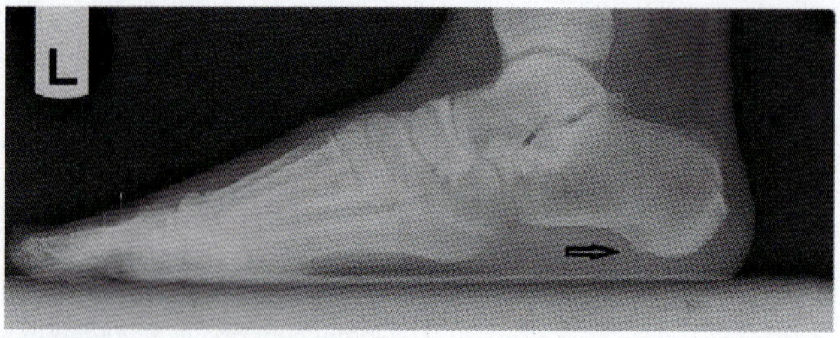

FIGURE 17.3 Lateral radiograph with small calcaneal spur (*arrow*). (From Johnson RE, Haas K, Lindow K, et al. Plantar fasciitis: what is the diagnosis and treatment? *Orthop Nurs* 2014;33(4):198–204.)

CLINICAL PEARLS

Bursitis and tendinitis of the ankle and foot may coexist with calcaneal spurs and may contribute to the patient's pain symptomatology. The judicious use of multiple imaging modalities will help improve the accuracy of diagnosis and help avoid clinical misadventures (Figs. 17.15, 17.21, and 17.22). The use of ultrasound-guided injection of calcaneal spurs with local anesthetic can serve as a diagnostic maneuver.

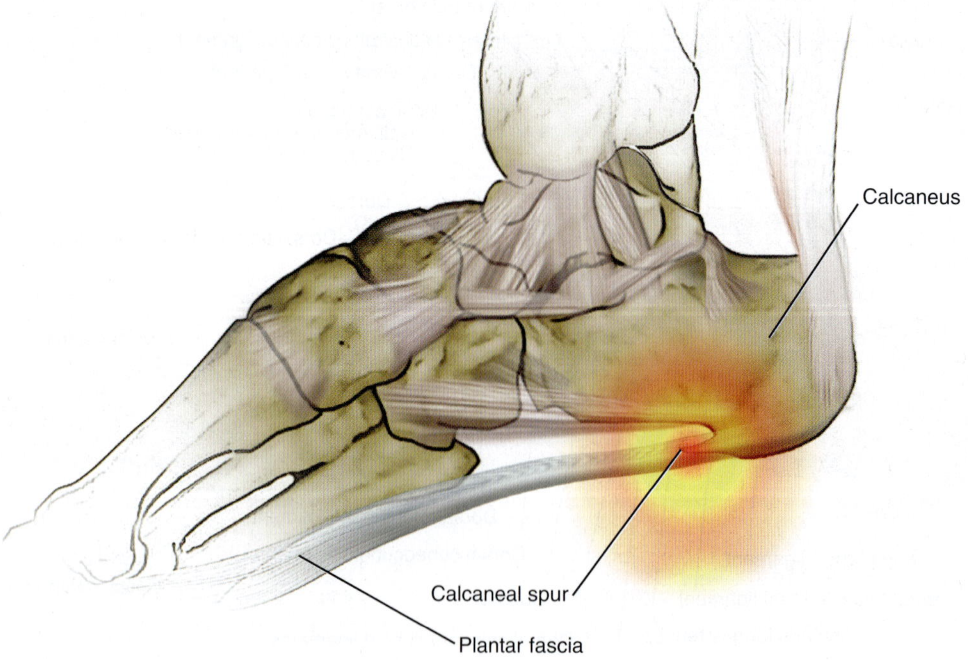

FIGURE 17.4 Calcaneal spurs are thought to be caused by an inflammation of the insertional fibers of plantar fascia onto the medial tuberosity of the calcaneus, although in some patients the cause is purelymechanical.

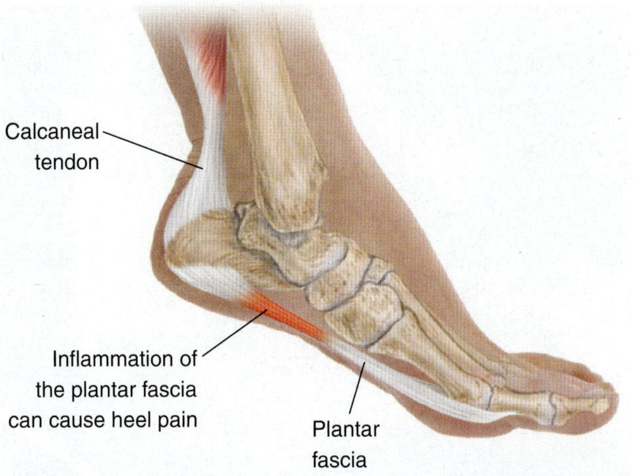

FIGURE 17.5 Inflammation of these insertional fibers of the plantar fascia can occur alone or can be part of a systemic inflammatory condition, such as rheumatoid arthritis, plantar fasciitis, Reiter syndrome, or gout, although in some patients the etiology is purely mechanical. (From Bucci C. *Condition-Specific Massage Therapy*. Baltimore, MD: Lippincott Williams & Wilkins; 2012.)

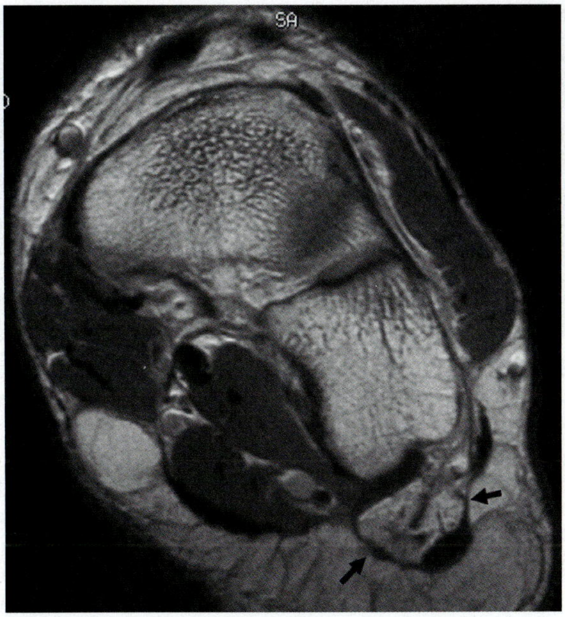

FIGURE 17.7 Chronic isolated denervation effect abductor digiti minimi, consistent with a lesion involving the LPN branch to abductor digiti minimi (inferior calcaneal nerve) (Baxter neuropathy). Coronal PD image demonstrates fatty atrophy of the abductor digiti minimi (*arrows*). (From Simmons DN, Lisle DA, Linklater JM. Imaging of peripheral nerve lesions in the lower limb. *Top Magn Reson Imaging* 2010;21(1):51–62.)

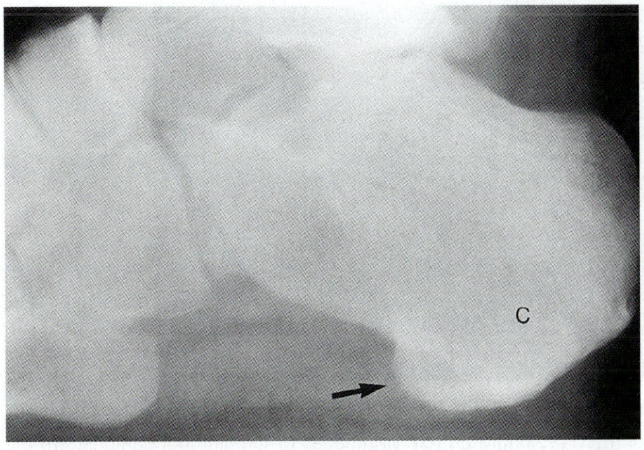

FIGURE 17.6 Lateral radiograph of the heel of a man with Reiter syndrome shows subtle cortical irregularity at the calcaneal insertion of the plantar aponeurosis (*arrow*). C, calcaneus. (From Koopman WJ, Moreland LW. *Arthritis and Allied Conditions: a Textbook of Rheumatology*. 15th ed. Philadelphia, PA: Lippincott Williams & Wilkins; 2005.)

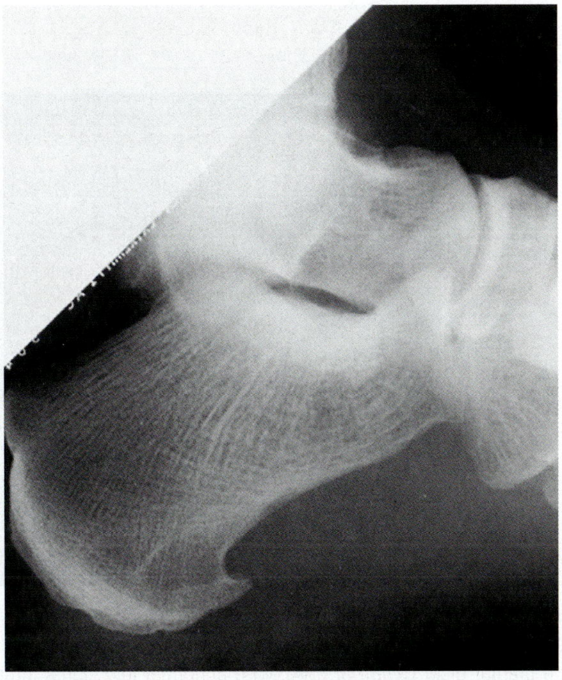

FIGURE 17.8 Lateral radiograph demonstrating a calcaneal spur. (From Koopman WJ, Moreland LW. *Arthritis and Allied Conditions: a Textbook of Rheumatology*. 15th ed. Philadelphia, PA: Lippincott Williams & Wilkins; 2005.)

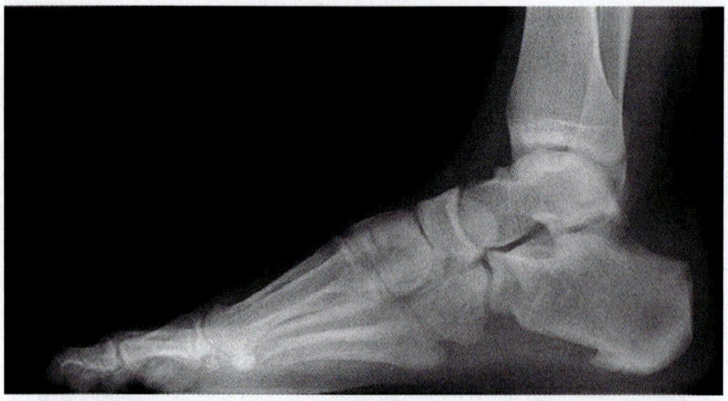

FIGURE 17.9 Lateral right foot radiograph shows increased opacification of Kager fat pad, which lies at the superior aspect of the posterior calcaneum and anterior to the Achilles tendon. This corresponds to the retrocalcaneal (subtendinous) bursal sac where the Achilles tendon attaches to the calcaneum. The increased attenuation within the soft tissues of Kager fat pad may be a consequence of the edema associated with either an inflammatory, infectious, or mechanical bursitis. There is also a plantar calcaneal spur seen on the plain radiograph, which without metabolic activity is of no diagnostic value with respect to confirming the presence of plantar fasciitis. Therefore, the radioisotope scan is of importance when diagnosing this condition. (From Breunung N, Barwick T, Fernando R, et al. Additional benefit of SPECT-CT in investigating heel pain. *Clin Nucl Med* 2008;33(10):705–706.)

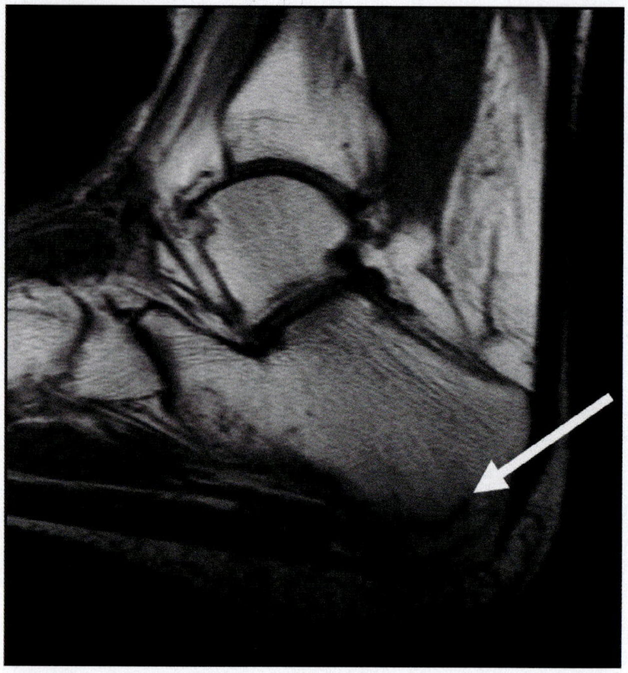

FIGURE 17.11 Calcaneal stress fracture. A recent army recruit presented with diffuse heel pain. This sagittal, T1-weighted MR image of the hindfoot shows a curvilinear, low signal intensity line extending parallel to the posterior surface of the calcaneus (*arrow*), with surrounding bone marrow edema, representing a stress fracture. (From Verma S, Feldman J, Mohsen N. MR imaging for evaluation of plantar pain. *Contemp Diagn Radiol* 2014;37(10):1–5.)

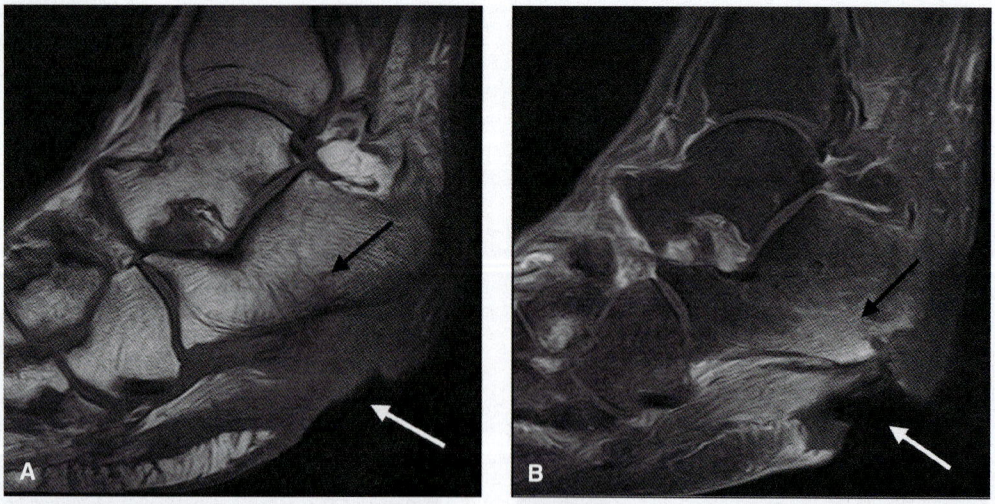

FIGURE 17.10 Osteomyelitis. A 35-year-old man presented with a large ulcer in the plantar soft tissues of the hindfoot beneath the calcaneus. The sagittal T1-weighted, precontrast **(A)** and sagittal T1-weighted, postcontrast, fat-saturated **(B)** MR images of the hindfoot demonstrate the large plantar ulcer (*white arrows*), with abnormal low signal intensity in the inferior calcaneus (*black arrow* in **A**) and calcaneal enhancement (*black arrow* in **B**) and the underlying soft tissues representing osteomyelitis with superimposed myositis and cellulitis. (From Verma S, Feldman J, Mohsen N. MR imaging for evaluation of plantar pain. *Contemp Diagn Radiol* 2014;37(10):1–5.)

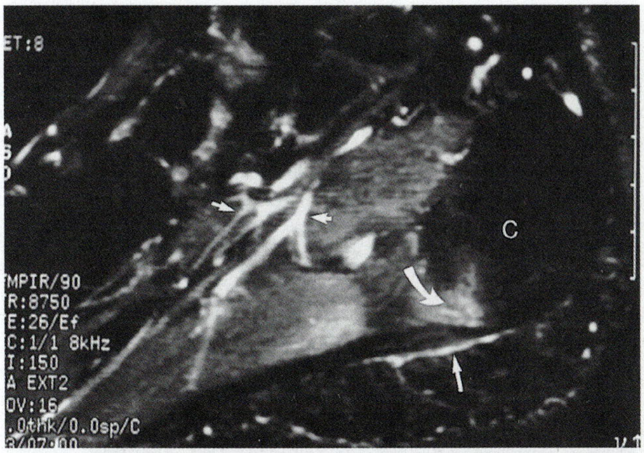

FIGURE 17.12 Sagittal, fast, multiplanar inversion recovery (FMPIR) image of the heel depicts water with high signal intensity and fat with low signal intensity, and thus shows edema in the local soft tissues and bone marrow (*curved arrow*) with extremely high sensitivity. Fluid can also be seen tracking along the plantar aponeurosis (*long straight arrow*) (plantar fasciitis). The arching high signal intensity structures (*short straight arrows*) are blood vessels. (From Koopman WJ, Moreland LW. *Arthritis and Allied Conditions: A Textbook of Rheumatology.* 15th ed. Philadelphia, PA: Lippincott Williams & Wilkins; 2005.)

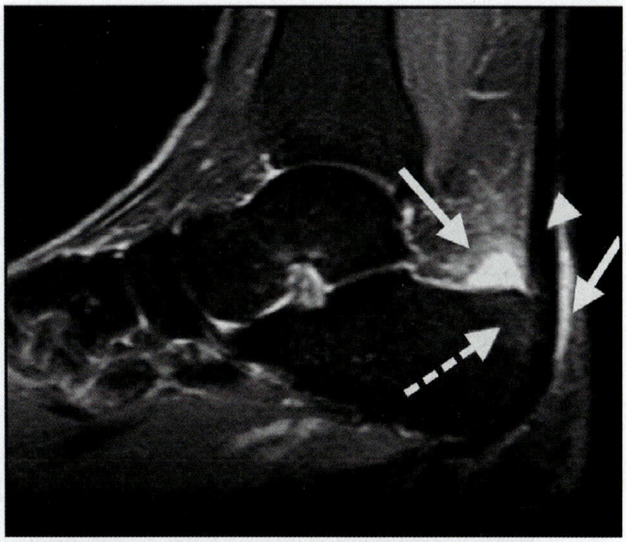

FIGURE 17.13 Haglund deformity. This runner presented with pain and swelling about the posterosuperior aspect of the calcaneus. This sagittal STIR MR image of the hindfoot shows bone marrow edema (*dashed arrow*) and mild bony protuberance at the calcaneal attachment of the Achilles tendon, fluid surrounding and within the distal Achilles tendon (*arrowhead*), and edema in the retrocalcaneal and retroachilles bursae (*solid arrows*). The MR findings are consistent with Haglund deformity. (From Verma S, Feldman J, Mohsen N. MR imaging for evaluation of plantar pain. *Contemp Diagn Radiol* 2014;37(10):1–5.)

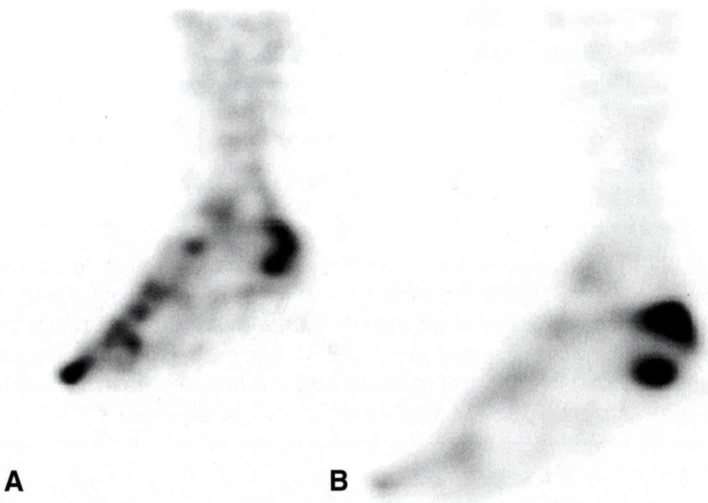

FIGURE 17.14 Early blood pool images **(A)** show marked increased vascularity in the superior and inferior aspects of the right calcaneus, with persistent uptake on the delayed images **(B)**. Characteristically on bone scintigraphy there is hyperemia on the blood pool images along the plantar fascia with more focal uptake at the inferior calcaneum on the delayed images. The tracer uptake superior to the right calcaneus is indicative of increased metabolic activity in the region of the retrocalcaneal bursa, which is consistent with bursitis. (From Breunung N, Barwick T, Fernando R, et al. Additional benefit of SPECT-CT in investigating heel pain. *Clin Nucl Med* 2008;33(10):705–706.)

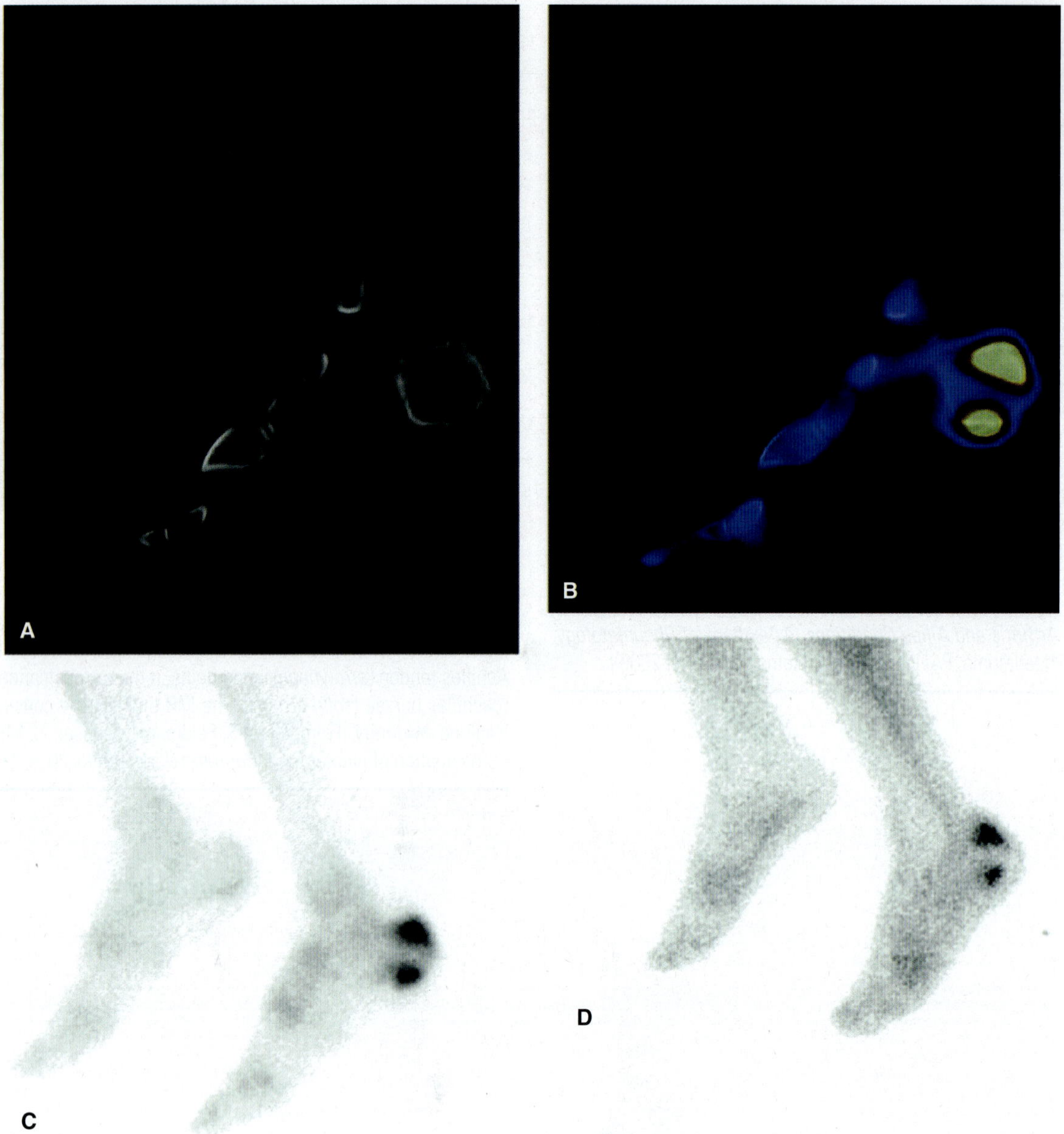

FIGURE 17.15 A,B,C and D: SPECT-CT highlights the usefulness of anatomic and functional image fusion. The increased tracer uptake on the SPECT study localizes to the superior and inferior aspects of the calcaneus on the CT component of the study. Soft tissue thickening related to Kager fat pad can be identified on the CT images. Plantar fascia thickening is also identified on the CT portion of the study. This imaging protocol enhances the diagnostic accuracy of pathology related to heel pain. SPECT-CT increases specificity when compared with using bone scintigraphy alone, especially when improving anatomic localization of metabolic activity in heel pain. (From Breunung N, Barwick T, Fernando R, et al. Additional benefit of SPECT-CT in investigating heel pain. *Clin Nuclear Med* 2008;33(10):705–706.)

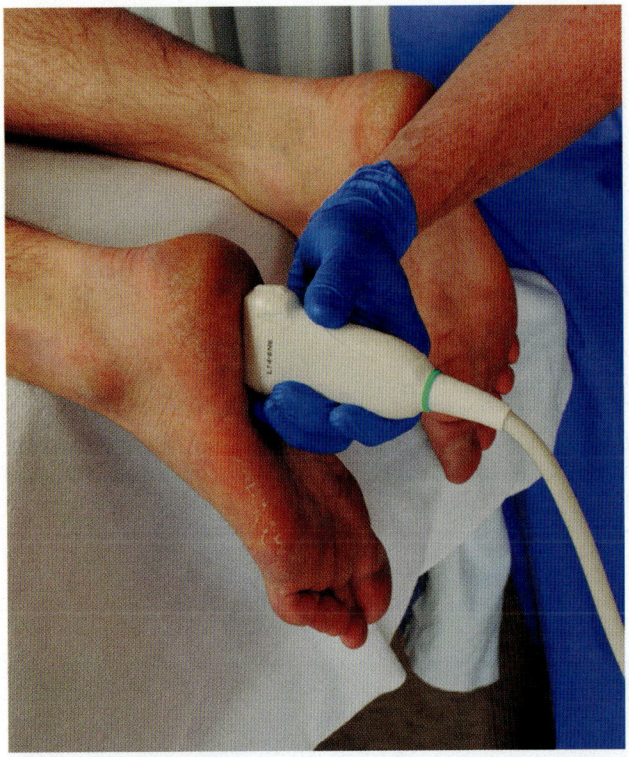

FIGURE 17.16 Proper longitudinal ultrasound transducer placement for ultrasound evaluation for calcaneal spurs.

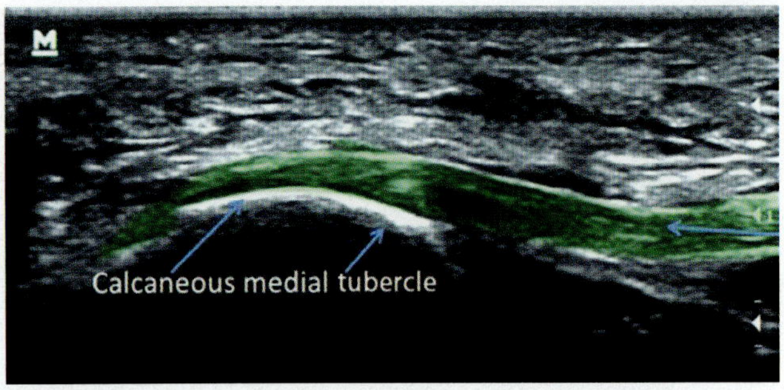

FIGURE 17.17 Longitudinal view of the plantar fascia (*green band*) and its calcaneal insertion.

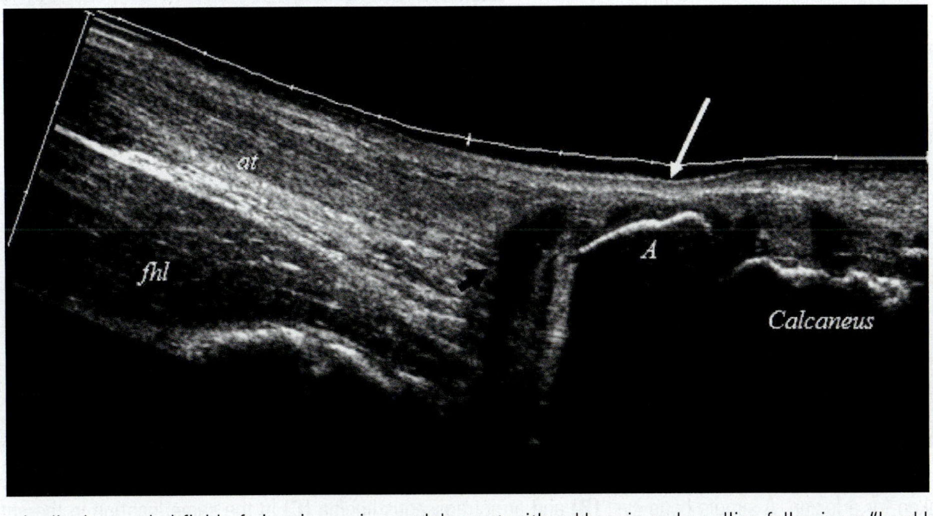

FIGURE 17.18 Longitudinal extended-field-of-view image in an adolescent with ankle pain and swelling following a "hard landing" during gymnastics. There is a moderately displaced fracture of the calcaneal apophysis (*a, arrow*). Moreover, a tear at the Achilles tendon (*at*) insertion can be seen (*short black arrow*) and is distal to the apophyseal fragment. The flexor hallucis long (*fhl*) and calcaneus are labeled for reference. (From Adler R, Sofka CM, Positano RG. *Atlas of Foot and Ankle Sonography*. Philadelphia, PA: Lippincott Williams & Wilkins; 2004:82.)

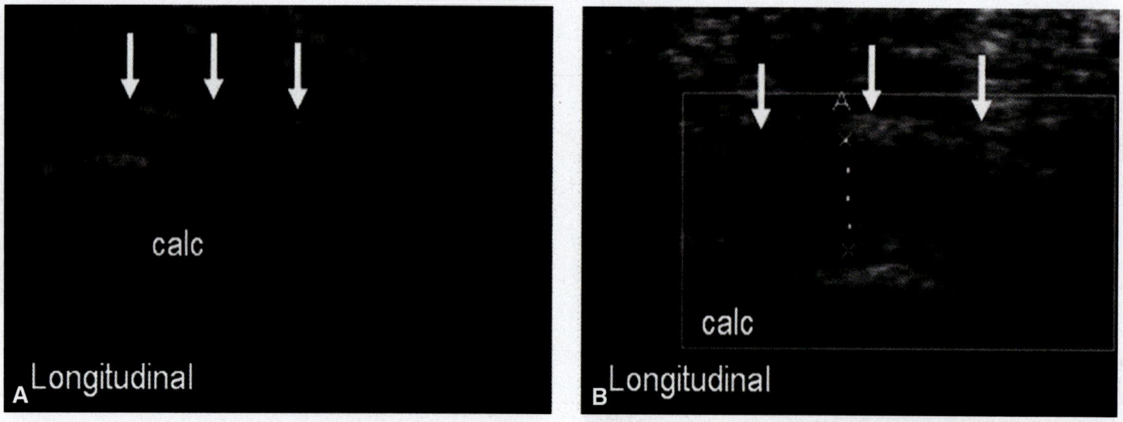

FIGURE 17.19 Longitudinal ultrasound images of normal plantar fascia (*arrows* in **A**) and plantar fasciitis **(B)**, demonstrating a thickened hypoechoic plantar fascia (*arrows*) inserting into the calcaneus (*calc*). (From Chew K, Stevens KJ, Wang T-G, et al. Introduction to diagnostic musculoskeletal ultrasound: part 2: examination of the lower limb. *Am J Phys Med Rehabil* 2008;87(3):238–248.)

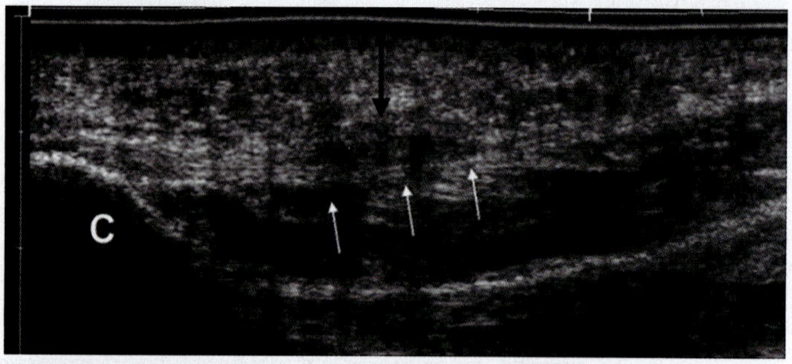

FIGURE 17.20 Superficial fibromatosis. A longitudinal gray scale image of the plantar foot shows a subcutaneous hypoechoic nodule (*black arrow*) within the plantar fascia (*white arrows*), separate from the calcaneal insertion (*c*). (From Hwang S, Adler RS. Sonographic evaluation of the musculoskeletal soft tissue masses. *Ultrasound Q* 2005;21(4):259–270.)

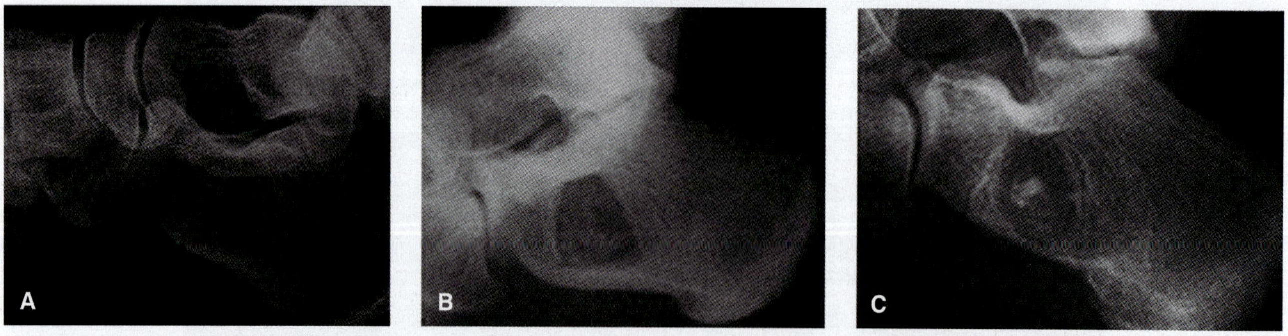

FIGURE 17.21 **A:** Lateral radiograph of the ankle showing an area of sparse trabeculae in the anterior calcaneus, known as Ward triangle. This should not be mistaken for a lesion. A simple bone cyst **(B)** and an intraosseous lipoma **(C)** in the same location in the anterior calcaneus are thought to occur because of the blood supply of this region and are secondary to infarction. (From Schatz J, Soper J, McCormack S, et al. Imaging of tumors in the ankle and foot. *Top Magn Reson Imaging* 2010;21(1):37–50.)

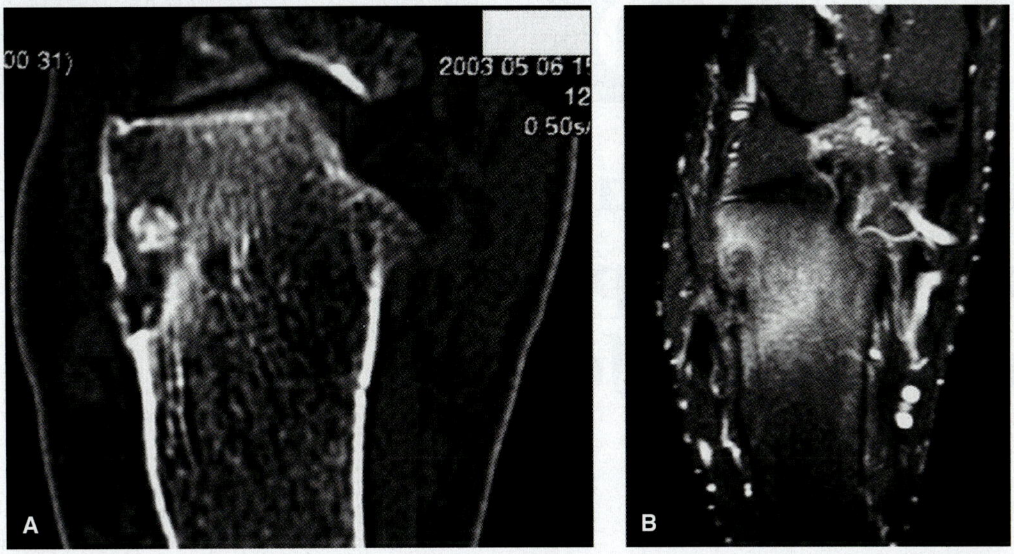

FIGURE 17.22 Osteoid osteoma. **A:** A radiolucent lesion with a central calcified nidus is seen on this axial CT scan of the calcaneus consistent with an osteoid osteoma. In cancellous bones such as this, reactive sclerosis is less marked. **B:** Fat-suppressed axial T2 MR image showing marked surrounding edema and a nidus of intermediate signal intensity. The nidus is less readily seen on the MR image compared to the CT scan in most cases. (From Schatz J, Soper J, McCormack S, et al. Imaging of tumors in the ankle and foot. *Top Magn Reson Imaging* 2010;21(1):37–50.)

Suggested Readings

Irving DB, Cook JL, Menz HB. Factors associated with chronic plantar heel pain: a systematic review. *J Sci Med Sport* 2006;9(1–2):11–22.

Onwuanyi ON. Calcaneal spurs and plantar heel pad pain. *Foot* 2000;10(4):182–185.

Smith S, Tinley P, Gilheany M, et al. The inferior calcaneal spur: anatomical and histological considerations. *Foot* 2007;17(1):25–31.

Thomas JL, Christensen JC, Kravitz SR, et al. The diagnosis and treatment of heel pain: a clinical practice guideline–revision 2010. *J Foot Ankle Surg* 2010; 49(3):S1–S19.

Waldman SD. Injection technique for calcaneal spurs. In: *Atlas of Pain Management Injection Techniques.* 3rd ed. Philadelphia, PA: Saunders; 2012:456–457.

Waldman SD, Campbell RSD. Calcaneal spurs. In: *Atlas of Common Pain Syndromes.* 3rd ed. Philadelphia, PA: Saunders; 2012:380–382.

CHAPTER 18

Arthritis and Other Abnormalities of the Metatarsophalangeal and Interphalangeal Joints

ANATOMIC CONSIDERATIONS

The metatarsophalangeal joints of the toes are condyloid joints characterized by the articulation of the rounded articular surfaces of the metatarsal heads into the shallow concavities of the articular surfaces of the proximal end of the first phalanges (Fig. 18.1). Each joint is lined with synovium and the ample synovial space allows for intra-articular placement of needles for injection and aspiration. The metatarsophalangeal joints have a dense joint capsule and strong plantar and collateral ligaments, although fracture and subluxation may still occur (Figs. 18.2 and 18.3). The metatarsophalangeal joints of the toes are also susceptible to overuse and misuse injuries with resultant inflammation and arthritis. The interphalangeal joints of the toes are ginglymoid hinge joints which have extensive flexion and more limited extension due to the limitation of the metatarsal and collateral ligaments (Figs. 18.2 and 18.4).

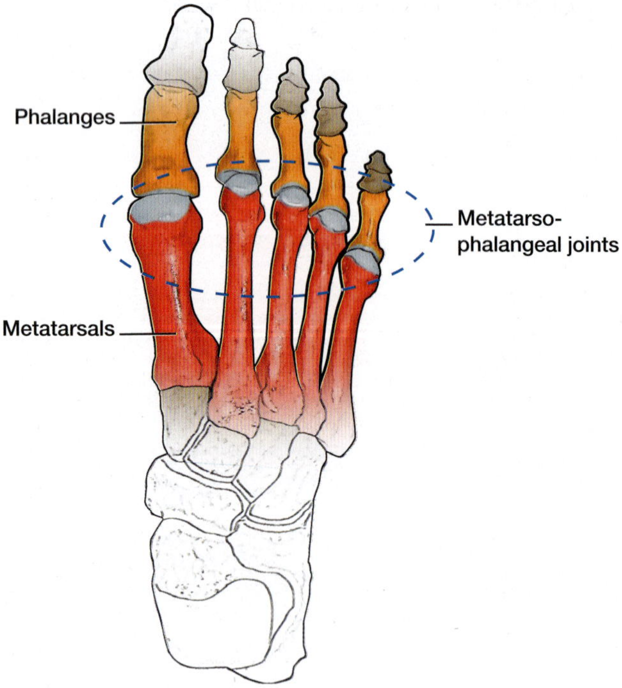

FIGURE 18.1 Anatomy of the metatarsophalangeal joints. (From Weber J, Kelley J. *Health Assessment in Nursing*. 2nd ed. Philadelphia, PA: Lippincott Williams & Wilkins; 2003.)

CLINICAL CORRELATES

The metatarsophalangeal joints of the toes are synovium lined condyloid joints characterized by the articulation of the rounded articular surfaces of the metatarsal heads into the shallow concavities of the articular surfaces of the proximal end of the first phalanges (Fig. 18.4). The primary function of the metatarsophalangeal and interphalangeal joints of the toes is to aid in the gripping function of the foot. The articular cartilage of the metatarsophalangeal and interphalangeal joints of the toes are susceptible to damage, which left untreated, will result in arthritis with its associated pain and functional disability. Osteoarthritis is seen in the metatarsophalangeal and interphalangeal joints of the toes which results in pain and functional disability, with rheumatoid arthritis, posttraumatic arthritis, and crystal arthropathy also causing arthritis of the metatarsophalangeal and interphalangeal joints of the toes. Gout selectively afflicts the metatarsophalangeal joint of the first toe and is called podagra (Figs. 18.5 and 18.6). Less common causes of arthritis-induced pain of the metatarsophalangeal and interphalangeal joints of the toes include other collagen vascular diseases, infection, psoriatic arthritis, villonodular synovitis, and Lyme disease (Figs. 18.7 and 18.8). Acute infectious arthritis of the metatarsophalangeal joints of the toes is best treated with early diagnosis, with culture and sensitivity of the synovial fluid, and prompt initiation of antibiotic therapy. The collagen vascular diseases generally manifest as a polyarthropathy rather than a monoarthropathy limited to the metatarsophalangeal and interphalangeal joints of the toes, although pain of the metatarsophalangeal and interphalangeal joints of the toes, secondary to the collagen vascular diseases, responds exceedingly well to ultrasound-guided intra-articular injection.

Patients with pain of the metatarsophalangeal and interphalangeal joints of the toes secondary to arthritis, gout, synovitis,

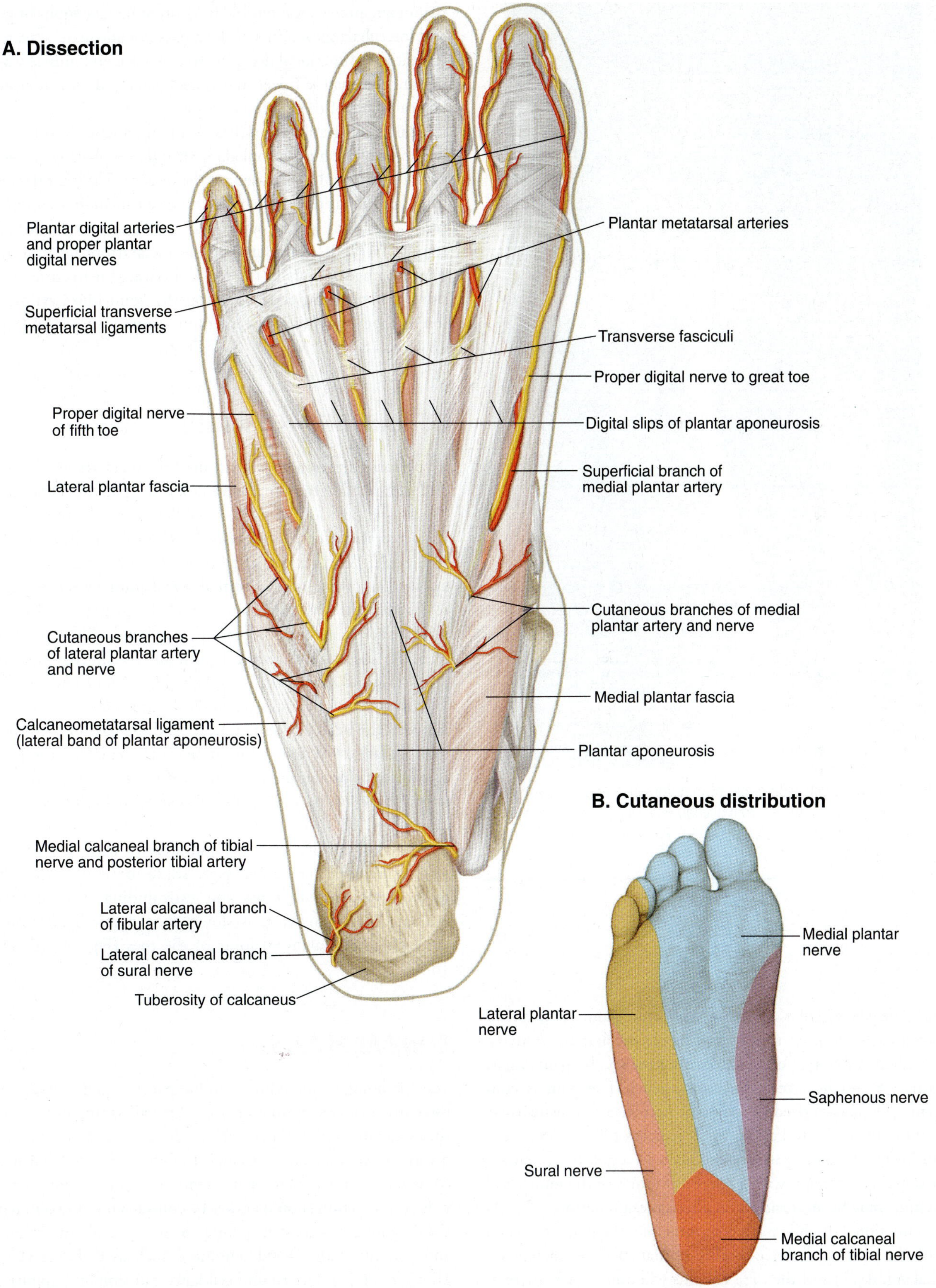

FIGURE 18.2 **A,B:** Cutaneous nerves of the sole of the foot. (From Tank PW, Gest TR. The lower limb. In: *Lippincott Williams & Wilkins Atlas of Anatomy*. Philadelphia, PA: Lippincott Williams & Wilkins; 2009:154.)

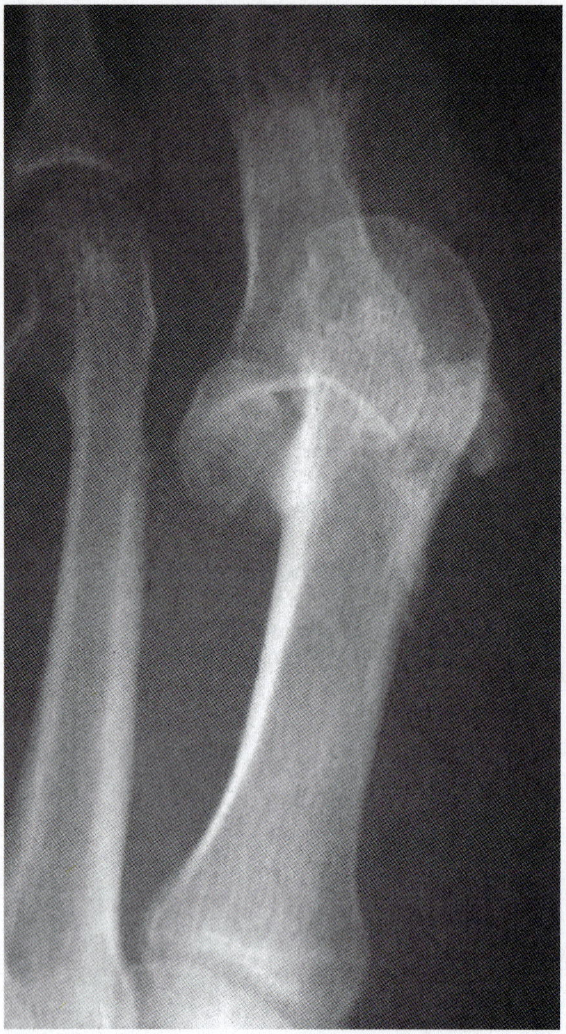

FIGURE 18.3 Plain radiograph of metatarsophalangeal joint showing a complete dislocation. (From Bucholz RW, Heckman JD. *Rockwood & Green's Fractures in Adults.* 5th ed. Philadelphia, PA: Lippincott Williams & Wilkins; 2001.)

and collagen vascular disease–related joint pain, complain of pain that is localized to the head of the metatarsals. Activity, including walking and weight bearing makes the pain worse, with rest and heat providing some relief. The pain is constant and characterized as aching in nature. Sleep disturbance is common with awakening when patients roll over onto the affected foot. Some patients complain of a grating, catching, or popping sensation with a range of motion of the joints, and crepitus may be appreciated on physical examination.

Functional disability often accompanies the pain associated with the many pathologic conditions that affect the metatarsophalangeal joints of the toes. Patients will often notice increasing difficulty in performing their activities of daily living and tasks that require standing, walking, or weight bearing. If the pathologic process responsible for pain of metatarsophalangeal and interphalangeal joints of the toes is not adequately treated, the patient's functional disability may worsen and muscle wasting and ultimately frozen metatarsophalangeal and interphalangeal joints of the toes may occur.

Plain radiographs are indicated in all patients who present with pain of the metatarsophalangeal and interphalangeal joints of the toes (Fig. 18.9). Based on the patient's clinical presentation, additional testing may be indicated including complete blood cell count, sedimentation rate, and antinuclear antibody testing. MRI or ultrasound of the metatarsophalangeal and interphalangeal joints of the toes is indicated if fracture, effusion, tendinopathy, crystal arthropathy, joint mice, synovitis, foreign body, bursitis, or ligamentous injury is suspected (Figs. 18.10 to 18.13).

ULTRASOUND TECHNIQUE

To perform ultrasound evaluation of the metatarsophalangeal and interphalangeal joints of the toes, the patient is placed in the supine position with the knee flexed so that the plantar surface of the affected foot rests comfortably on the examination table. With the patient in the above position, the dorsal surface of the metatarsophalangeal joint of the affected toe is identified by palpation. A high-frequency small linear ultrasound transducer is placed in a longitudinal position over the metatarsophalangeal joint of the affected toe and an ultrasound survey scan is taken (Figs. 18.14 and 18.15). The hypoechic metatarsophalangeal joint space is identified between the head of the metatarsal and the base of the proximal phalanges. When the joint space is identified, the joint is evaluated for the presence of arthritis, synovitis, effusion, crystal deposition, and abnormal masses including ganglion cysts (Figs. 18.16 to 18.25). Ultrasound and color Doppler are used to identify synovitis and areas of neovascularity in healing tendons and joints (Figs. 18.26 to 18.30). After the metatarsophalangeal joints and surrounding structures are evaluated the transducer is slowly moved distally to evaluate each interphalangeal joint of the toes (Figs. 18.31 and 18.32).

CLINICAL PEARLS

Toe pathology—including tendinopathy, occult fractures, osteoarthritis, rheumatoid arthritis, crystal arthropathies, bursitis, synovitis, and impingement syndromes—may coexist with disease of the metatarsophalangeal joints of the toes and may contribute to the patient's pain symptoms. Foreign body synovitis and infection should always be considered in the differential diagnosis of persistent plantar pain, especially in children and patients with altered sensation, such as diabetics (Figs. 18.33 to 18.35). Ultrasound guidance can simplify aspiration and injection of the metatarsophalangeal and interphalangeal joints of the toes.

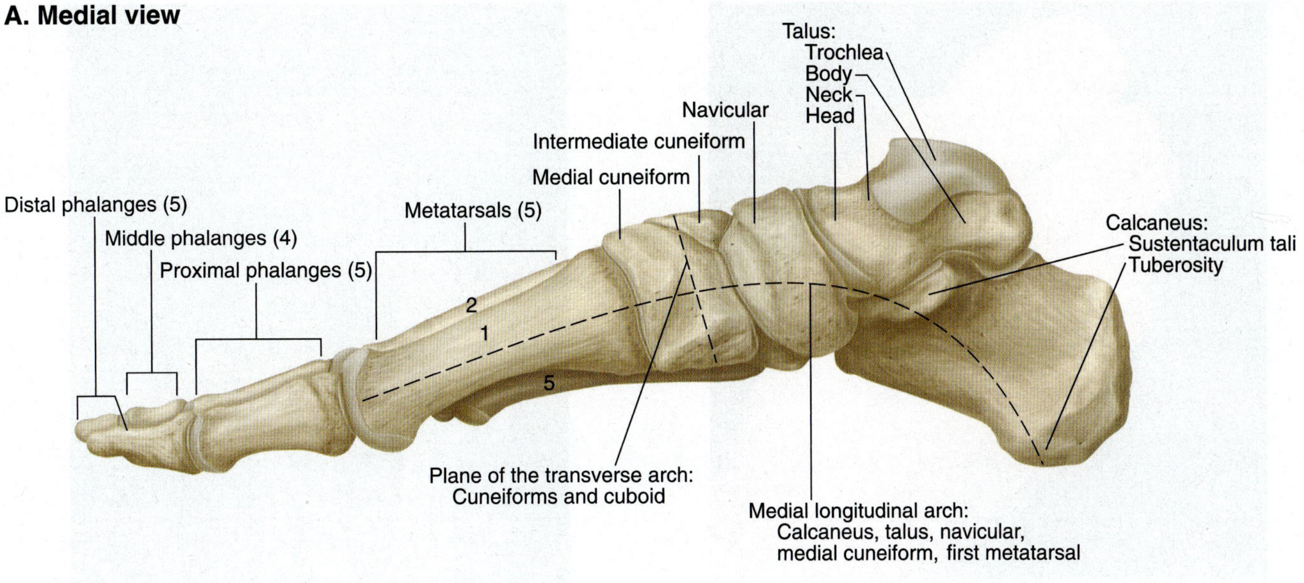

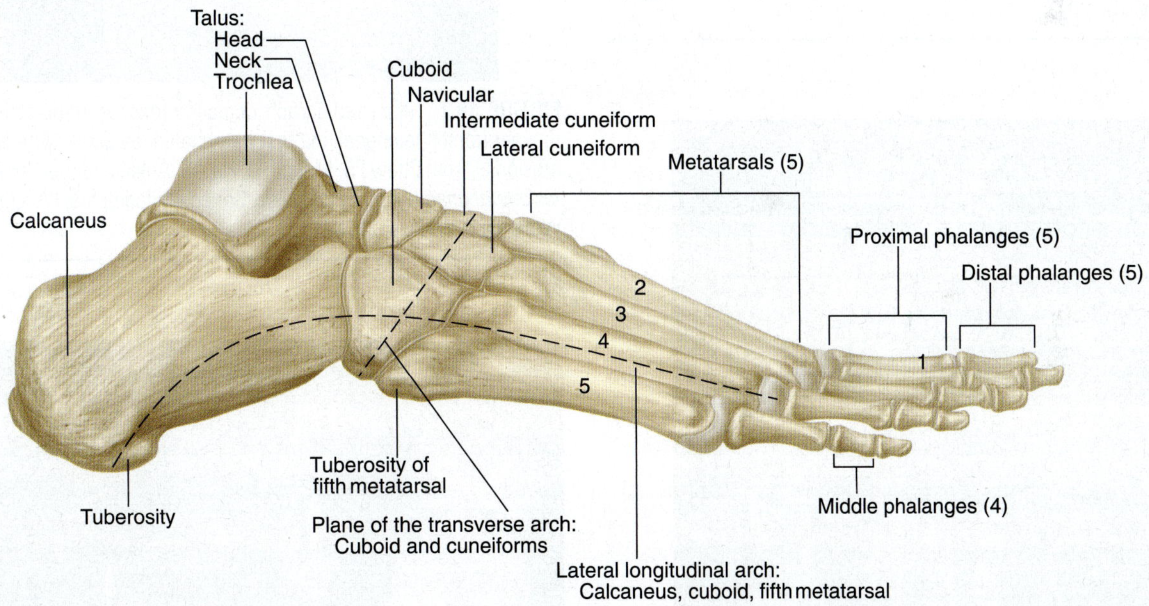

FIGURE 18.4 **A,B:** The metatarsophalangeal joints of the toes are also susceptible to overuse and misuse injuries with resultant inflammation and arthritis. The interphalangeal joints of the toes are ginglymoid hinge joints which have extensive flexion and more limited extension due to the limitation of the plantar and collateral ligaments. (From Tank PW, Gest TR. The lower limb. In: *Lippincott Williams & Wilkins Atlas of Anatomy*. Philadelphia, PA: Lippincott Williams & Wilkins; 2009:127.)

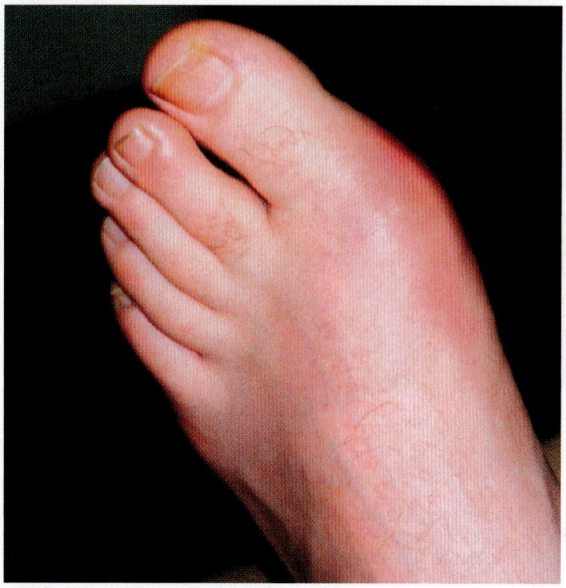

FIGURE 18.5 Gout frequently afflicts the first metatarsophalangeal joint and is called podagra. (From Barker LR, Burton JR, Zieve, PD. *Principles of Ambulatory Medicine*. 4th ed. Baltimore, MD: Williams & Wilkins; 1995:935.)

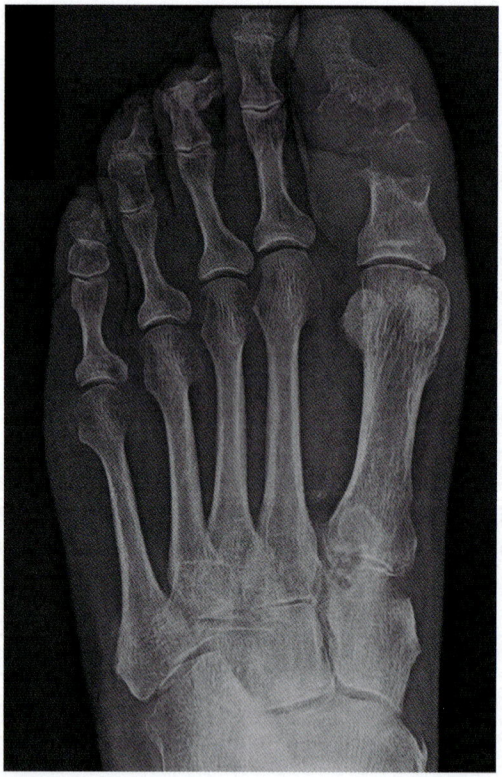

FIGURE 18.6 Plain radiograph demonstrating tophaceous gout of the first interphalangeal and tarsometatarsal joint. Note that the erosions have sclerotic edges and overhanging edges. (From Chew FS, Mulcah H, Ha AS. Ankle and foot. In: *Musculoskeletal Imaging: a Teaching File*. 3rd ed. Philadelphia, PA: Lippincott Williams & Wilkins; 2012.)

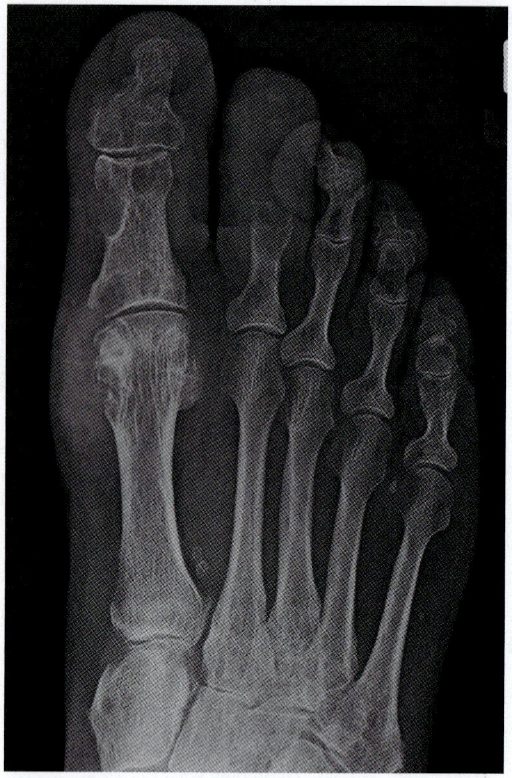

FIGURE 18.7 Plain radiograph demonstrating psoriatic arthritis of the metatarsophalangeal and first interphalangeal joint. Note articular erosions. (From Chew FS, Mulcah H, Ha AS. Ankle and foot. In: *Musculoskeletal Imaging: a Teaching File*. 3rd ed. Philadelphia, PA: Lippincott Williams & Wilkins; 2012.)

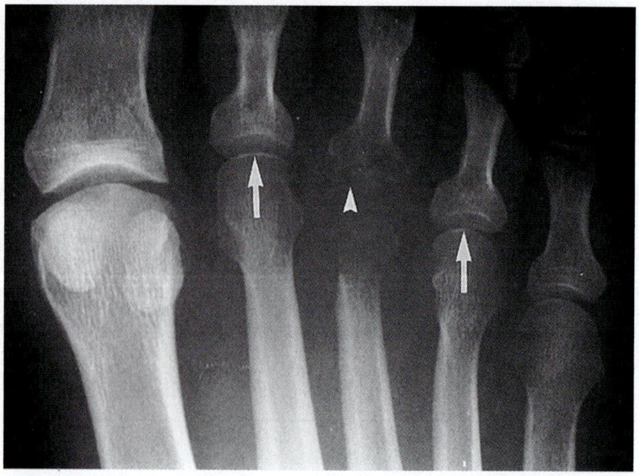

FIGURE 18.8 Posteroanterior radiograph of the toes shows septic arthritis of the metatarsophalangeal joint. At the third joint there is loss of the normal articular cortical bone of both the metatarsal head and base of the proximal phalanx (*arrowhead*). Observe the localized loss of bone density (osteopenia) of the same bones. Compare these changes with the adjacent unaffected joints (*arrows*). (From Rowe LJ, Yochum TR. Normal skeletal anatomy and radiographic positioning. In: *Yochum and Rowes' Essentials of Skeletal Radiology*. Vol 1. 3rd ed. Philadelphia, PA: Lippincott Williams & Wilkins; 2005:127.)

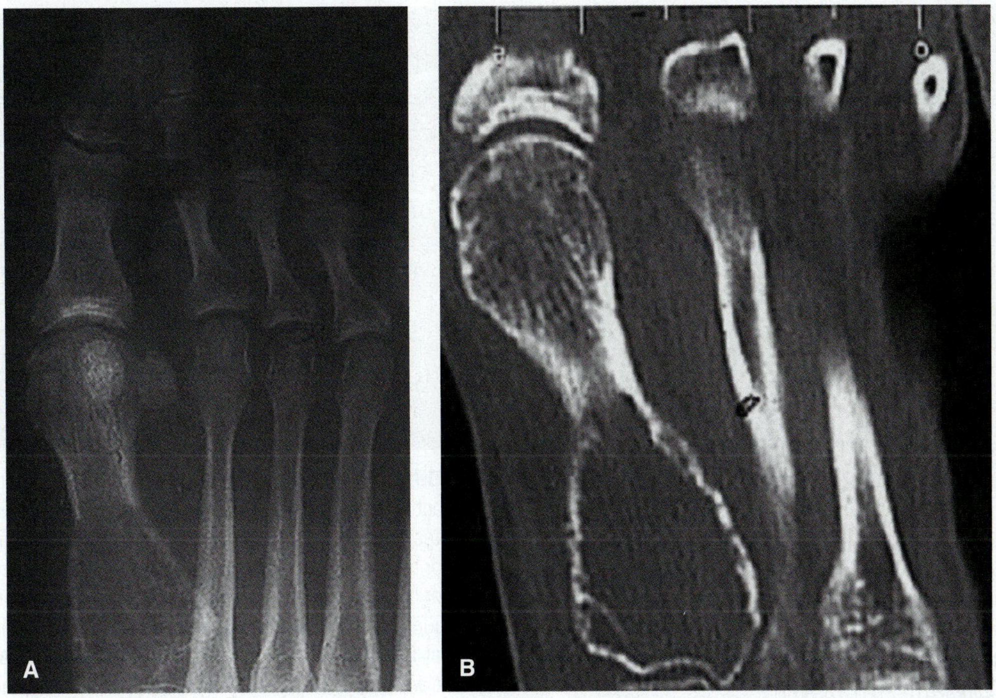

FIGURE 18.9 Giant cell tumor. Anteroposterior radiograph **(A)** and axial CT scan **(B)** revealing a radiolucent, expanded lesion in the base of the first metatarsal with a well-defined but nonsclerotic margin, typical of a GCT. (From Schatz J, Soper J, McCormack S, et al. Imaging of tumors in the ankle and foot. *Top Magn Reson Imaging* 2010;21(1):37–50.)

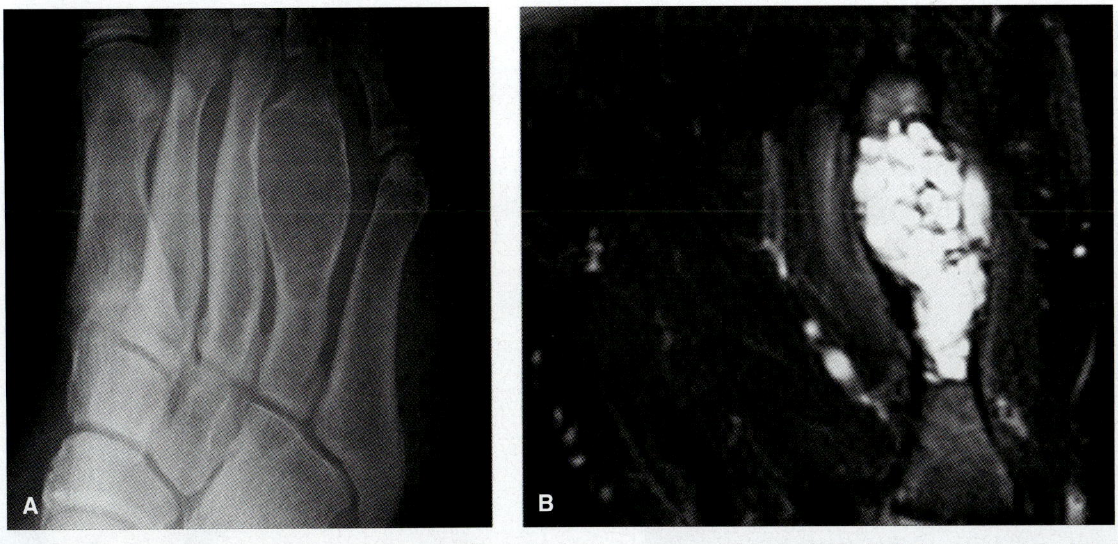

FIGURE 18.10 Aneurysmal bone cyst. **A:** Anteroposterior radiograph showing an expanded lucent lesion in the fourth metatarsal shaft, sharply defined but no sclerotic rim. Fine internal bony trabeculae can be seen. **B:** Fat-suppressed T2-weighted MR image showing the lesion having multiple lobules of fluid signal intensity, traversed by low-signal bony septae. (From Schatz J, Soper J, McCormack S, et al. Imaging of tumors in the ankle and foot. *Top Magn Reson Imaging* 2010;21(1):37–50.)

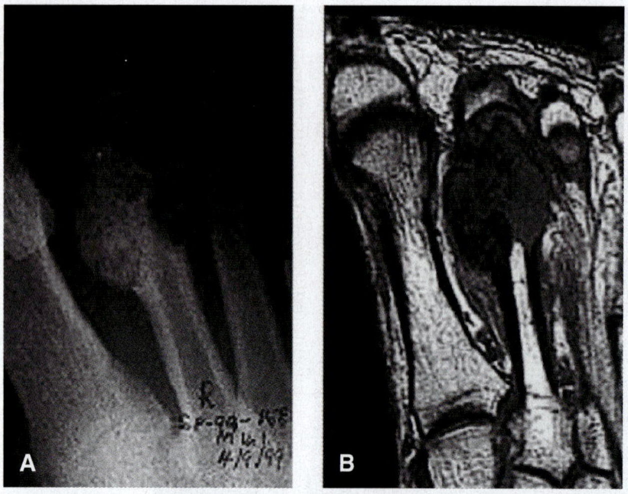

FIGURE 18.11 Osteosarcoma. **A:** Aggressive lesion in the distal metaphysis of the second metatarsal exhibiting cortical destruction laterally and sclerotic soft tissue extension projecting medially. **B:** Axial PD MR image demonstrating the hypointense component medially that represents tumor bone formation. (From Schatz J, Soper J, McCormack S, et al. Imaging of tumors in the ankle and foot. *Top Magn Reson Imaging* 2010;21(1):37–50.)

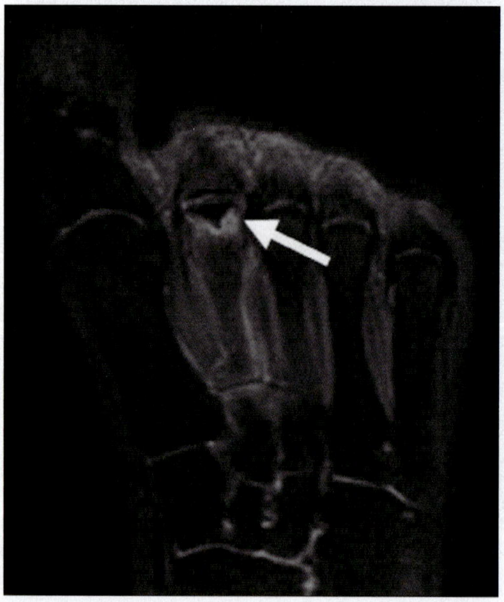

FIGURE 18.12 Freiberg infarction. This coronal, T2-weighted, fat-saturation MR image of the forefoot shows an area of low signal intensity in the head of the second metatarsal with associated flattening of the head and adjacent serpiginous edema (*arrow*), representing Freiberg infarction. (From Verma S, Feldman J, Mohsen N. MR imaging for evaluation of plantar pain. *Contemp Diagn Radiol* 2014;37(10):1–5.)

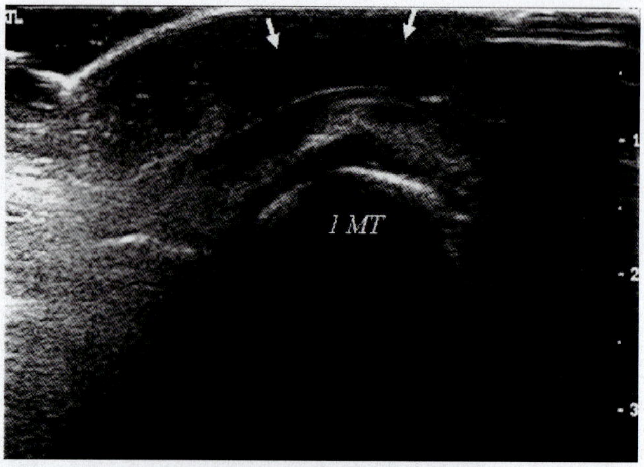

FIGURE 18.13 Longitudinal ultrasound image along the plantar aspect of the foot at the level of the first metatarsal head demonstrates an encapsulated, mildly heterogeneous collection superficial to flexor hallucis longus tendon consistent with an adventitial bursa. The flexor hallucis longus tendon is immediately below the collection, and portions of the proximal phalanx are present to the left of the metatarsal head (1 MT). (From Adler R, Sofka CM, Positano RG. *Atlas of Foot and Ankle Sonography*. Philadelphia, PA: Lippincott Williams & Wilkins; 2004:23.)

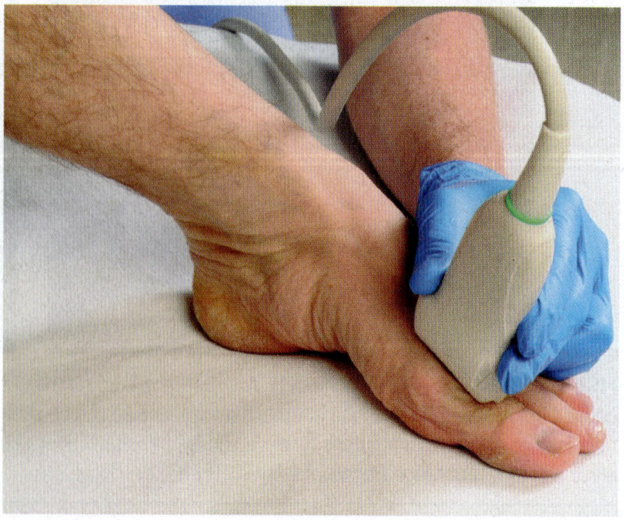

FIGURE 18.14 Correct longitudinal position for ultrasound transducer for ultrasound evaluation of the metatarsophalangeal and interphalangeal joints of the toes.

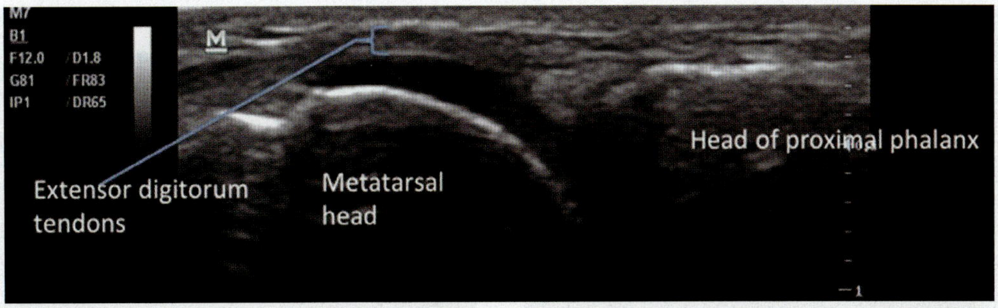

FIGURE 18.15 Longitudinal ultrasound view of the metatarsophalangeal joint space. Note the well-defined joint space and smooth articular surface.

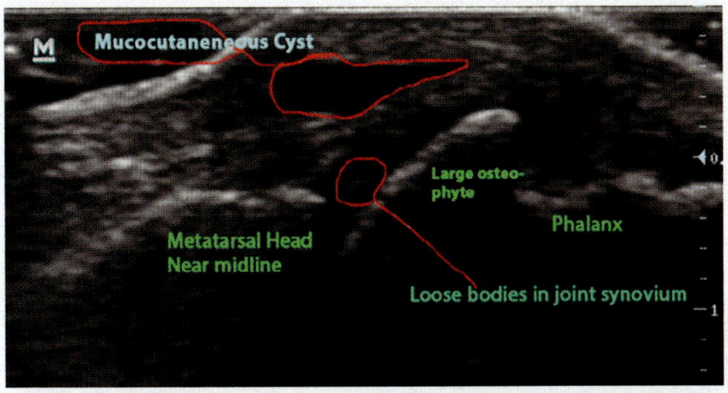

FIGURE 18.16 Longitudinal ultrasound image of the great toe demonstrating a large osteophyte with associated intra-articular joint mice of the right first metatarsophalangeal joint. Note the mucocutaneous cyst.

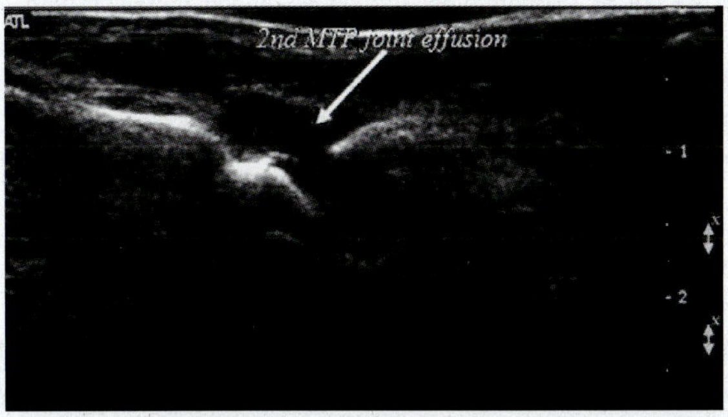

FIGURE 18.18 Longitudinal ultrasound image of the second metatarsophalangeal (MTP) joint demonstrates a small effusion with thickening of the dorsal joint capsule (*arrow*). (From Adler R, Sofka CM, Positano RG. *Atlas of Foot and Ankle Sonography*. Philadelphia, PA: Lippincott Williams & Wilkins; 2004:27.)

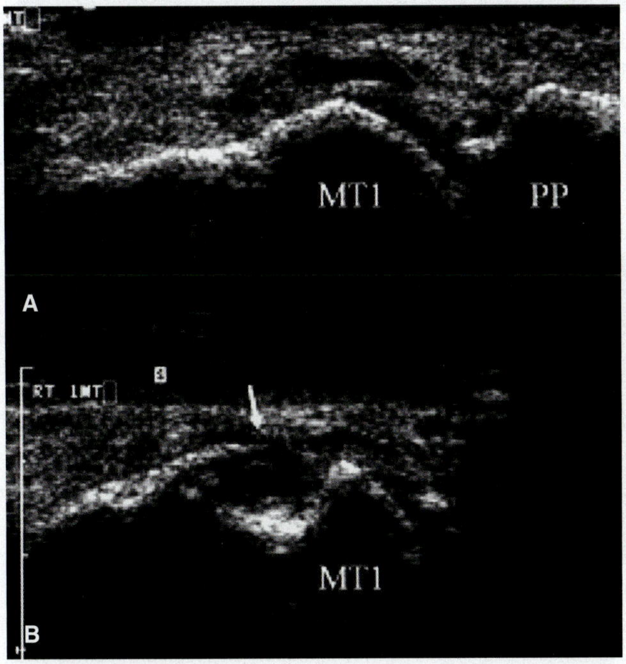

FIGURE 18.17 **A:** Longitudinal image of the first metatarsophalangeal (MTP) joint in a patient with hallux valgus deformity demonstrating a small effusion. The first metatarsal (MT1) and proximal phalanx (PP) are labeled. **B:** Long-axis view of the first MTP joint in the same patient, scanned along the medial joint line, demonstrates cystic change in the first metatarsal head (*arrow*). (From Adler R, Sofka CM, Positano RG. *Atlas of Foot and Ankle Sonography*. Philadelphia, PA: Lippincott Williams & Wilkins; 2004:30.)

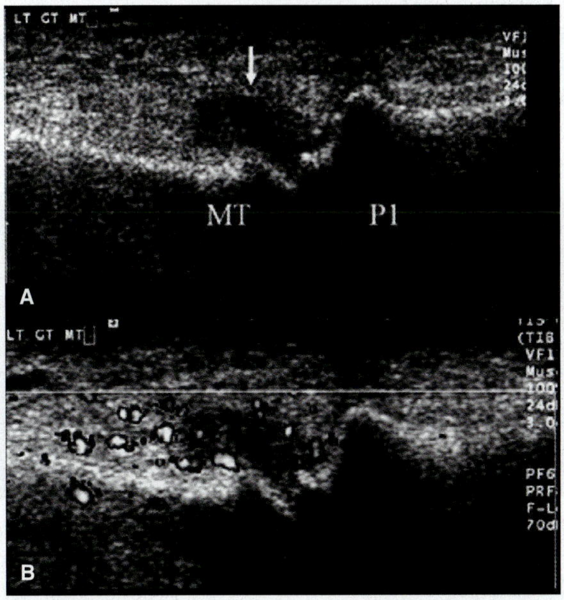

FIGURE 18.19 **A:** Longitudinal view of the first metatarsophalangeal (MTP) joint in a patient with pain and swelling and clinical concern of gout. Hypoechoic debris is seen distending the joint space (*arrow*). The metatarsal head (MT) and proximal phalanx (P1) are labeled. **B:** There is marked regional hyperemia when power Doppler is applied, consistent with inflammation. (From Adler R, Sofka CM, Positano RG. *Atlas of Foot and Ankle Sonography*. Philadelphia, PA: Lippincott Williams & Wilkins; 2004:27.)

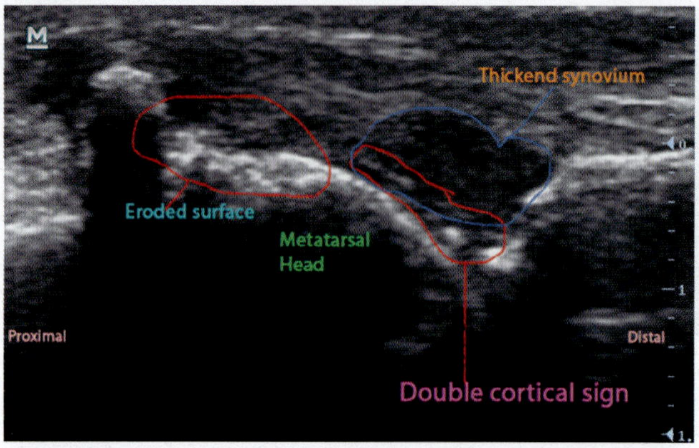

FIGURE 18.20 Longitudinal ultrasound image demonstrating erosion of the articular cartilage consistent with gouty arthritis and associated synovitis of the right first metatarsophalangeal joint. Note the double cortical sign.

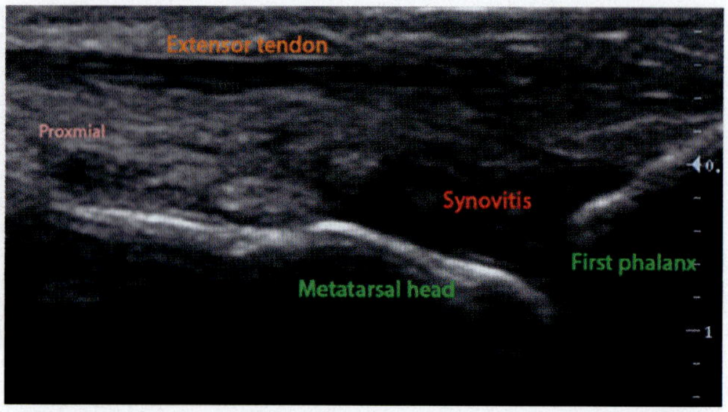

FIGURE 18.21 Longitudinal ultrasound image demonstrating synovitis in a patient with active rheumatoid arthritis presenting with an inflamed metatarsophalangeal joint.

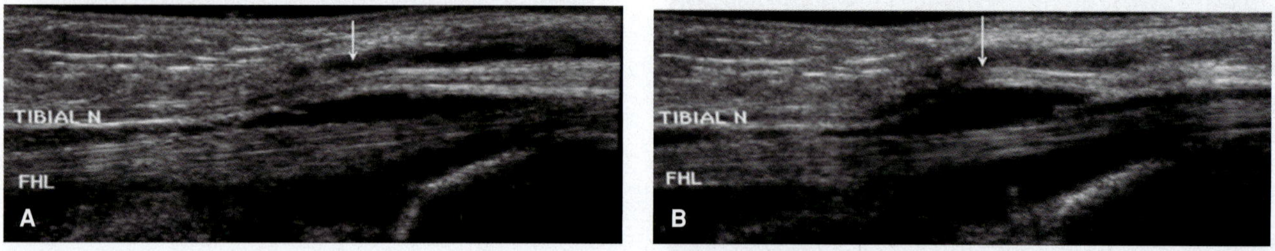

FIGURE 18.22 **A:** Longitudinal ultrasound image demonstrating tenosynovitis of flexor hallucis longus with an effusion in the tendon sheath. **B:** On plantar flexion of the big toe the fluid in the sheath moves proximally and displaces the tibial nerve. (From Simmons DN, Lisle DA, Linklater JM. Imaging of peripheral nerve lesions in the lower limb. *Top Magn Reson Imaging* 2010;21(1):51–62.)

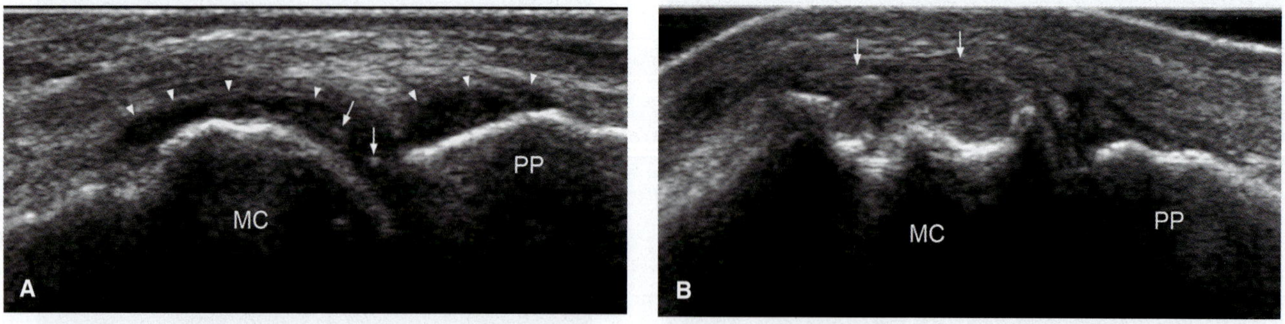

FIGURE 18.23 Longitudinal ultrasound of first metatarsophalangeal joint. **A:** Dorsal aspect of joint showing a small- to moderate-sized effusion/synovial proliferation (*arrowheads*). There are several discrete echogenic foci within the joint consistent with crystal aggregates (*arrows*). **B:** Medial aspect of the joint. There is a wide, deep erosion (*arrows*) with overhanging edges consistent with a gouty or crystal arthropathy. MC, metacarpal; PP, proximal phalanx. (From Lee R, Griffith J. Foot and ankle. In: Beggs I, ed. *Musculoskeletal Ultrasound.* Philadelphia, PA: Lippincott Williams & Wilkins; 2014:172.)

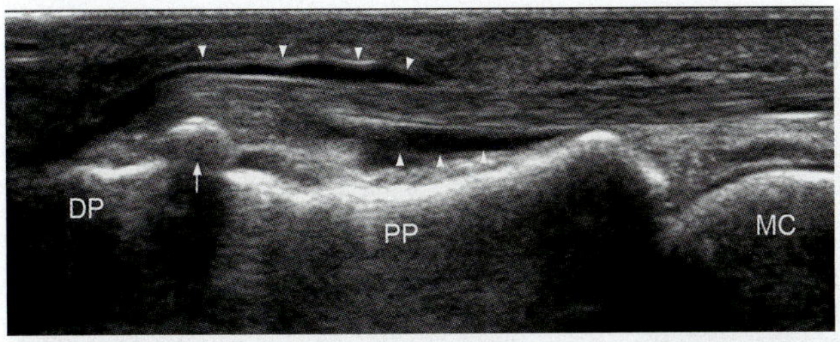

FIGURE 18.24 Longitudinal ultrasound of the big toe showing a moderate tenosynovitis (*arrowheads*) of the FHL tendon with a tendon sheath effusion surrounding a mildly swollen but otherwise normal tendon. Note the sesamoid bone (*arrow*) overlying the distal interphalangeal joint. MC, metatarsal; PP, proximal phalanx; DP, distal phalanx. (From Lee R, Griffith J. Foot and ankle. In: Beggs I, ed. *Musculoskeletal Ultrasound*. Philadelphia, PA: Lippincott Williams & Wilkins; 2014:172.)

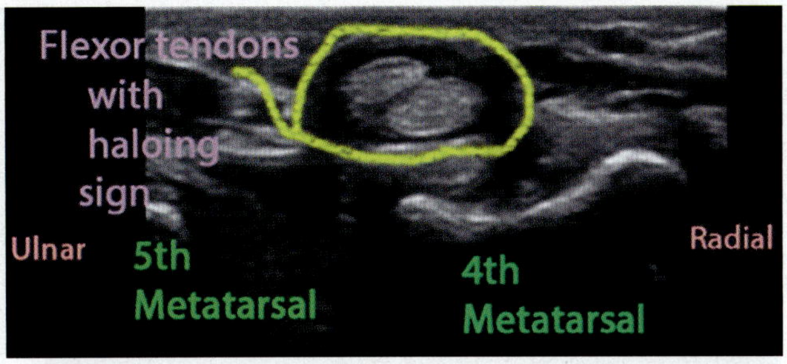

FIGURE 18.26 Transverse ultrasound image demonstrating tendinitis with significant effusion involving the flexor tendons of the toes. Note the positive halo sign indicating fluid around the affected tendons.

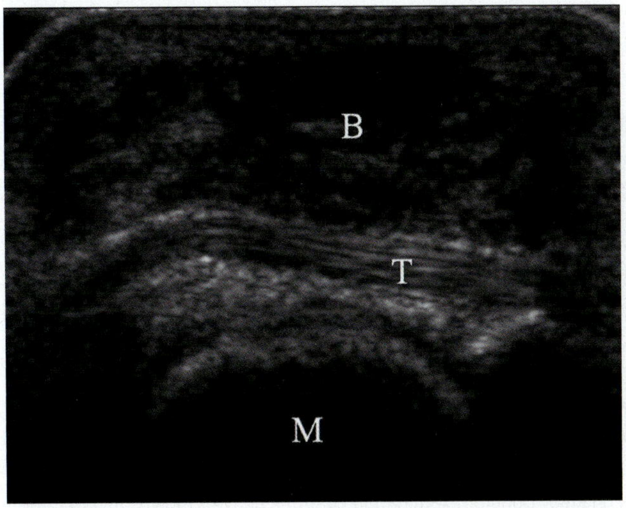

FIGURE 18.25 Rheumatoid bursitis superficial to first metatarsophalangeal joint. Longitudinal ultrasound scan shows enlarged hypoechoic bursa (B) superficial to flexor hallucis longus tendon (T) and first metatarsal head (M). (From Court-Payen M, Szkudlarek M, Beggs I. Inflammatory joint diseases. In: Beggs I, ed. *Musculoskeletal Ultrasound*. Philadelphia, PA: Lippincott Williams & Wilkins; 2014:227.)

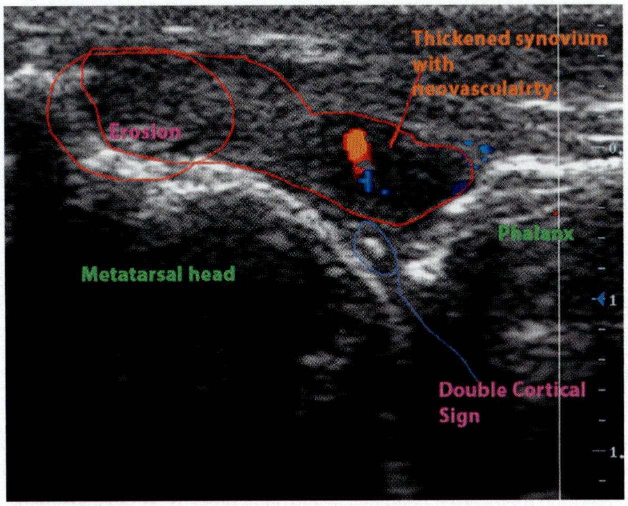

FIGURE 18.27 Longitudinal color Doppler image demonstrating synovitis of the right first metatarsophalangeal joint. Note the neovascularity.

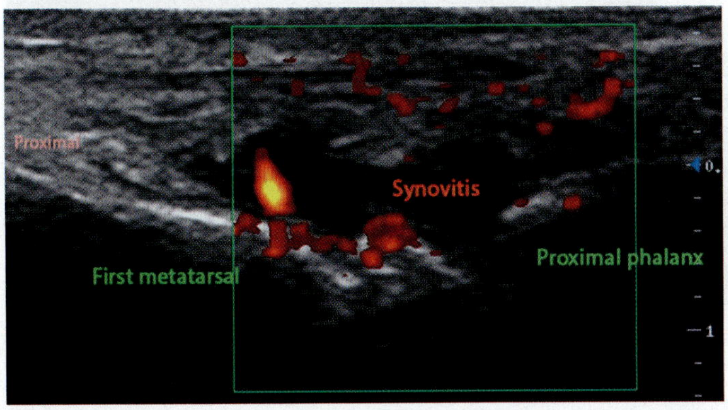

FIGURE 18.28 Longitudinal color Doppler image of the first metarsophalangeal joint demonstrating synovitis in a patient with active rheumatoid arthritis. Note the significant neovascularity.

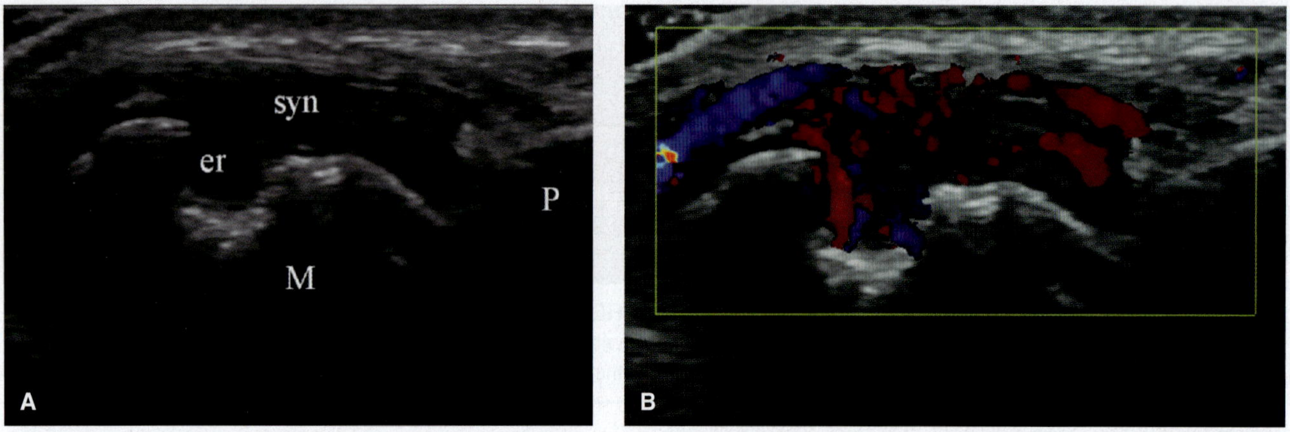

FIGURE 18.29 Dorsal longitudinal scans of second MTP joint in patient with RA. **A:** Synovial hypertrophy (syn) with erosion of metatarsal head (er). M, metatarsal head; P, proximal phalanx. **B:** Synovial hyperemia on color Doppler examination confirms active synovitis. (From Court-Payen M, Szkudlarek M, Beggs I. Inflammatory joint diseases. In: Beggs I, ed. *Musculoskeletal Ultrasound.* Philadelphia, PA: Lippincott Williams & Wilkins; 2014:223.)

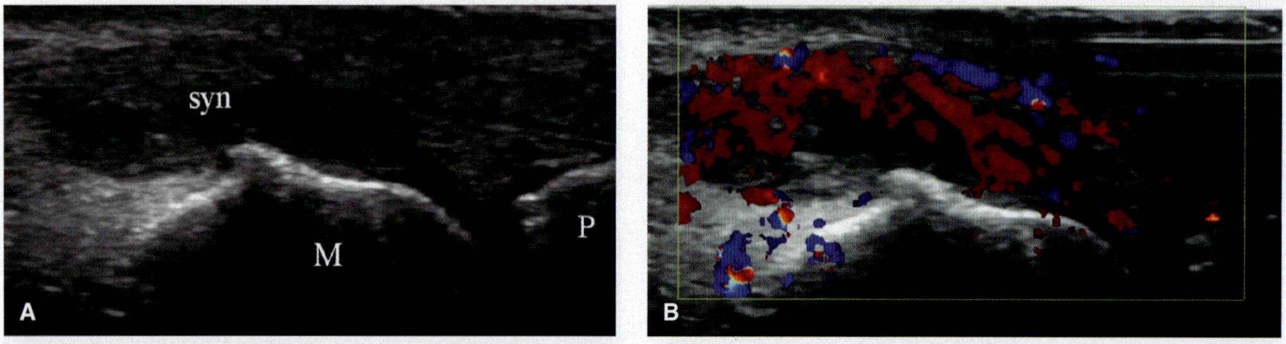

FIGURE 18.30 **A:** Dorsal longitudinal ultrasound scan of the third MCP joint shows synovial thickening (syn) extending from the joint line and along the metacarpal head (M). P, proximal phalanx. **B:** Synovial hyperemia on color Doppler examination confirms active synovitis. (From Court-Payen M, Szkudlarek M, Beggs I. Inflammatory joint diseases. In: Beggs I, ed. *Musculoskeletal Ultrasound.* Philadelphia, PA: Lippincott Williams & Wilkins; 2014:222.)

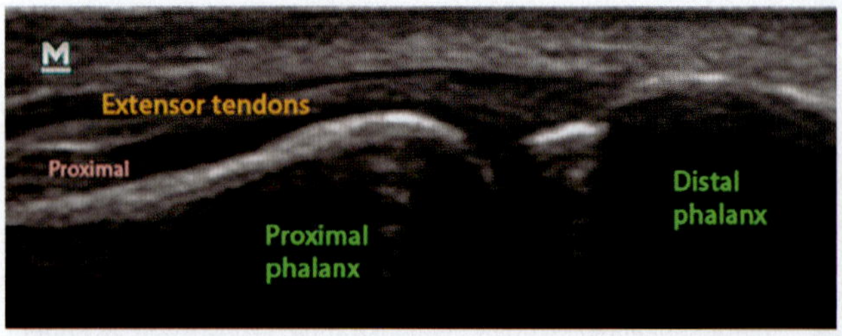

FIGURE 18.31 Longitudinal ultrasound image of a normal interphalangeal joint of the first toe.

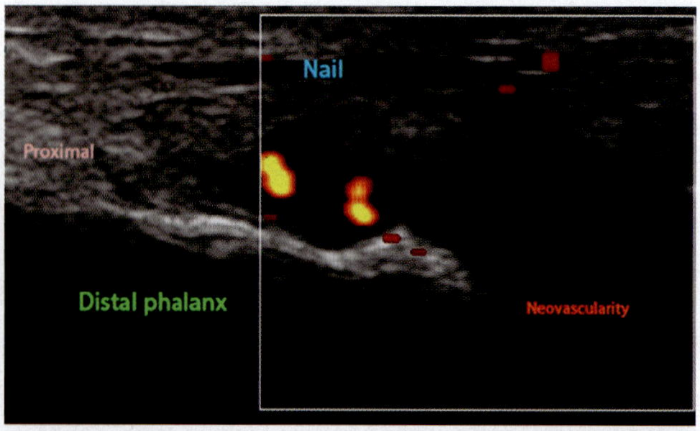

FIGURE 18.32 Longitudinal color Doppler image demonstrating acute inflammation of the distal interphalangeal joint.

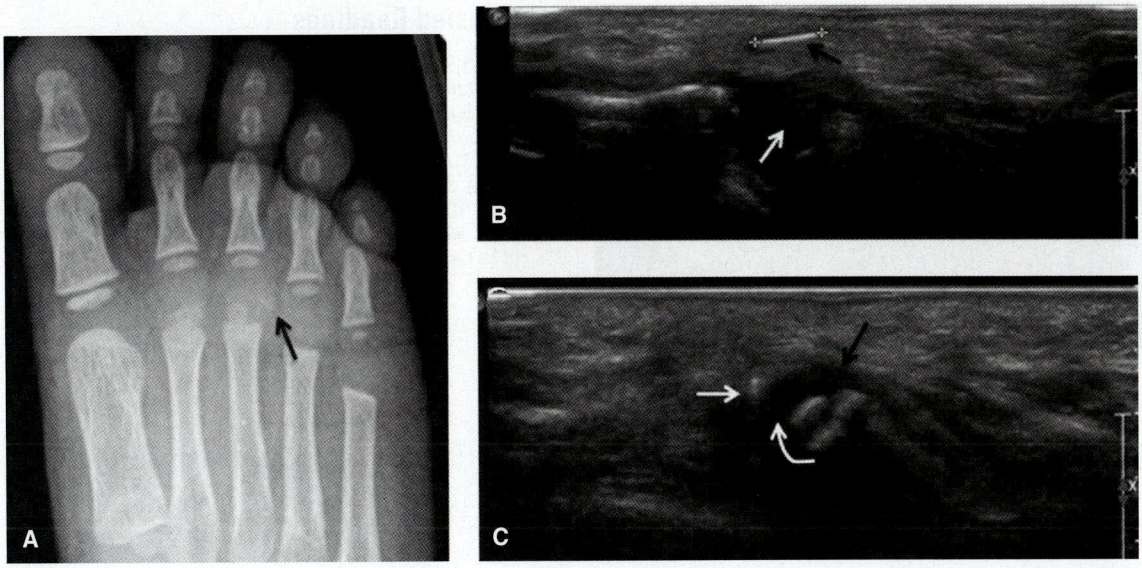

FIGURE 18.33 **A:** Oblique radiograph of the right foot in a 2-year-old patient showing two perpendicular, faint, linear, dense structures in the region of the third metatarsal head (*arrow*). **B:** Sagittal ultrasound image at the plantar foot revealing a 5-mm linear structure consistent with a foreign body (*black arrow*) in the subcutaneous tissues over the third metatarsal head (*white arrow*). **C:** Sagittal ultrasound image showing 2-mm linear object (*straight white arrow*) embedded in a tendon (*black arrow*) overlying the third metatarsal head (*curved white arrow*). (From Nwawka K, Kabutey NK, Locke CM, et al. Ultrasound-guided needle localization to aid foreign body removal in pediatric patients. *J Foot Ankle Surg* 2014;53(1):67–70.)

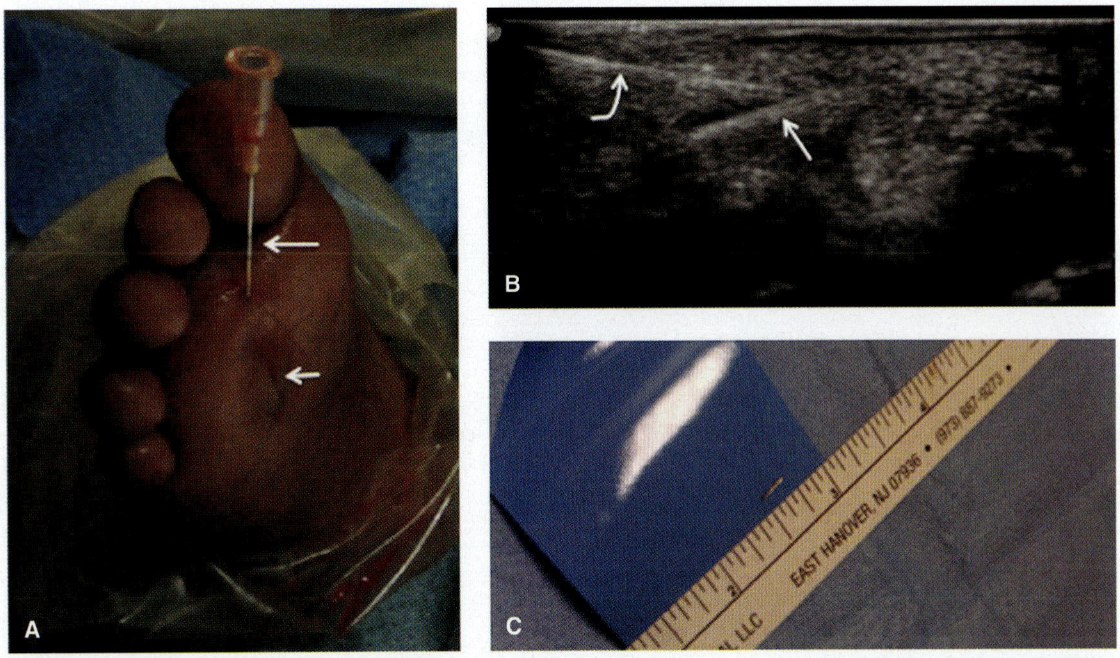

FIGURE 18.34 **A:** Right foot of a 2-year-old patient during the foreign body removal procedure. A small vertical incision (*short arrow*) for focal dissection was created directly inferior to the needle (*long arrow*) at the region of the needle tip. **B:** Sagittal image from high-frequency ultrasound-guided needle localization showing the needle (*curved arrow*) with its tip at the foreign object (*straight arrow*). **C:** The retrieved foreign body, a 5-mm shard of glass. (From Nwawka K, Kabutey NK, Locke CM, et al. Ultrasound-guided needle localization to aid foreign body removal in pediatric patients. *J Foot Ankle Surg* 2014;53(1):67–70.)

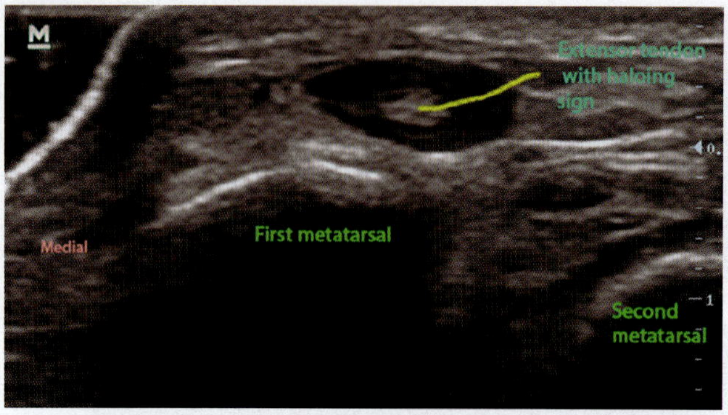

FIGURE 18.35 Transverse ultrasound image demonstrating tenosynovitis of the extensor tendon of the great toe. Note the positive halo sign caused by effusion around the tendon.

Suggested Readings

De Zordo T, Mur E, Bellmann-Weiler R, et al. US guided injections in arthritis. *Eur J Radiol* 2009;71(2):197–203.

Grassi W, Salaffi F, Filippucci E. Ultrasound in rheumatology. *Best Practice Res Clin Rheumatol* 2005;19(3):467–485.

Waldman SD. Intra-articular injection of the toe joints. In: *Pain Review.* Philadelphia, PA: Saunders; 2009:591–592.

Waldman SD. Technique for intra-articular injection of the toe joints. In: *Atlas of Pain Management Injection Techniques.* 3rd ed. Philadelphia, PA: Saunders; 2012:419–421.

CHAPTER 19

Hallux Valgus Deformity

ANATOMIC CONSIDERATIONS

The metatarsophalangeal joints are condyloid joints characterized by the articulation of the rounded articular surfaces of the metatarsal heads into the shallow concavities of the articular surfaces of the proximal end of the first phalanges (Fig. 19.1). Each joint is lined with synovium and the ample synovial space allows for intra-articular placement of needles for injection and aspiration. The metatarsophalangeal joints have a dense joint capsule and strong plantar and collateral ligaments, although fracture and subluxation may still occur (Figs. 19.2 and 19.3). The metatarsophalangeal joints are also susceptible to overuse and misuse injuries with resultant inflammation and arthritis (Fig. 19.4).

CLINICAL CORRELATES

Bunion, which is also known as the hallux valgus, refers to a constellation of symptoms including soft tissue swelling over the first metatarsophalangeal joint associated with abnormal angulation of the joint that results in a prominent first metatarsal head (Fig. 19.5). Ultimately, the first metatarsophalangeal joint may sublux, and the overlapping of the first and second toes worsens, resulting in a painful condition known as the hallux valgus deformity (Fig. 19.6). The metatarsocuneiform joint may also play a role in the evolution of hallux valgus (Fig. 19.7). Frequently an inflamed adventitious bursa may coexist with the bunion, further exacerbating the pain and cosmetic deformity (Fig. 19.8). More common in women, bunion is usually the result of wearing shoes with a too-tight toe box, with the wearing of high-heeled shoes exacerbating the problem.

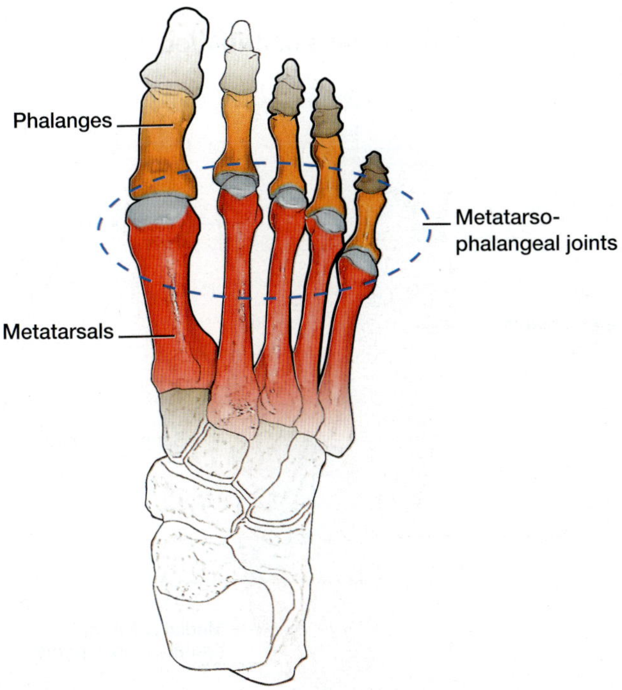

FIGURE 19.1 Anatomy of the metatarsophalangeal joints.

Most patients who present with bunion also present with the complaint of pain that is localized to the affected first metatarsophalangeal joint and the inability to get shoes to fit. Walking makes the pain worse, with rest and heat providing some relief. The pain is constant and is characterized as aching and may interfere with sleep. Some patients complain of a grating or popping sensation with use of the joint, and crepitus may be present on physical examination. In addition to the just-mentioned pain, patients who suffer with bunions develop the characteristic hallux valgus deformity, which consists of a prominent first metatarsal head and improper angulation of the joint, with overlapping first and second toes.

Functional disability often accompanies the pain of the hallux valgus joint. Patients will often notice increasing difficulty in performing their activities of daily living and tasks that require standing, walking, or weight bearing. If the pathologic process responsible for pain of hallux valgus is not adequately treated, the patient's functional disability may worsen and muscle wasting and ultimately a frozen first metatarsophalangeal joint may occur.

Plain radiographs are indicated in all patients who present with pain of the hallux valgus (Fig. 19.9). Based on the patient's clinical presentation, additional testing may be indicated including complete blood cell count, sedimentation rate, and antinuclear antibody testing. MRI or ultrasound of the hallux valgus joint is indicated if fracture, effusion, tendinopathy, crystal arthropathy, joint mice, synovitis, foreign body, bursitis, or ligamentous injury is suspected (Fig. 19.10).

ULTRASOUND TECHNIQUE

To perform ultrasound evaluation of hallux valgus, the patient is then placed in the supine position with the knee flexed so that the plantar surface of the affected foot rests comfortably on the examination table. With the patient in the above position,

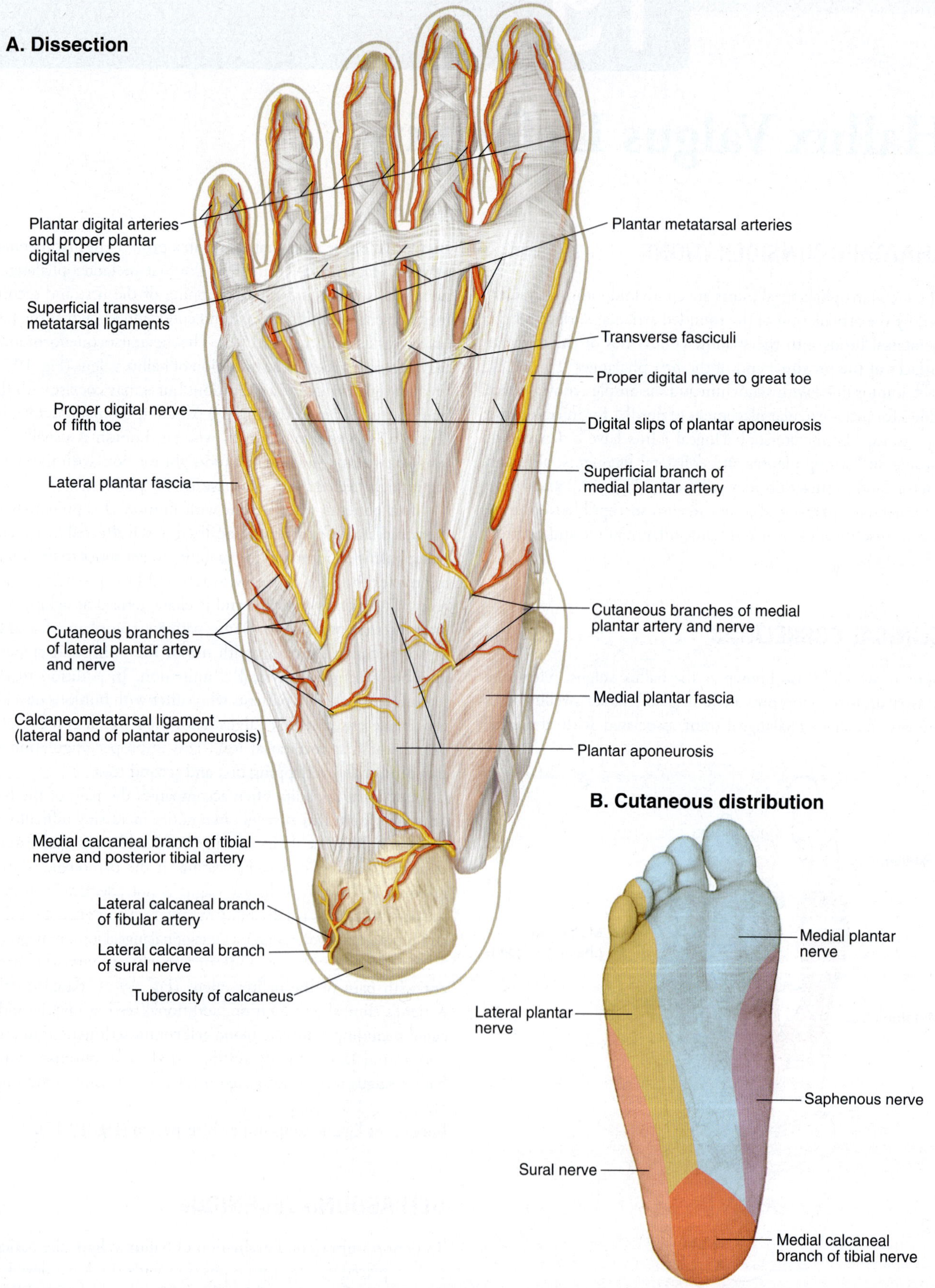

FIGURE 19.2 **A,B:** Cutaneous nerves of the sole of the foot. (From Tank PW, Gest TR. The lower limb. In: *Lippincott Williams & Wilkins Atlas of Anatomy.* Philadelphia, PA: Lippincott Williams & Wilkins; 2009:134.)

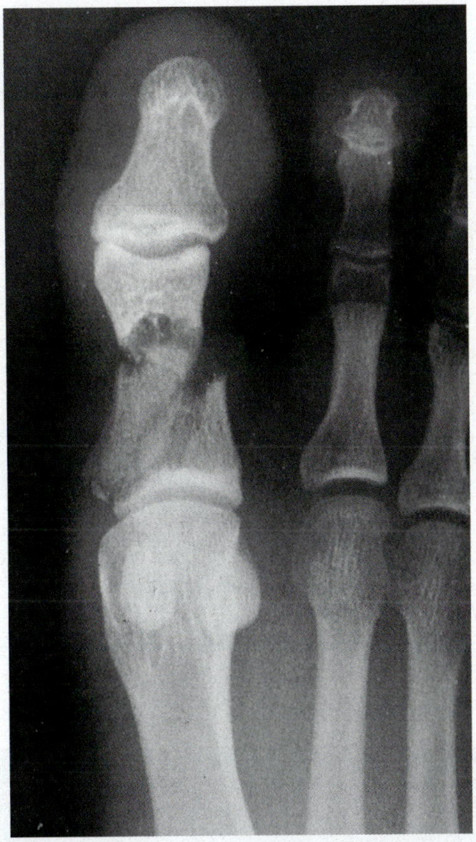

FIGURE 19.3 Posteroanterior radiograph of the foot shows a comminuted fracture through the shaft of the proximal phalanx of the great toe, extending immediately distal to the proximal articular surface of the phalanx. (From Rowe LJ, Yochum TR, Maola CJ. Trauma. In: *Yochum and Rowes' Essentials of Skeletal Radiology*. Vol 1. 3rd ed. Philadelphia, PA: Lippincott Williams & Wilkins; 2005:793.)

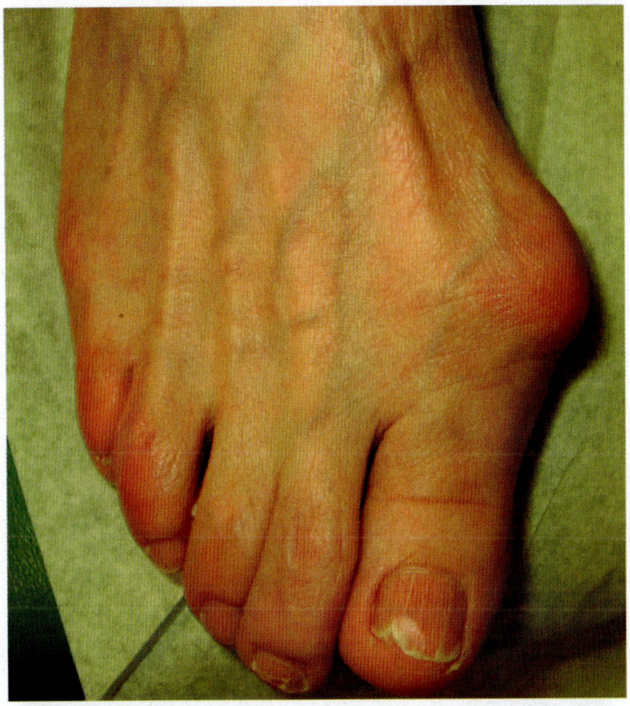

FIGURE 19.5 The classic appearance of hallux valgus deformity. (Image provided by Stedman's Medical Dictionary, 2013.)

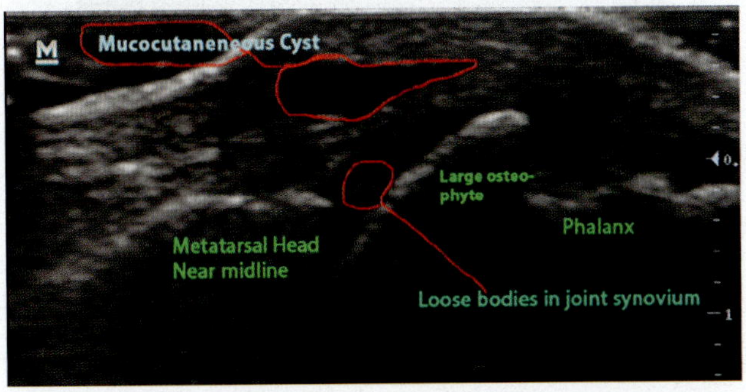

FIGURE 19.4 Longitudinal ultrasound image of the great toe demonstrating a large osteophyte with associated intra-articular joint mice of the right first metatarsophalangeal joint. Note the mucocutaneous cyst.

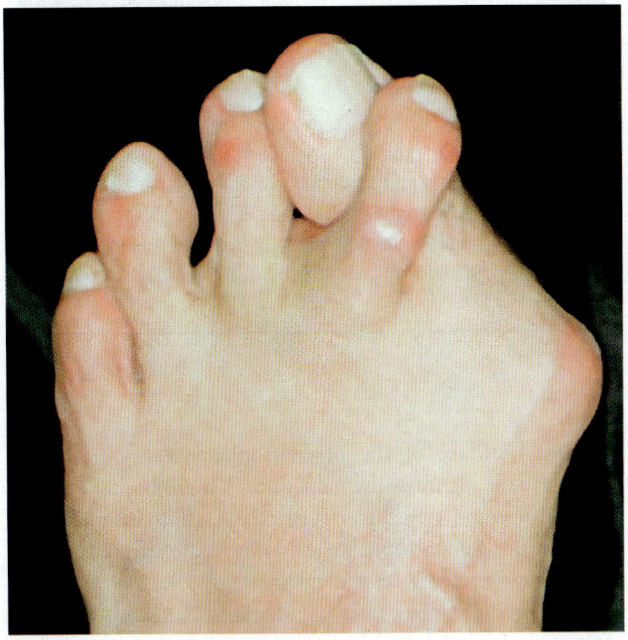

FIGURE 19.6 The hallux valgus deformity with subluxation of the first metatarsophalangeal joint resulting in the overlapping of the first and second toes. (From Weber J, Kelley J. *Health Assessment in Nursing*. 2nd ed. Philadelphia, PA: Lippincott Williams & Wilkins; 2003.)

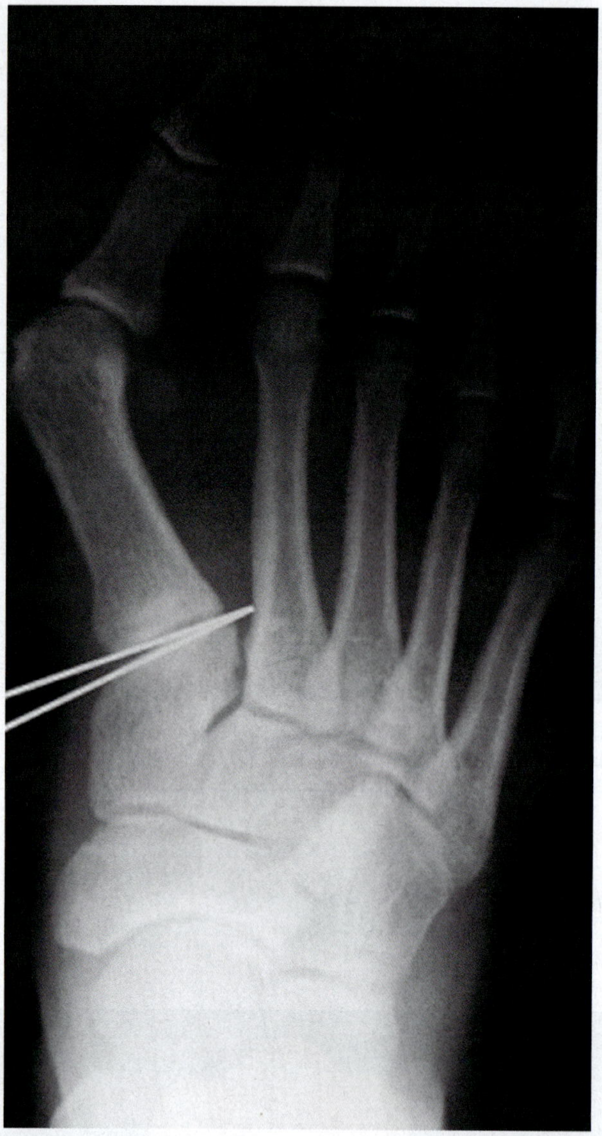

FIGURE 19.7 Plain radiograph demonstrating the angle between the base of the first metatarsal joint and the articular surface of the medial cuneiform. (From Jung HG, Lopez RGL, Lee SH, et al. Proximal reverse chevron metatarsal osteotomy and lateral release through 1 medial incision for hallux valgus correction. *Techn Foot Ankle Surg* 2014; 13(3):145–149.)

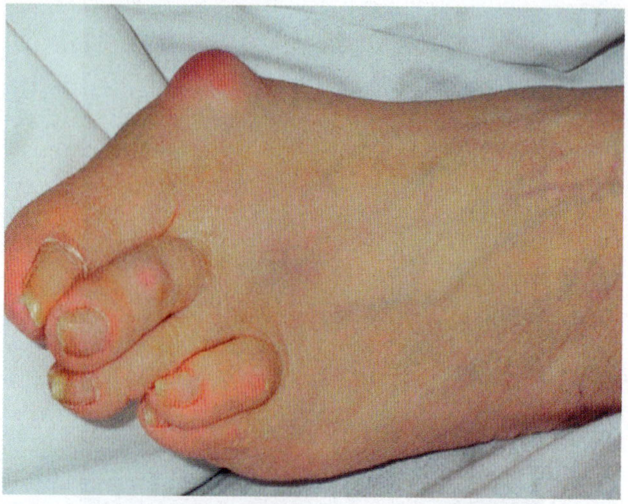

FIGURE 19.8 An inflamed adventitial bursa frequently accompanies the pain and functional disability associated with bunion. (From Berg D, Worzala K. *Atlas of Adult Physical Diagnosis*. Philadelphia, PA: Lippincott Williams & Wilkins; 2006.)

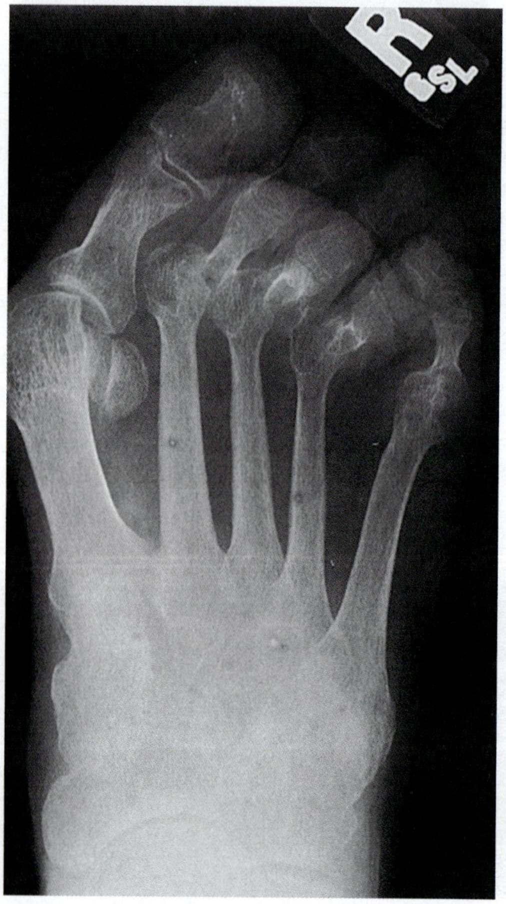

FIGURE 19.9 Plain radiograph of the hallux valgus deformity. (From Koopman WJ, Moreland LW. *Arthritis and Allied Conditions: a Textbook of Rheumatology*. 15th ed. Philadelphia, PA: Lippincott Williams & Wilkins; 2005.)

the dorsal surface of the metatarsophalangeal joint of the affected toe is identified by palpation. A high-frequency small linear ultrasound transducer is placed in a longitudinal position over the metatarsophalangeal joint of the affected toe and an ultrasound survey scan is taken (Figs. 19.11 and 19.12). The hypoechoic joint space is identified between the head of the metatarsal and the base of the proximal phalanges. When the joint space is identified, the joint is assessed for degenerative changes, synovitis, effusion, crystal arthropathy as well as the angle between the articular surfaces of both joints (Fig. 19.13). The integrity of the plantar plate is also evaluated (Fig. 19.14).

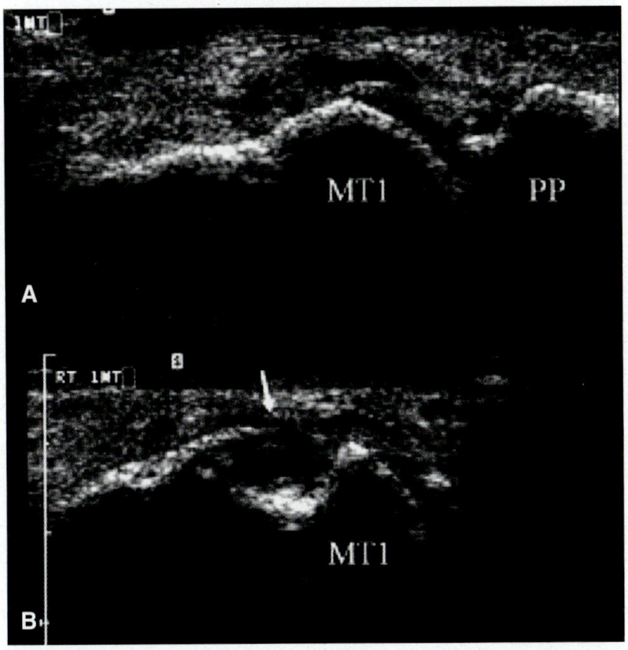

FIGURE 19.10 **A:** Longitudinal of the first metatarsophalangeal (MTP) joint in a patient with hallux valgus deformity demonstrating a small effusion. The first metatarsal (MT1) and proximal phalanx (PP) are labeled. **B:** Long-axis view of the first MTP joint in the same patient scanned along the medial joint line, demonstrates cystic change in the first metatarsal head (*arrow*). (From Adler R, Sofka CM, Positano RG. *Atlas of Foot and Ankle Sonography*. Philadelphia, PA: Lippincott Williams & Wilkins; 2004:29.)

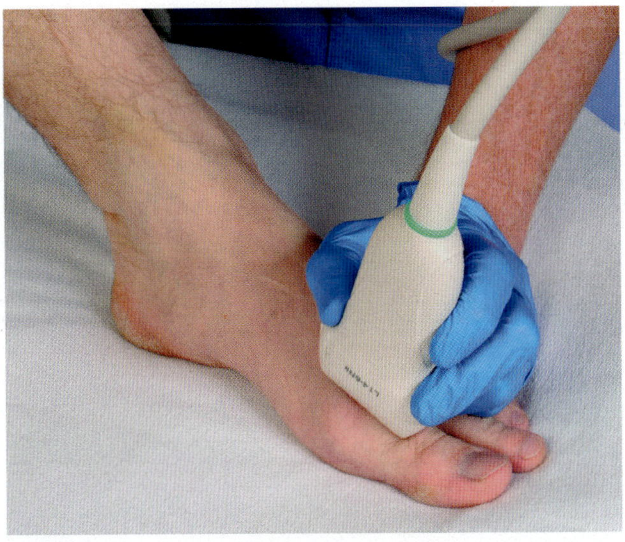

FIGURE 19.11 Correct longitudinal position for ultrasound transducer for ultrasound evaluation of the first metatarsophalangeal joint.

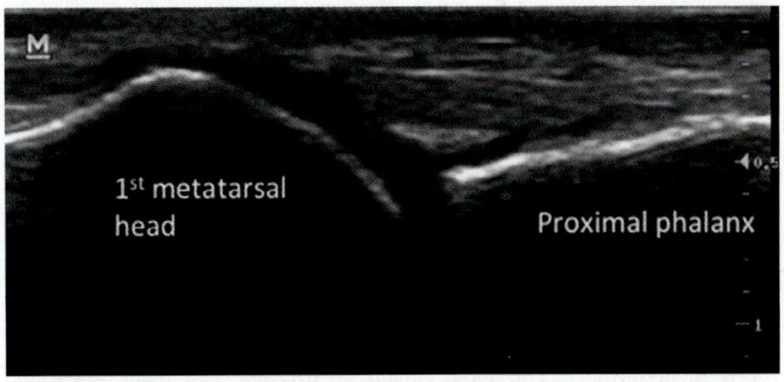

FIGURE 19.12 Longitudinal ultrasound view of the metatarsophalangeal joint space of the great toe.

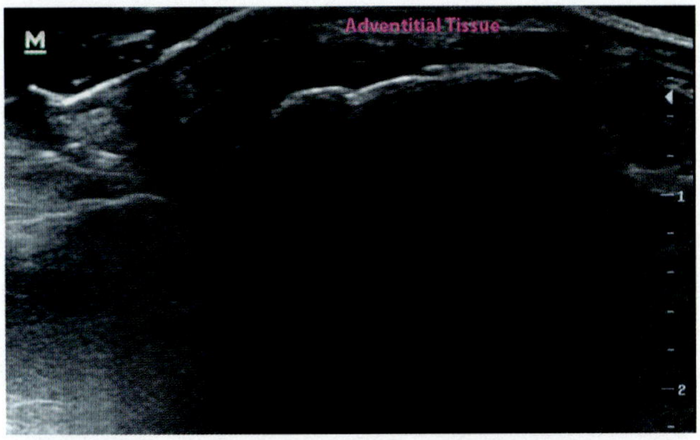

FIGURE 19.13 Longitudinal ultrasound view of hallux valgus. Note the significant adventitial tissue over the lateral great toe.

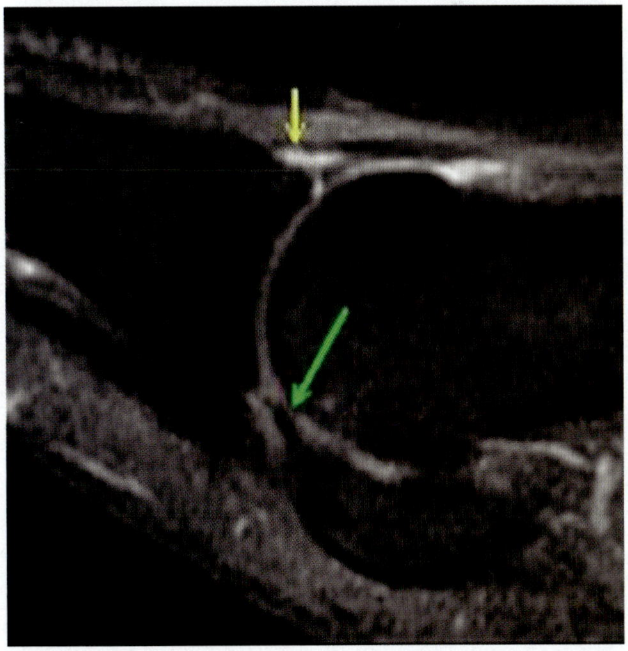

FIGURE 19.14 Longitudinal ultrasound image demonstrating the plantar plate of the first metatarsophalangeal joint. Green arrow, plantar plate; yellow arrow, small effusion.

CLINICAL PEARLS

Toe pathology including tendinopathy, occult fractures, osteoarthritis, rheumatoid arthritis, crystal arthropathies, avascular necrosis bursitis, synovitis, and impingement syndromes may coexist with disease of the hallux valgus and may contribute to the patient's pain symptoms.

Suggested Readings

Albert A, Leemrijse T. The dorsal bunion: an overview. *Foot Ankle Surg* 2005; 11(2):65–68.

Kennedy JG, Collumbier JA. Bunions in dancers. *Clin Sports Med* 2008;27(2): 321–328.

Mann R. Bunion deformity in elite athletes. In: Porter DA, Schon LC, eds. *Baxter's the Foot and Ankle in Sport.* 2nd ed. St Louis, MO: Mosby; 2008: 435–443.

Mann RA, Horton GA. Management of the foot and ankle in rheumatoid arthritis. *Rheum Dis Clin North Am* 1996;22(3):457–476.

Motta-Valencia K. Dance-related injury. *Phys Med Rehab Clin N Am* 2006;17(3): 697–723.

Waldman SD. Intra-articular injection of the toe joints. In: *Pain Review.* Philadelphia, PA: Saunders; 2009:591–592.

Waldman SD. Technique for intra-articular injection of the toe joints. In: *Atlas of Pain Management Injection Techniques.* 3rd ed. Philadelphia, PA: Saunders; 2012:419–421.

CHAPTER 20

Bunionette

ANATOMIC CONSIDERATIONS

The metatarsophalangeal joints are condyloid joints characterized by the articulation of the rounded articular surfaces of the metatarsal heads into the shallow concavities of the articular surfaces of the proximal end of the first phalanges (Fig. 20.1). Each joint is lined with synovium and the ample synovial space allows for intra-articular placement of needles for injection and aspiration. The metatarsophalangeal joints have a dense joint capsule and strong plantar and collateral ligaments, although fracture and subluxation may still occur (Figs. 20.2 to 20.4). The metatarsophalangeal joints are also susceptible to overuse and misuse injuries with resultant inflammation and arthritis.

CLINICAL CORRELATES

Bunionette, which is also known as the tailor's bunion, refers to a constellation of symptoms including soft tissue swelling over the fifth metatarsophalangeal joint associated with abnormal angulations of the joint that results in a prominent fifth metatarsal head (Fig. 20.5). Ultimately, the fifth metatarsophalangeal joint may sublux, and a corn overlying the metatarsal head will develop along with an inflamed adventitious bursa may coexist with the bunionette, further exacerbating the pain and cosmetic deformity (Figs. 20.6 and 20.7). Occurring more commonly in women, bunionette is most commonly the result of wearing shoes with a too-tight toe box, with the wearing of high-heeled shoes exacerbating the problem.

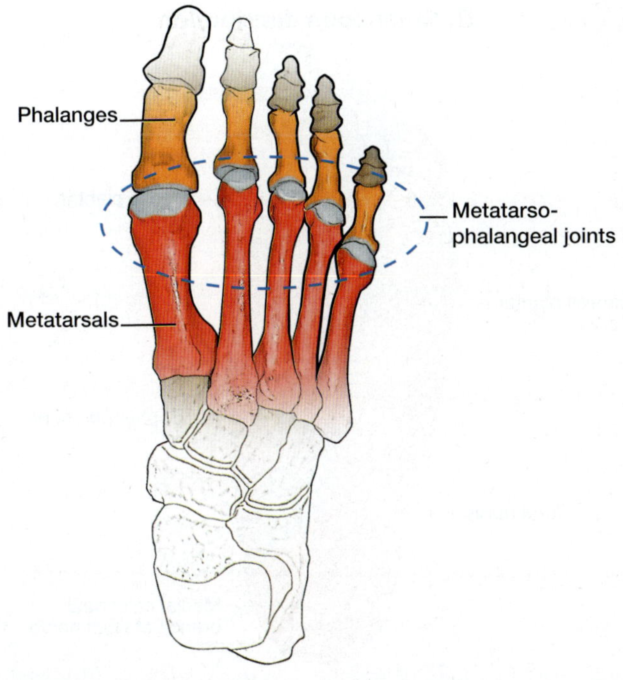

FIGURE 20.1 Anatomy of the metatarsophalangeal joints.

Most patients who present with bunionette also present with the complaint of pain that is localized to the affected fifth metatarsophalangeal joint and the inability to get shoes to fit. Walking makes the pain worse, with rest and heat providing some relief. The pain is constant and is characterized as aching and may interfere with sleep. Some patients complain of a grating or popping sensation with use of the joint and crepitus may be present on physical examination. In addition to the just-mentioned pain, patients who suffer with bunionette develop the characteristic bunionette deformity, which consists of a prominent fifth metatarsal head and improper angulation of the fifth metatarsal (Fig. 20.8).

Functional disability often accompanies the pain of the bunionette joint. Patients will often notice increasing difficulty in performing their activities of daily living and tasks that require standing, walking, or weight bearing. If the pathologic process responsible for pain of bunionette is not adequately treated, the patient's functional disability may worsen and muscle wasting and ultimately a frozen fifth metatarsophalangeal joint may occur.

Plain radiographs are indicated in all patients who present with pain of the bunionette (Figs. 20.9 and 20.10). Based on the patient's clinical presentation, additional testing may be indicated, including complete blood cell count, sedimentation rate, and antinuclear antibody testing. MRI or ultrasound of the bunionette joint is indicated if fracture, effusion, tendinopathy, crystal arthropathy, joint mice, synovitis, foreign body, bursitis, or ligamentous injury is suspected (Fig. 20.11).

ULTRASOUND TECHNIQUE

To perform ultrasound evaluation of the fifth metatarsophalangeal joint the patient is placed in the supine position with

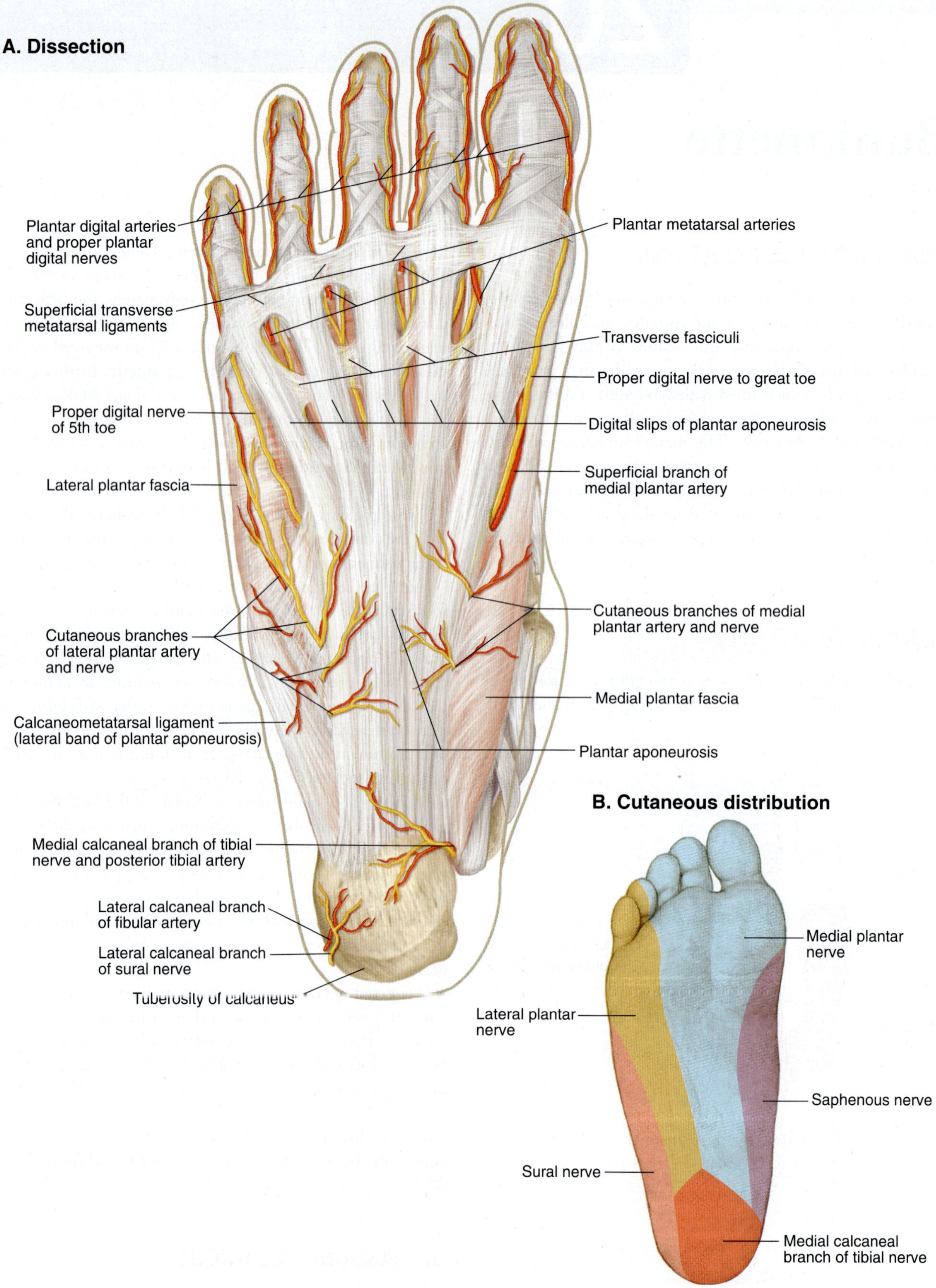

FIGURE 20.2 **A,B:** Cutaneous nerves of the sole of the foot. (From Tank PW, Gest TR. The lower limb. In: *Lippincott Williams & Wilkins Atlas of Anatomy*. Philadelphia, PA: Lippincott Williams & Wilkins; 2009:134.)

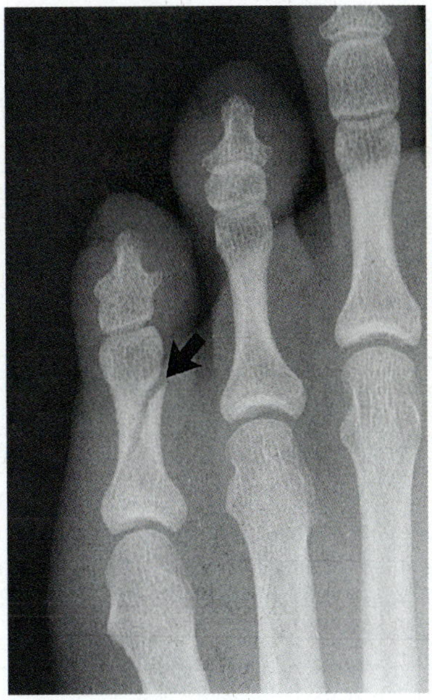

FIGURE 20.3 Radiograph of bedroom fracture of the dorsoplantar toes. Note the oblique fracture of the shaft of the proximal phalanx of the fifth toe (*arrow*), which occurred after striking a hard object. (Courtesy of Gaylord H. Hanssen, DC, Doniphan, Nebraska. From Rowe LJ, Yochum TR, Maola CR. Trauma. In: *Yochum and Rowes' Essentials of Skeletal Radiology*. Vol 1. 3rd ed. Philadelphia, PA: Lippincott Williams & Wilkins; 2005:884.)

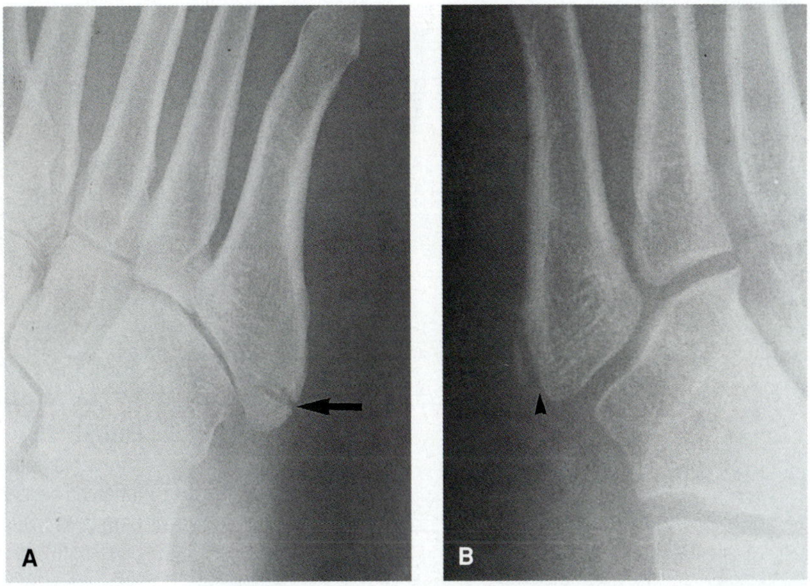

FIGURE 20.4 **A:** Jones fracture of the medial oblique foot. Note the characteristic transverse orientation of the fracture line of the base of the fifth metatarsal (*arrow*). **B:** Normal. Note the apophysis for the base of the fifth metatarsal separated by a longitudinally oriented lucent cleft (*arrowhead*). With skeletal maturation, this radiolucent cleft will eventually ossify and become united to the base of the fifth metatarsal. (From Rowe LJ, Yochum TR, Maola CR. Trauma. In: *Yochum and Rowes' Essentials of Skeletal Radiology*. Vol 1. 3rd ed. Philadelphia, PA: Lippincott Williams & Wilkins; 2005:884.)

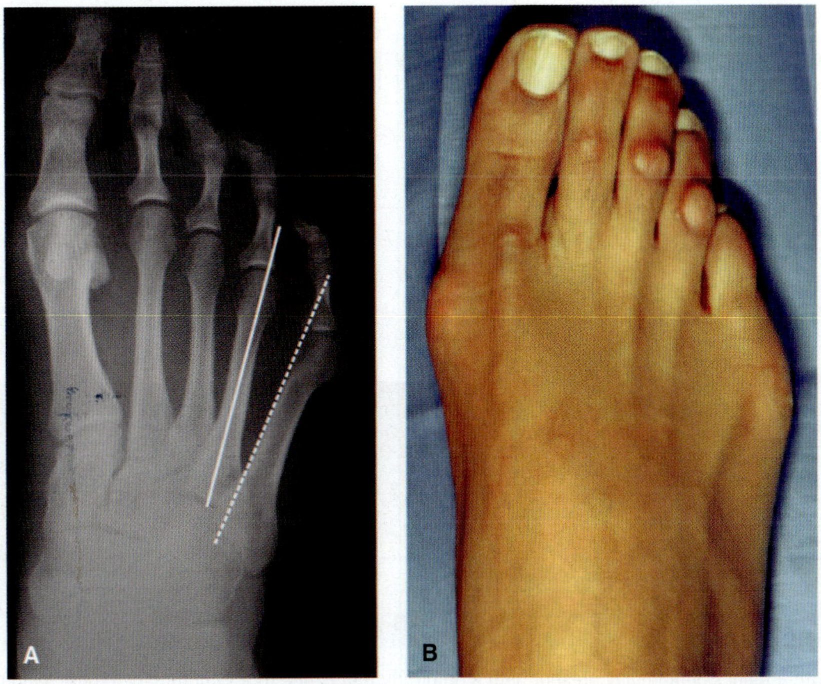

FIGURE 20.5 Tailor's bunion deformity. **A:** Plain radiograph demonstrating bunionette deformity. **B:** Clinically, the patient generally presents with symptoms occurring laterally or plantar laterally, often with an adduction of the fifth toe. (From Thomas JL, Blitch EL 4th, Chaney DM, et al. Diagnosis and treatment of forefoot disorders. Section 4. Tailor's bunion. *J Foot Ankle Surg* 2009;48(2):257–263; Fig. 1.)

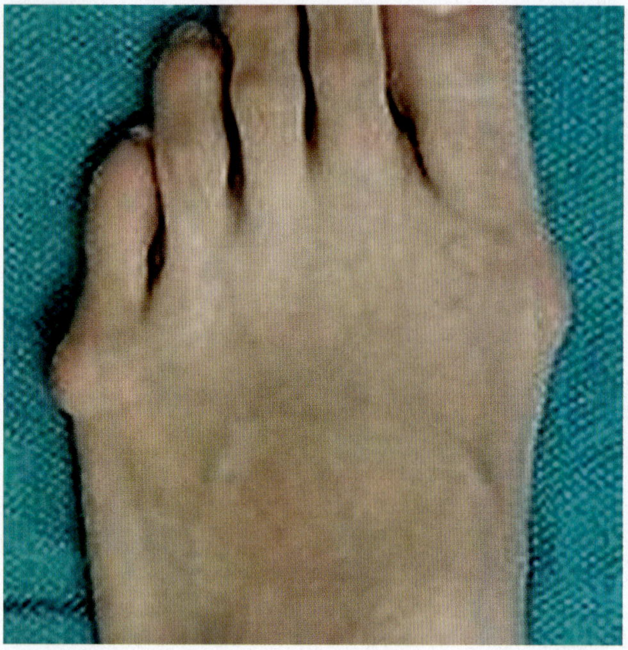

FIGURE 20.6 Significant corn and adventitial bursitis development can accompany the bunionette deformity.

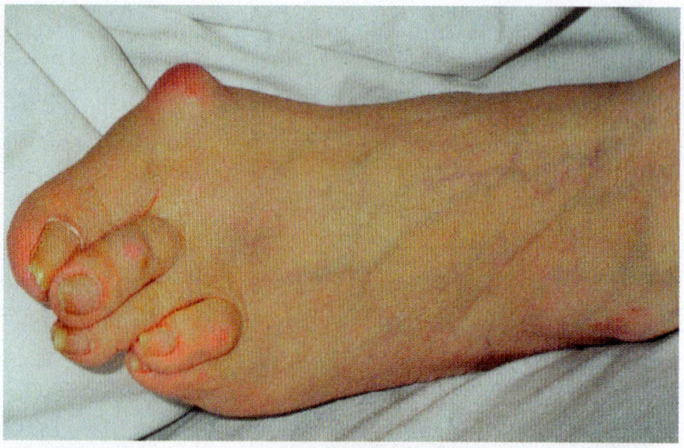

FIGURE 20.7 Bunionette affects the fifth metatarsophalangeal joint. This patient also suffers from hallux valgus with a significantly inflamed adventitial bursa of the first metatarsophalangeal joint. (From Berg D, Worzala K. *Atlas of Adult Physical Diagnosis*. Philadelphia, PA: Lippincott Williams & Wilkins; 2006.)

the knee flexed so that the plantar surface of the affected foot rests comfortably on the examination table. With the patient in the above position, the dorsal surface of the metatarsophalangeal joint of the affected toe is identified by palpation. A high-frequency small linear ultrasound transducer is placed in a longitudinal position over the metatarsophalangeal joint of the affected toe and an ultrasound survey scan is taken (Figs. 20.12 and 20.13). The hypoechic joint space is identified between the head of the metatarsal and the base of the proximal phalanges. When the joint space is identified, the adjacent articular surfaces are evaluated for degenerative changes, synovitis, effusion, crystal arthropathy as well as the angle between the articular surfaces of both affected joints.

CLINICAL PEARLS

Toe pathology including tendinopathy, occult fractures, osteoarthritis, rheumatoid arthritis, crystal arthropathies, avascular necrosis bursitis, synovitis, and impingement syndromes may

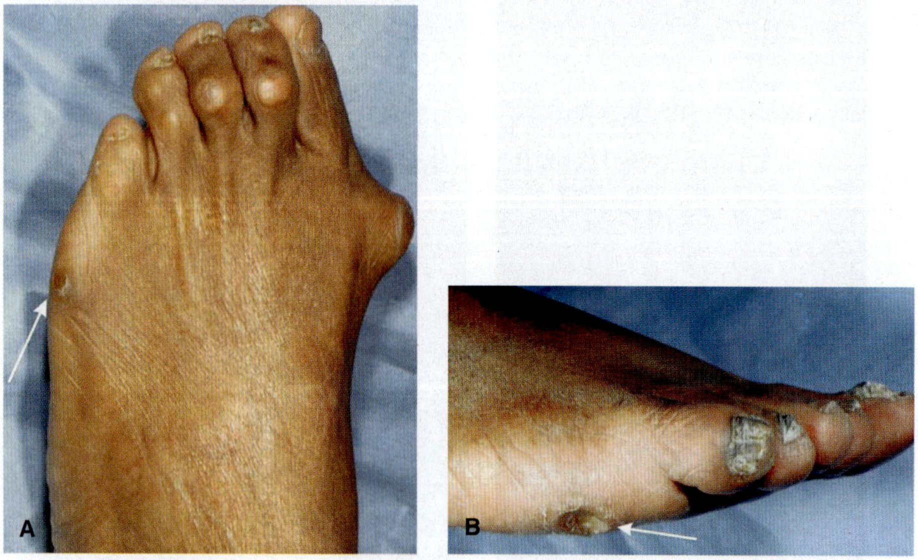

FIGURE 20.8 Patients with a tailor's bunion may present with a deformity that is due to a symptomatic lateral lesion **(A)** or a plantar keratotic lesion **(B)**. (From Thomas JL, Blitch EL 4th, Chaney DM, et al. Diagnosis and treatment of forefoot disorders. Section 4. Tailor's bunion. *J Foot Ankle Surg* 2009;48(2):257–263.)

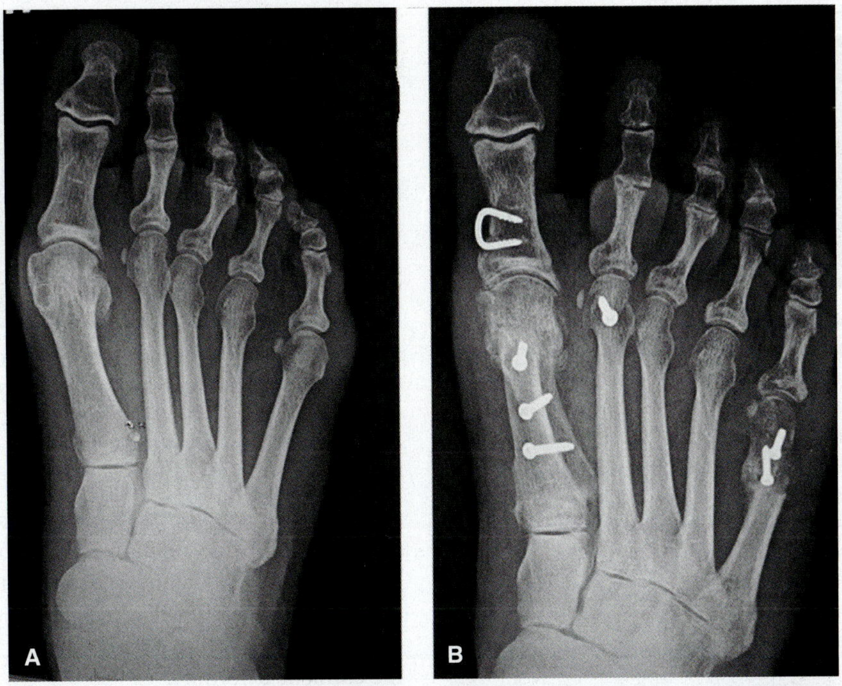

FIGURE 20.9 **A,B:** Anteroposterior radiographof bunionette deformity. (From Cooper MT, Coughlin MJ. Subcapital oblique osteotomy for correction of bunionette deformity: modification of technique and expanded indications. *Tech Foot Ankle Surg* 2014;13(3):140–144.)

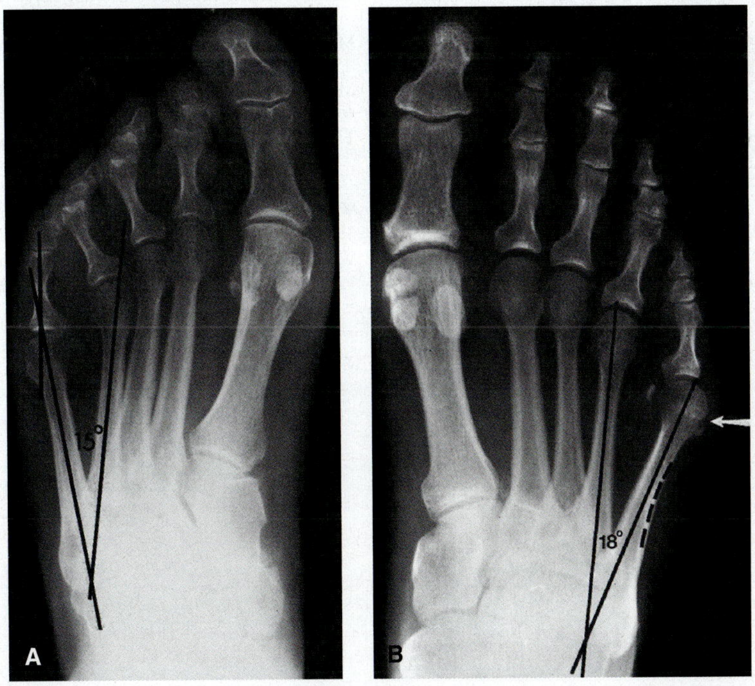

FIGURE 20.10 Bunionette deformities. **A:** Bunionette deformity with a fourth–fifth metatarsal angle of 15 degrees. **B:** More severe bunionette deformity with prominence of the metatarsal head and bone erosion (*arrow*), lateral bowing (*broken line*), and a fourth–fifth metatarsal angle of 18 degrees. (From Berquist TH, Whalen JL. Reconstructive procedures: preoperative and postoperative imaging. In: *Imaging of the Foot and Ankle*. 3rd ed. Philadelphia, PA: Lippincott Williams & Wilkins; 2011:620.)

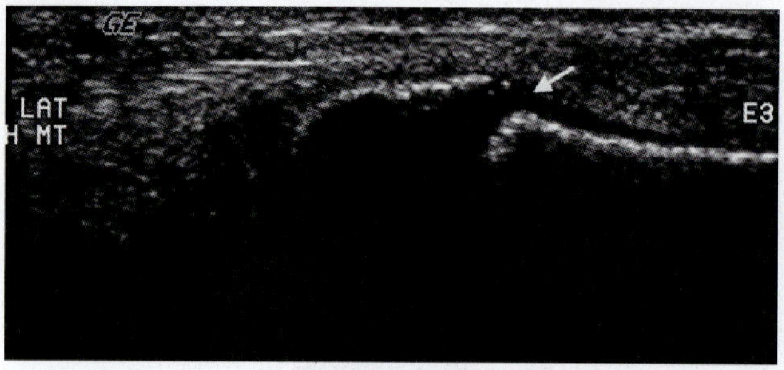

FIGURE 20.11 Patient with lateral midfoot pain following an inversion injury. A cortical stepoff and subperiosteal hematoma are evident (*arrow*) at the site of a minimally displaced fracture of the base of the fifth metatarsal. A minimally displaced fracture was confirmed radiographically (not shown). (From Adler R, Sofka CM, Positano RG. *Atlas of Foot and Ankle Sonography*. Philadelphia, PA: Lippincott Williams & Wilkins; 2004:37.)

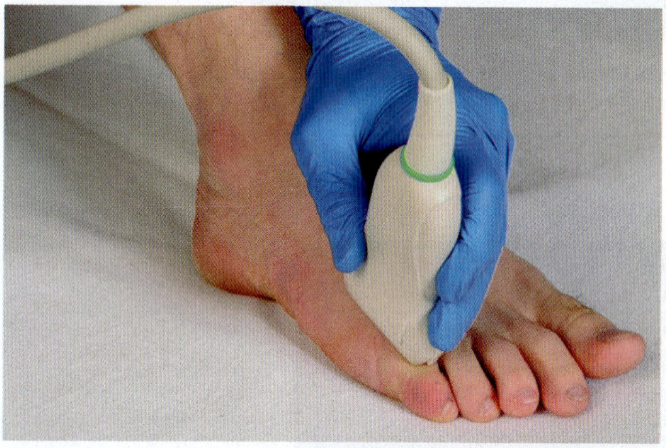

FIGURE 20.12 Correct longitudinal position for ultrasound transducer for ultrasound evaluation of bunionette deformity.

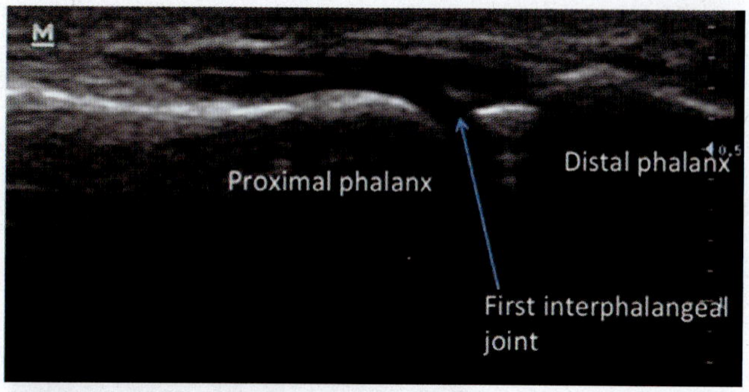

FIGURE 20.13 Longitudinal ultrasound view of the metatarsophalangeal joint space of the great toe. Dorsal aspect of the foot: Metatarsophalangeal joint digit 2 and extensor digitorum tendon longitudinal.

coexist with disease of the bunionette and may contribute to the patient's pain symptoms. Ultrasound-guided injection of the bunionette deformity with local anesthetic and anti-inflammatory steroid will often provide dramatic symptomatic improvement, but surgery will usually be required to correct the cosmetic deformity.

Suggested Readings

Ajis A, Koti M, Maffulli N. Tailor's bunion: a review. *J Foot Ankle Surg* 2005; 44(3):236–245.

Cooper MT. The bunionette deformity: overview and classification. *Tech Foot Ankle Surg* 2010;9(1):2–4.

Mann RA, Horton GA. Management of the foot and ankle in rheumatoid. *Rheum Dis Clin North Am* 1996;22(3):457–476.

Motta-Valencia K. Dance-related injury. *Phys Med Rehabil Clin N Am* 2006;17(3): 697–723.

Thomas JL, Blitch EL 4th, Chaney DM, et al. Diagnosis and treatment of forefoot disorders. Section 2. Central metatarsalgia. *J Foot Ankle Surg* 2009;48(2): 239–272.

Waldman SD. Intra-articular injection of the toe joints. In: *Pain Review.* Philadelphia, PA: Saunders; 2009:591–592.

Waldman SD. Injection technique for bunionette. In: *Atlas of Pain Management Injection Techniques.* 3rd ed. Philadelphia, PA: Saunders; 2012:446–448.

CHAPTER 21

Hammer Toe, Claw Toe, and Mallet Toe Pain Syndromes

ANATOMIC CONSIDERATIONS

The interphalangeal joints of the foot are ginglymoid joints (Fig. 21.1). Each joint has its own capsule. The articular surface of these joints is covered with hyaline cartilage that is susceptible to arthritis. The toe joint capsules are lined with a synovial membrane that attaches to the articular cartilage. The deep transverse ligaments connect the joints of the five toes and provide majority of strength to the toe joints (Fig. 21.2). The muscles of the toe joint and their attaching tendons are susceptible to trauma and to wear and tear from overuse and misuse. These joints are also susceptible to overuse and misuse injuries with resultant inflammation, arthritis, and deformity (Fig. 21.3).

CLINICAL CORRELATES

Hammertoe refers to a constellation of symptoms including a painful flexion deformity of the proximal interphalangeal joint with the middle and distal phalanges flexed down onto the proximal phalange. Hammertoe deformity almost always involves the second toe and the condition is almost always bilateral (Figs. 21.4 and 21.5). Significant dorsal corns may develop further exacerbating the deformity (Fig. 21.6). Over time the affected joints may become ankylosed, making the proper fitting of shoes next to impossible (Fig. 21.7). Occurring more commonly in women, like hallux valgus, hammertoe is most commonly the result of wearing shoes with a too-tight toe box, with the wearing of high-heeled shoes exacerbating the problem (Fig. 21.8).

Most patients who present with hammertoe complain of pain localized to the affected proximal interphalangeal joint and of being unable to get shoes to fit. Walking makes the pain worse, with rest and heat providing some relief. The pain is constant and is characterized as aching and may interfere with sleep. Some patients complain of a grating or popping sensation with use of the joint and crepitus may be present on physical examination. In addition to the just-mentioned pain, patients who suffer with hammertoes develop the characteristic hammertoe deformity, which consists of a painful flexion deformity of the proximal interphalangeal joint with the middle and distal phalanges flexed down onto the proximal phalange (Fig. 21.3). Functional disability often accompanies the pain of the hammertoe joint. Patients will often notice increasing difficulty in performing their activities of daily living and tasks that require standing, walking, or weight bearing. If the pathologic process responsible for pain of hammertoe is not adequately treated, the patient's functional disability may worsen and muscle wasting and ultimately a frozen interphalangeal joint may occur.

Claw toe is a common toe deformity that is the result of hyperextension of the metatarsophalangeal joint with significant flexion at both the proximal and distal interphalangeal joints (Fig. 21.9). Claw toe is a disease of the later decades, occurring five times more frequently in women. Frequently associated with neurologic diseases including Charcot–Marie–Tooth disease, Charcot joint, cerebral palsy, and multiple sclerosis as well as inflammatory arthropathies, if untreated the deformity will become permanent, making wearing shoes difficult if not impossible. Patients suffering from claw toe will complain of pain over the dorsal aspect of the proximal interphalangeal joint, which is raised like a bird's claw, causing impingement on the top of the shoe. Coexistent pain on the tip of the affected toe is often present as the toe tip is forced against the inside bottom of the shoe. This toe-tip pain is made worse with walking. Callus formation over the points of impingement are common as is nail deformity (Fig. 21.10).

Mallet toe is the result of a flexion contracture of the distal interphalangeal joint, occurring most commonly in the second toe (Figs. 21.3 and 21.11). Causes include hyperextension injuries to the toes which result in avulsion of the distal insertion of the extensor tendon as well as inflammatory arthropathies (Fig. 21.12). The patient will complain of pain at the distal interphalangeal joint and the tip of the toe. As with claw toe, pressure from the inside of the patient's shoe may cause corn and callus formation as well as pressure ulcers, especially in insensate feet. With time the flexion deformity becomes ankylosed further worsening the pain and deformity. Nail abnormality from constant downward pressure is also a common finding in patients suffering from mallet toe.

Plain radiographs are indicated in all patients who present with pain and deformity of hammertoe, claw toe, and mallet toe (Figs. 21.13 to 21.15). Based on the patient's clinical presentation, additional testing may be indicated including complete blood cell count, sedimentation rate, and antinuclear antibody testing. MRI or ultrasound of the affected joint is indicated if fracture, effusion, tendinopathy, crystal arthropathy, joint mice, synovitis, foreign body, bursitis, or ligamentous injury is suspected.

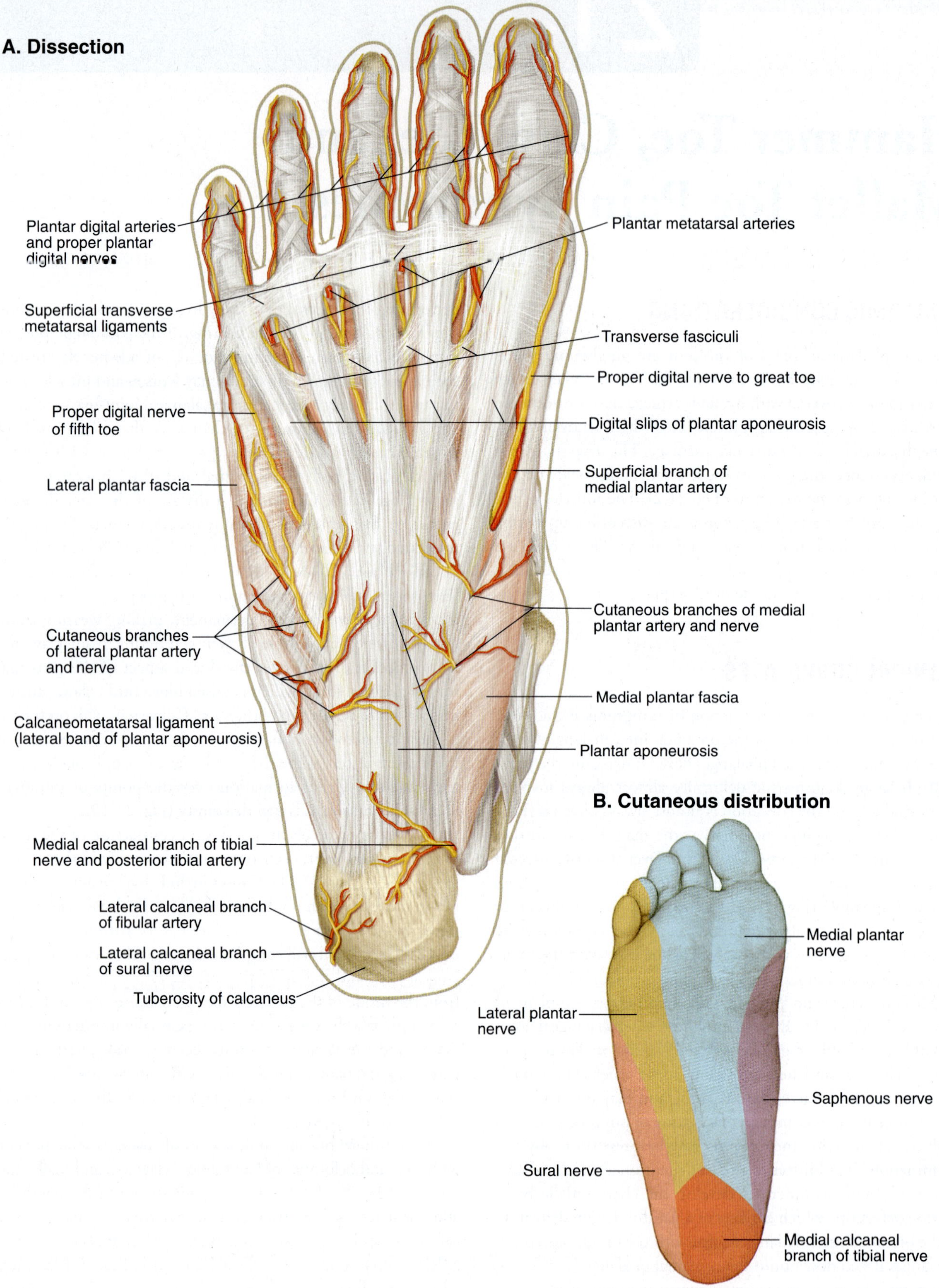

FIGURE 21.1 **A,B:** Cutaneous nerves of the sole of the foot. (From Tank PW, Gest TR. The lower limb. In: *Lippincott Williams & Wilkins Atlas of Anatomy*. Philadelphia, PA: Lippincott Williams & Wilkins; 2009:134.)

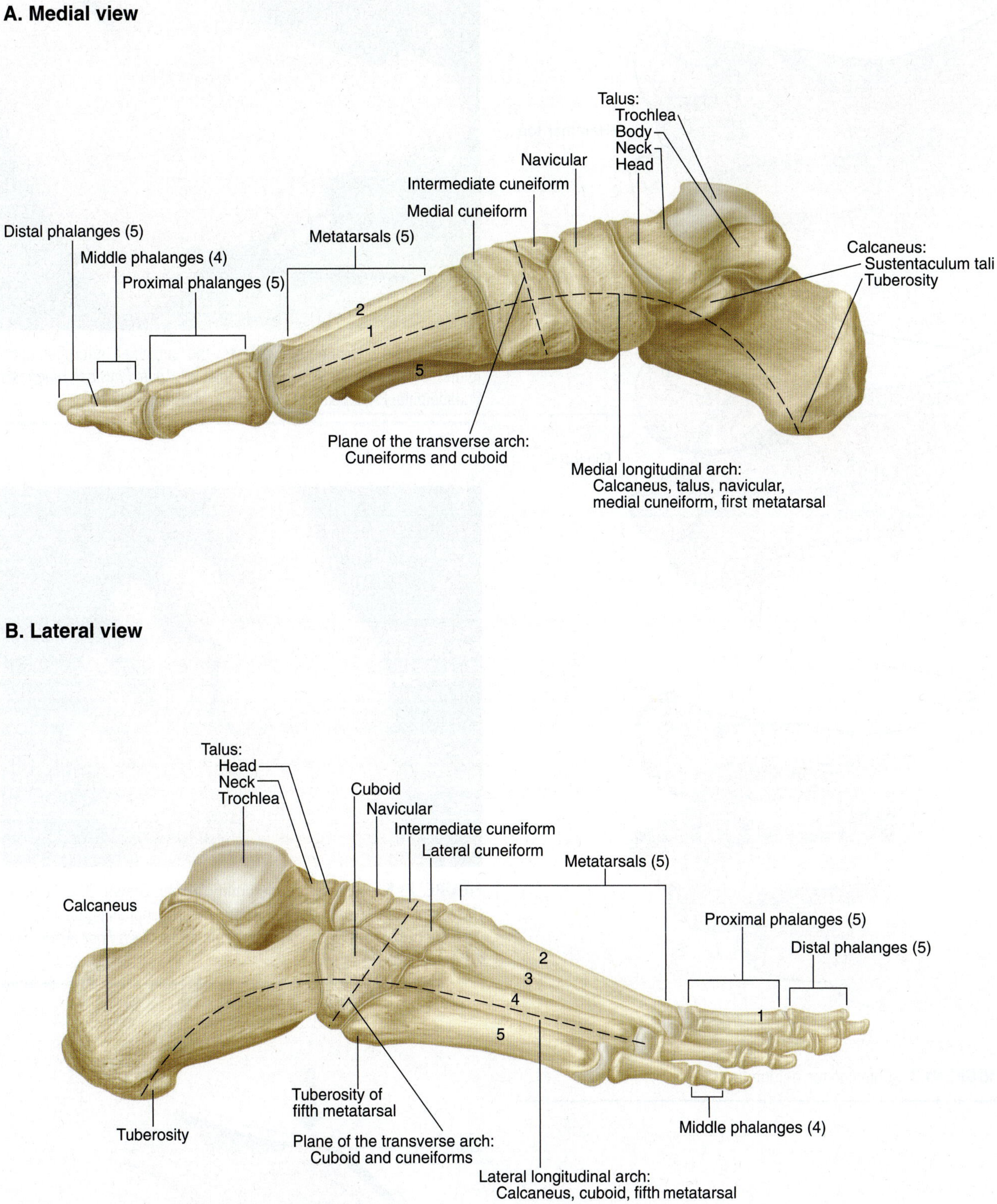

FIGURE 21.2 **A,B:** The metatarsophalangeal joints of the toes are also susceptible to overuse and misuse injuries with resultant inflammation and arthritis. The interphalangeal joints of the toes are ginglymoid joints which have extensive flexion and more limited extension due to the limitation of the plantar and collateral ligaments. (From Tank PW, Gest TR. The lower limb. In: *Lippincott Williams & Wilkins Atlas of Anatomy*. Philadelphia, PA: Lippincott Williams & Wilkins; 2009:127.)

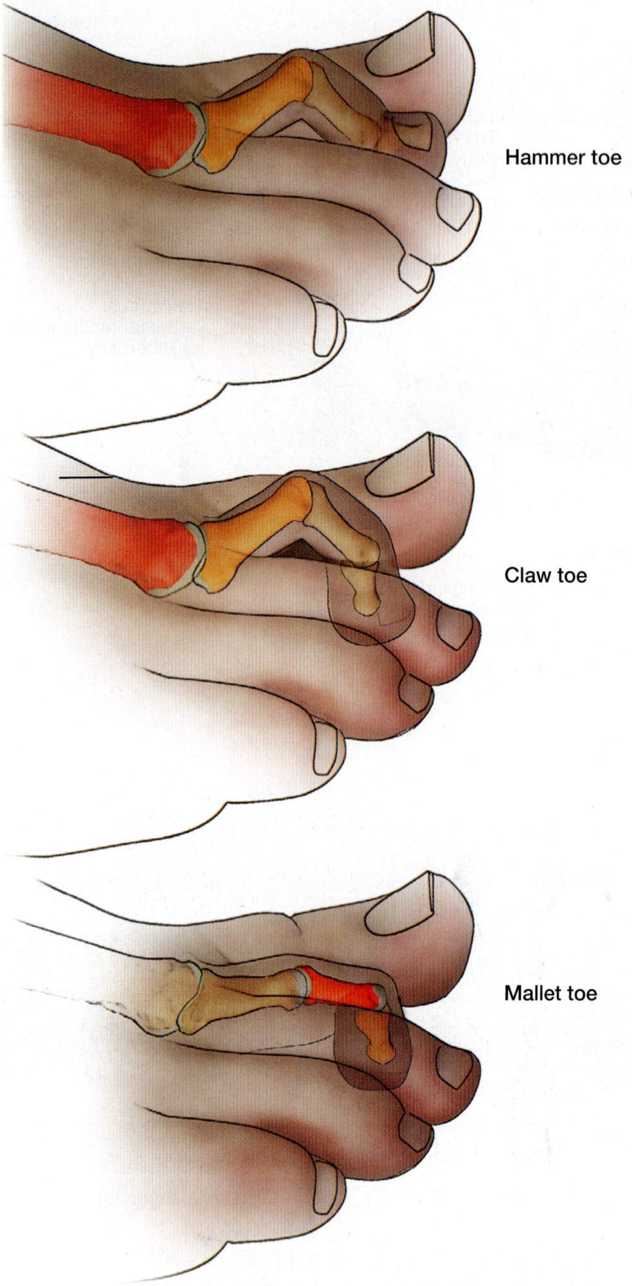

FIGURE 21.3 Common toe deformities.

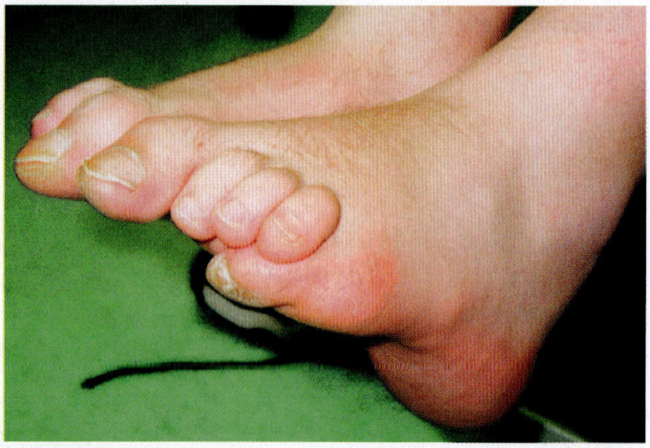

FIGURE 21.4 Hammertoe affects the proximal interphalangeal joints. (From Berg D, Worzala K. *Atlas of Adult Physical Diagnosis*. Philadelphia, PA: Lippincott Williams & Wilkins; 2006.)

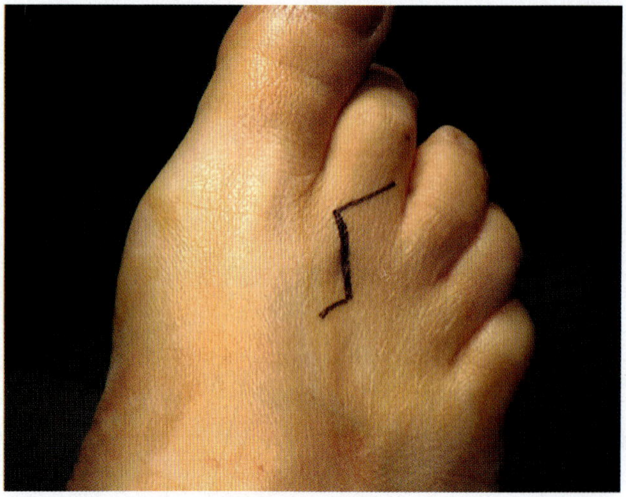

FIGURE 21.5 Hammertoe deformity. (From Grawe BM, Amis J. Resection arthroplasty of the lesser metatarsophalangeal joint for correction of the severe complex hammertoe. *Tech Foot Ankle Surg* 2011;10(1):40–46.)

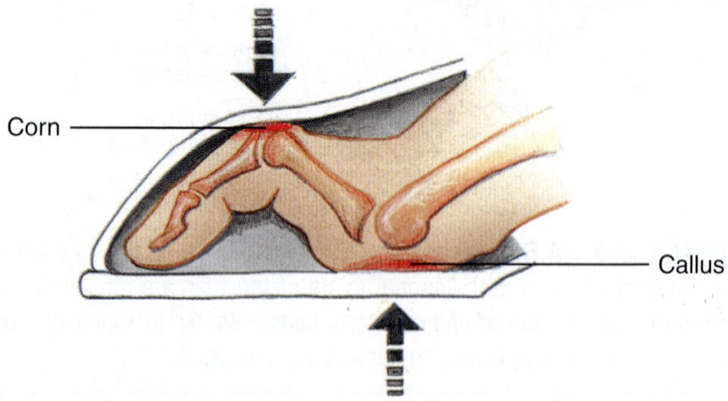

FIGURE 21.6 Significant callus development can accompany the hammertoe deformity. (Anatomical Chart Company, 2013.)

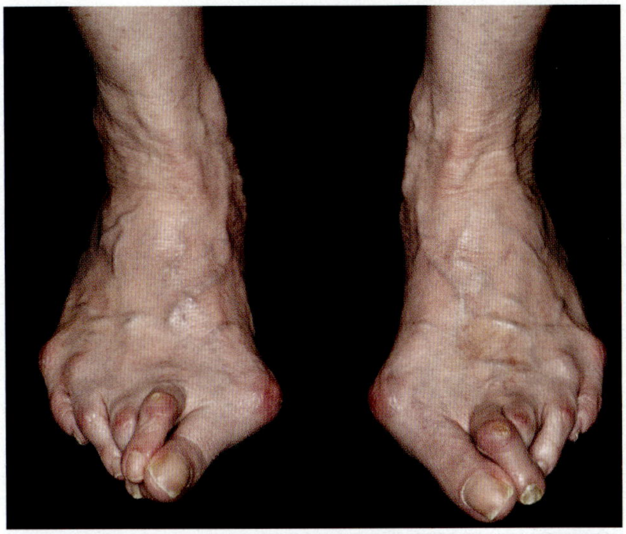

FIGURE 21.7 Severe hallux valgus and associated crossover and hammertoes. (From Davies MB. Common disorders of the adult foot and ankle. *Surg Oxford* 2013;31(9):488–494.)

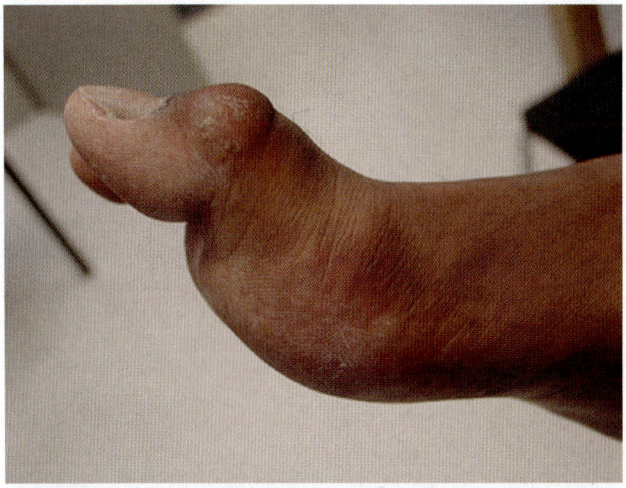

FIGURE 21.9 Claw toe deformity is a common toe deformity that is the result of hyperextension of the metatarsophalangeal joint with significant flexion at both the proximal and distal interphalangeal joints. (From Nicholson CW, Anderson RW. Turf toe injuries. In: Wiesel SW, ed. *Operative Techniques in Orthopaedic Surgery*. Vol 4. Philadelphia, PA: Lippincott Williams & Wilkins; 2011:3665–3673.)

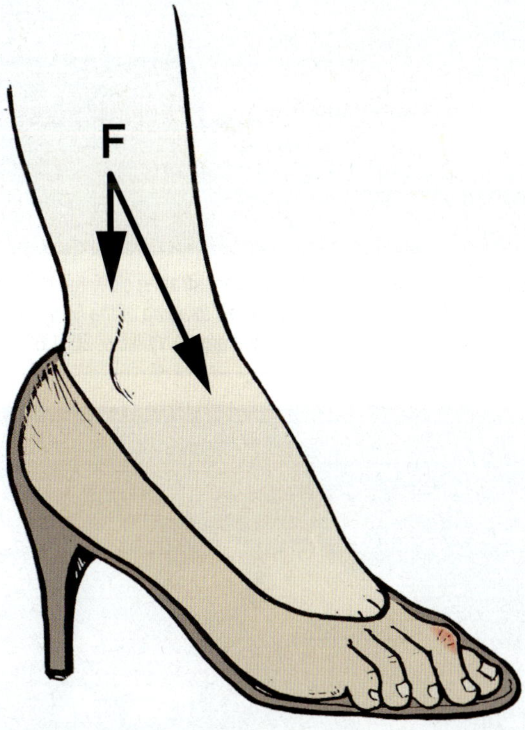

FIGURE 21.8 Poor-fitting shoe with a narrow toe box which forces proximal phalanx into extension and proximal interphalangeal joint into flexion and an excessively high heel, which allows the toes to slide forward into the narrow toe box. (From Koval KJ, Zuckerman JD. *Atlas of Orthopaedic Surgery: A Multimedia Reference*. Philadelphia, PA: Lippincott Williams & Wilkins; 2004.)

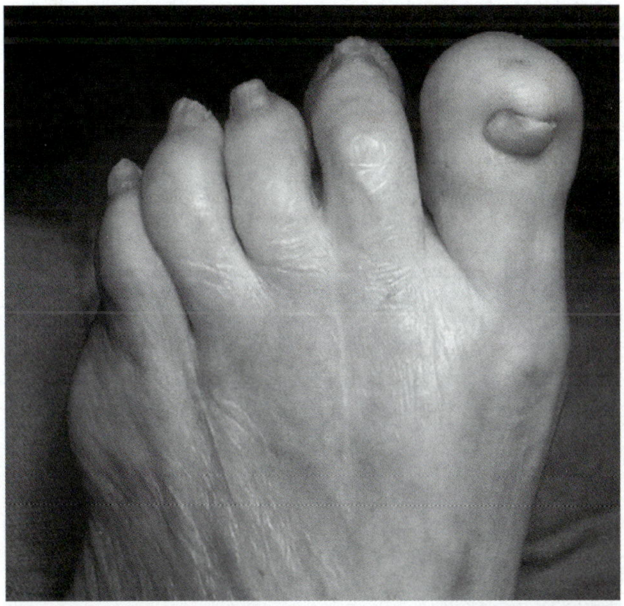

FIGURE 21.10 Example of claw toe deformity with prior metatarsophalangeal joint surgery. Note nail deformities. (From Johnson JT. Treatment of fixed deformities of the distal interphalangeal and proximal interphalangeal joints of the lesser toes. *Techn Foot Ankle Surg* 2004;3(2):100–105.)

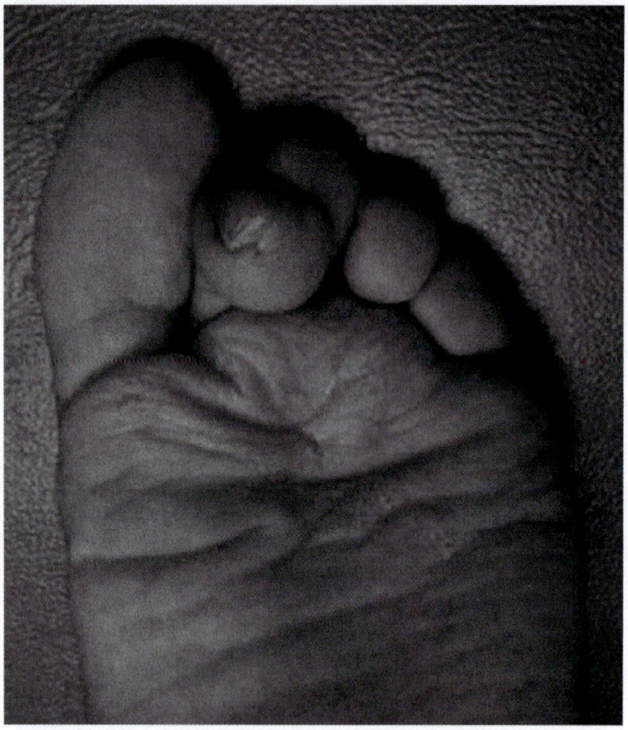

FIGURE 21.11 Mallet toe is the result of a flexion contracture of the distal interphalangeal joint, occurring most commonly in the second toe. This example has extreme plantar prominence. (From Stevens PM, Stotts AK. Toe deformities. In: McCarthy JJ, Drennan JC. *Drennan's The Child's Foot and Ankle*. Philadelphia, PA: Lippincott Williams & Wilkins; 2010:280–289.)

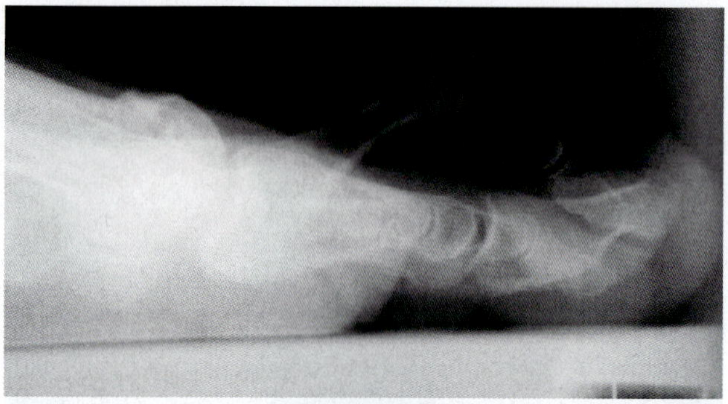

FIGURE 21.13 Lateral radiograph demonstrating the flexion deformity associated with hammertoe. (From Koval KJ, Zuckerman JD. *Atlas of Orthopaedic Surgery: A Multimedia Reference*. Philadelphia, PA: Lippincott Williams & Wilkins; 2004.)

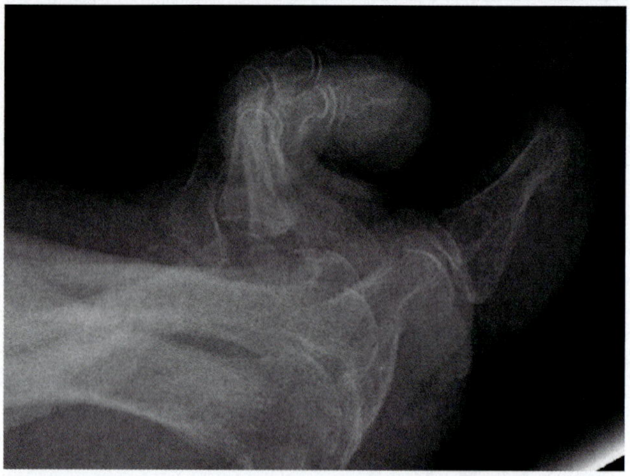

FIGURE 21.14 Lateral radiograph demonstrating claw toe deformities of all of the lesser toes. (From Berquist TH. *Imaging of the Foot and Ankle*. 3rd ed. Philadelphia, PA: Lippincott Williams & Wilkins; 2011:618.)

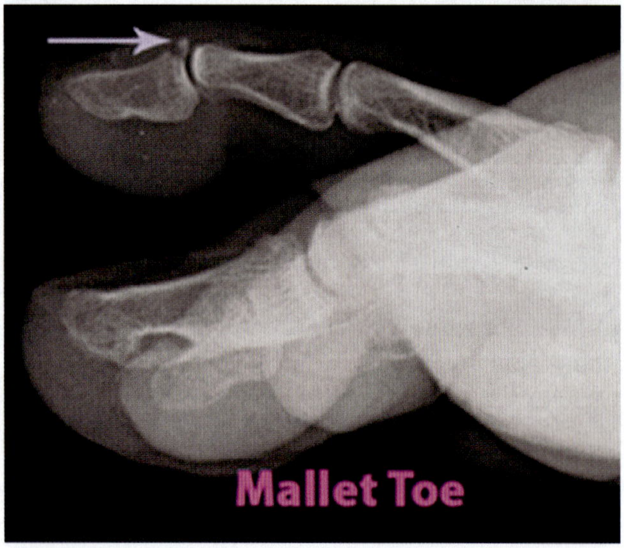

FIGURE 21.12 Mallet toe following acute injury. Lateral x-ray showing avulsed fragment.

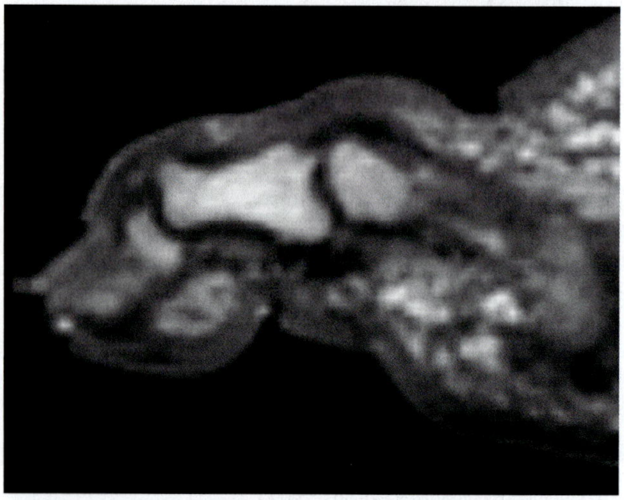

FIGURE 21.15 Mallet toe. Sagittal T1-weighted MR image demonstrating flexion deformity of the distal interphalangeal joint. (From Berquist TH. *Imaging of the Foot and Ankle*. 3rd ed. Philadelphia, PA: Lippincott Williams & Wilkins; 2011:618.)

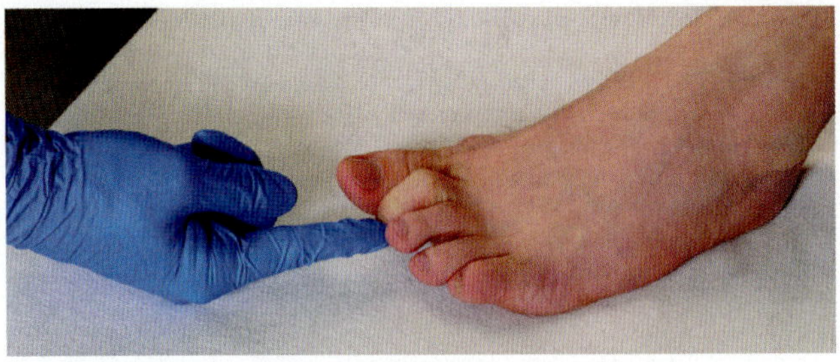

FIGURE 21.16 Inspection of the hammertoe to determine whether the joint is ankylosed.

ULTRASOUND TECHNIQUE

To perform ultrasound evaluation for toe deformities, the patient is then placed in the supine position with the knee flexed so that the plantar surface of the affected foot rests comfortably on the examination table. With the patient in the above position, the dorsal surface of the metatarsophalangeal joint of the affected toe is identified by palpation and the deformity is inspected to assess the degree of ankylosis (Fig. 21.16). A high-frequency small linear ultrasound transducer is placed in a longitudinal position over the proximal interphalangeal joint of the affected toe and an ultrasound survey scan is taken (Figs. 21.17 and 21.18). The hypoechic joint space is identified between the interphalangeal joints.

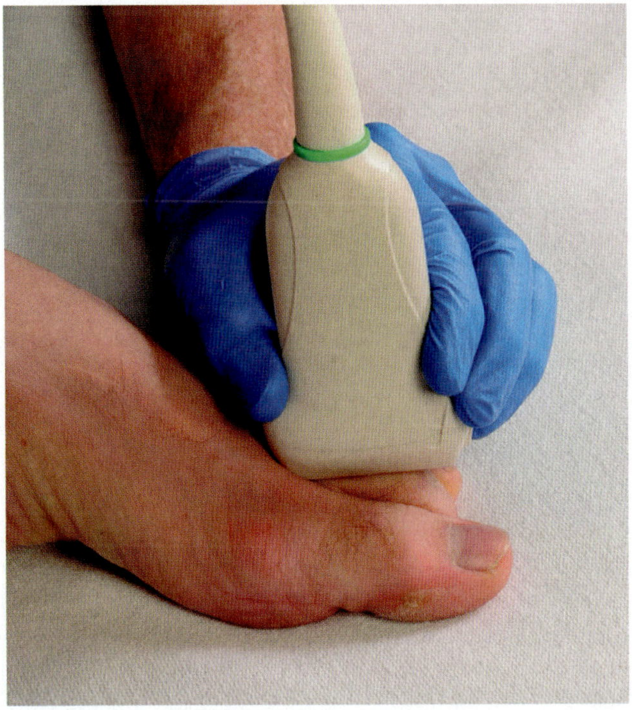

FIGURE 21.17 Correct longitudinal position for ultrasound transducer for ultrasound evaluation of joint deformities.

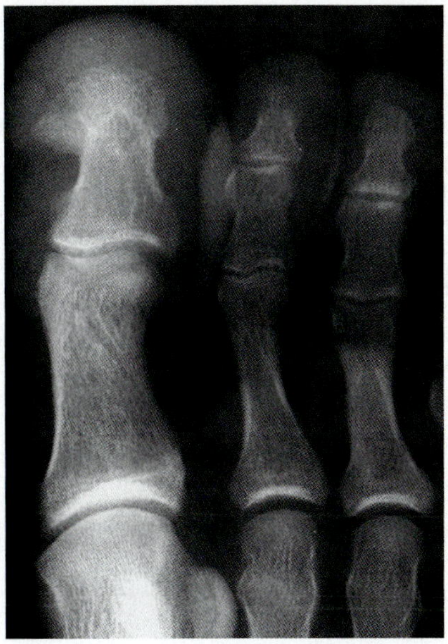

FIGURE 21.18 Subungual exostosis. Radiograph showing an ossified lesion arising from the bone surface deep into the nail bed of the great toe. Note that the underlying cortex is intact. (From Schatz J, Soper J, McCormack S, et al. Imaging of the tumors in the ankle and foot. *Top Magn Reson Imaging* 2010;21(1):37–50.)

When the joint space is identified, the joint is evaluated for degenerative changes, synovitis, effusion, crystal arthropathy as well as the angle between the articular surfaces of both affected joints.

CLINICAL PEARLS

Toe pathology—including tendinopathy, occult fractures, osteoarthritis, rheumatoid arthritis, crystal arthropathies, avascular necrosis bursitis, synovitis, and impingement syndromes—may coexist with disease of the hammertoe and may contribute to the patient's pain symptoms (Fig. 21.19). Given

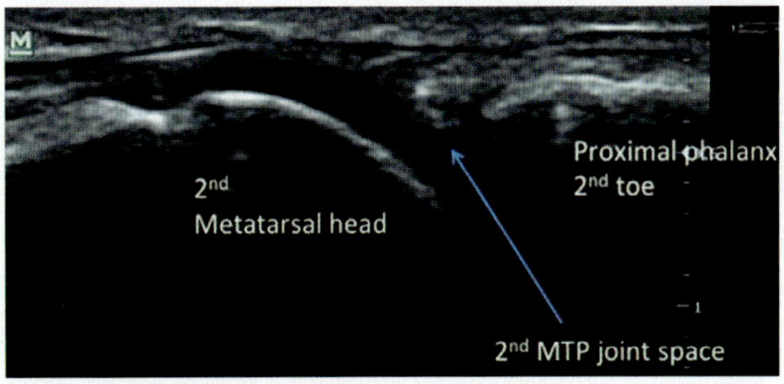

FIGURE 21.19 Longitudinal ultrasound view of the metatarsophalangeal joint space of the great toe. Dorsal aspect of the foot: Metatarsophalangeal joint digit 2 and extensor digitorum tendon longitudinal.

the constant pressure on the skin overlying the abnormally positioned joints, infection remains an ever present possibility. Ultrasound-guided injection of the toe deformity with local anesthetic and anti-inflammatory steroid will often provide dramatic symptomatic improvement, but surgery will usually be required to correct the cosmetic deformity.

Suggested Readings

Mann RA, Horton GA. Management of the foot and ankle in rheumatoid arthritis. *Rheum Dis Clin North Am* 1996;22(3):457–476.

Motta-Valencia K. Dance-related injury. *Phys Med Rehabil Clin N Am* 2006;17(3):697–723.

Thomas JL, Blitch EL 4th, Chaney DM, et al. Diagnosis and treatment of forefoot disorders. Section 2. Central metatarsalgia. *J Foot Ankle Surg* 2009;48(2):239–250.

Waldman SD. Intra-articular injection of the toe joints. In: *Pain Review.* Philadelphia, PA: Saunders; 2009:591–592.

Waldman SD. Injection technique for hammertoe. In: *Atlas of Pain Management Injection Techniques.* 3rd ed. Philadelphia, PA: Saunders; 2012:471–472.

CHAPTER 22

Morton Neuroma Syndrome

ANATOMIC CONSIDERATIONS

In a manner analogous to that of the digital nerves of the hand, the digital nerves of the foot travel through the intrametatarsal space to innervate each toe. The plantar digital nerves, which are derived from the posterior tibial nerve, provide sensory innervation to the major portion of the plantar surface (Fig. 22.1). These nerves are subject to entrapment and resultant development of perineural fibrosis and degeneration resulting in the clinical syndrome known as Morton neuroma (Fig. 22.2). The dorsal aspect of the foot is innervated by terminal branches of the deep and superficial peroneal nerves. The overlap of the innervation of these nerves may be considerable.

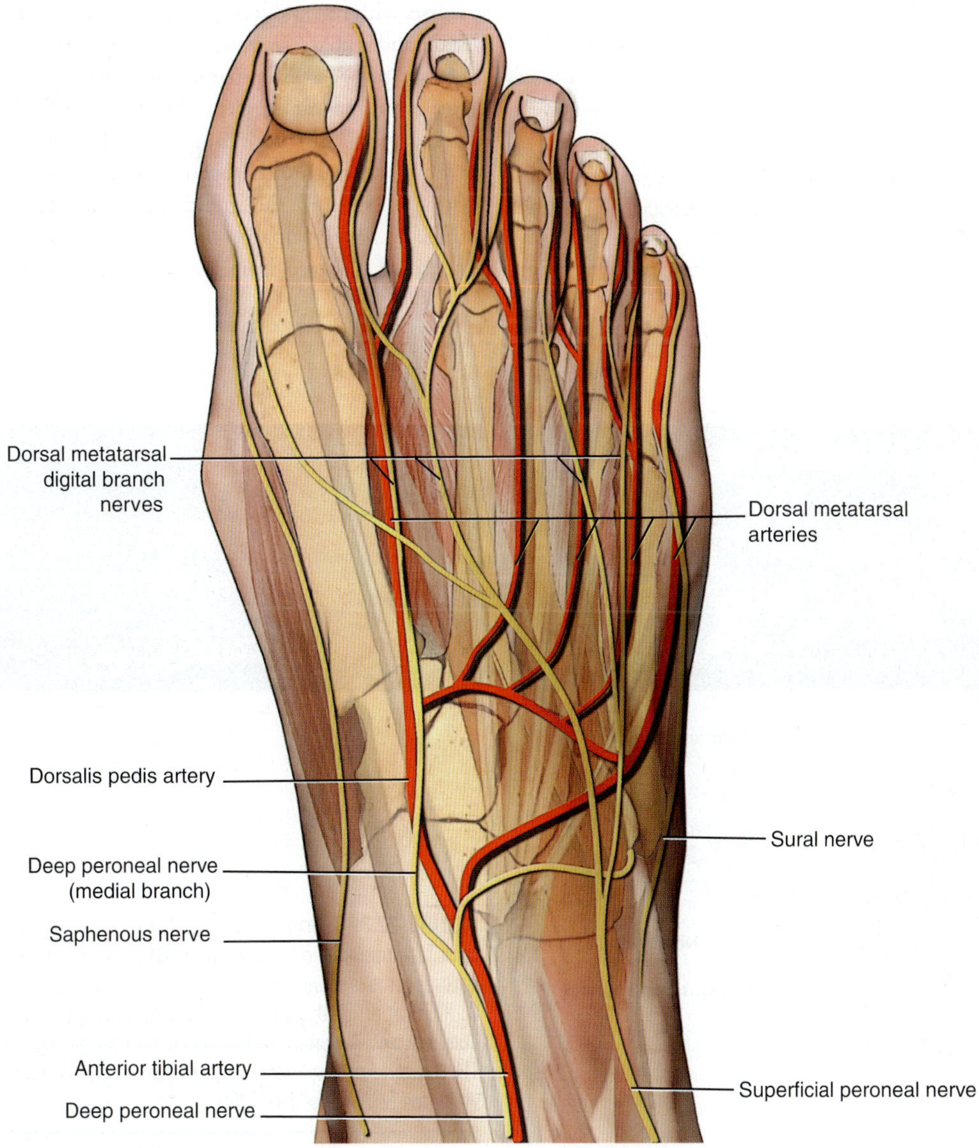

FIGURE 22.1 Anatomy of the metatarsophalangeal and digital nerves.

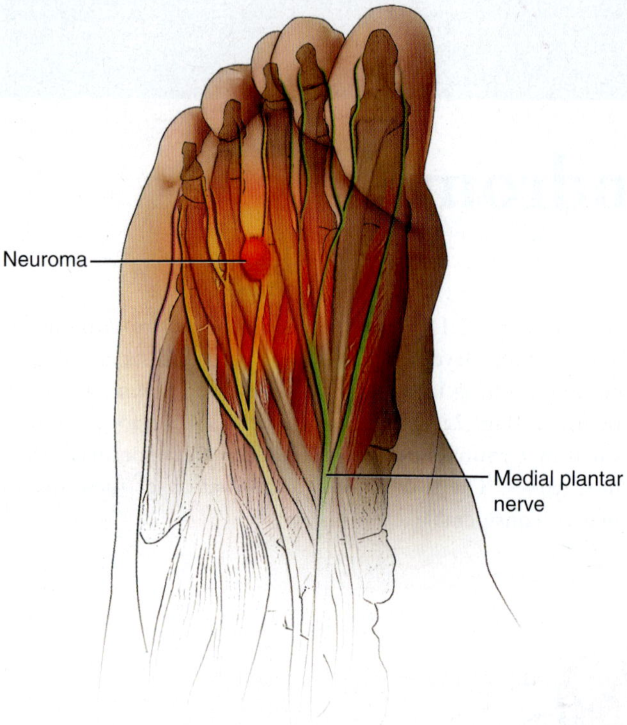

FIGURE 22.2 Patients suffering from Morton neuroma present with the complaint of pain in the plantar surface with associated dysesthesias radiating into the adjacent toes.

CLINICAL CORRELATES

Morton neuroma, which was first described by Thomas Morton in 1876 refers to a constellation of symptoms including tenderness and burning pain in the plantar surface of the forefoot, with associated painful dysesthesias into the affected two toes. This pain syndrome is thought to be caused by perineural fibrosis of the interdigital nerves (Fig. 22.3). There is often coexistent intermetatarsal bursitis as the pathogenesis of both pathologic conditions is similar (Fig. 22.4). Although the nerves between the third and fourth toes most often are affected, the second and third toes and, rarely, the fourth and fifth toes can be affected.

Most patients with Morton neuroma present with the complaint of pain in the plantar surface with associated dysesthesias radiating into the adjacent toes. Patients commonly complain that it feels like they are walking with a stone caught in their shoe. Walking, standing, or wearing tight shoes makes the pain worse, with rest and heat providing some relief. The pain is constant and is characterized as aching and may interfere with sleep.

On physical examination, the pain associated with Morton neuroma can be reproduced by performing the Mulder maneuver. This is accomplished by firmly squeezing the two metatarsal heads together with one hand while placing firm pressure on the interdigital space with the other hand (Fig. 22.5). A palpable click may also be appreciated as the neuroma is forced from between the metatarsals. The patient

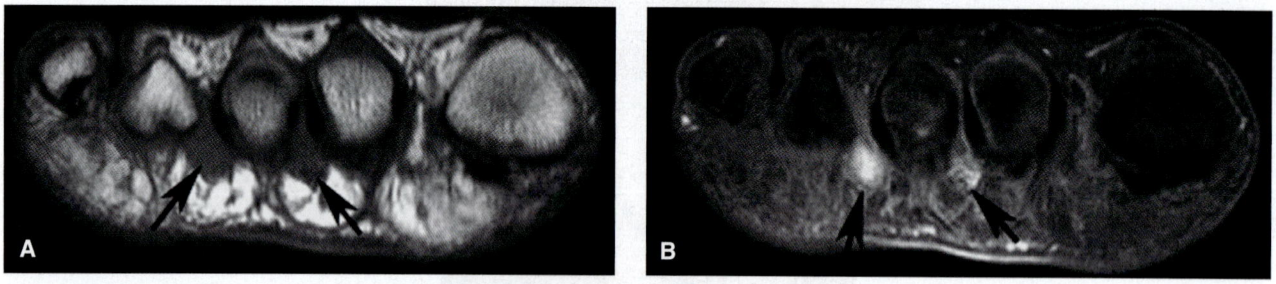

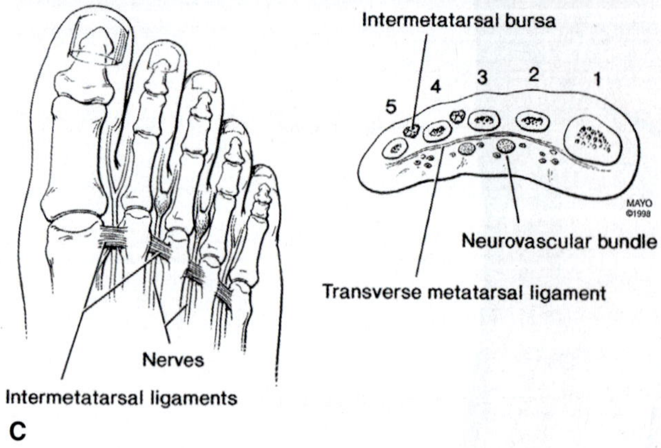

FIGURE 22.3 Morton neuroma. Axial T1-weighted **(A)** and postcontrast fat-suppressed T1-weighted **(B)** images demonstrating neuromas between the second and third and third and fourth metatarsal bases. **C:** Illustration of the location of Morton neuromas and intermetatarsal bursae with relation to the transverse metatarsal ligament. (From Berquist TH. *Imaging of the Foot and Ankle*. 3rd ed. Philadelphia, PA: Lippincott Williams & Wilkins; 2011:200.)

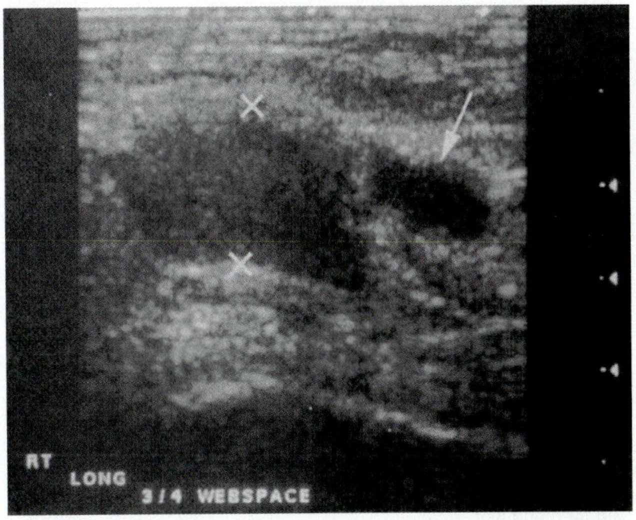

FIGURE 22.4 Morton neuroma change with an associated small effusion in the intermetatarsal bursa. Anechoic fluid (*arrow*) is seen within the bursa at the proximal dorsal aspect of typical Morton web space change (*area between X's*). Distal is to the left of the image. (From Read JW, Noakes JB, Kerr D, et al. Morton's metatarsalgia: sonographic findings and correlated histopathology. *Foot Ankle Int* 1999;20(3): 153–161.)

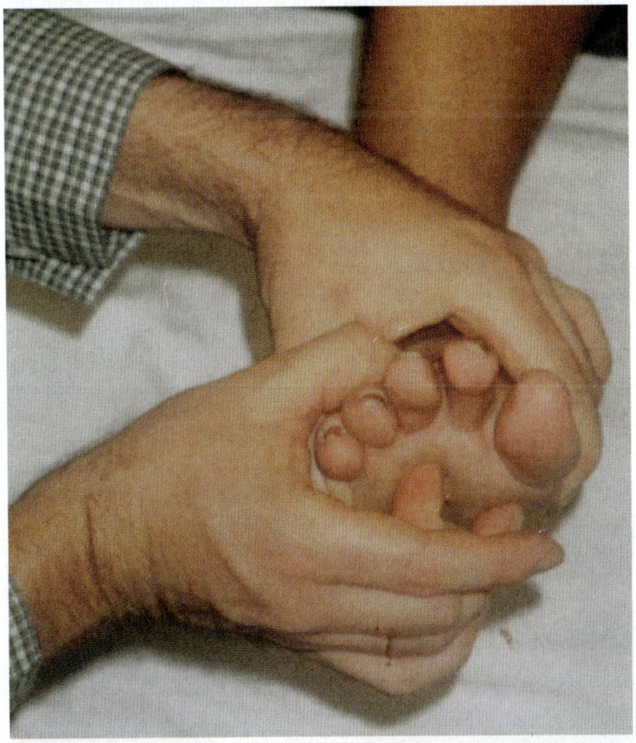

FIGURE 22.5 Mulder maneuver is accomplished by firmly squeezing the two metatarsal heads together with one hand while placing firm pressure on the interdigital space with the other hand. (From Berg D, Worzala K. *Atlas of Adult Physical Diagnosis*. Philadelphia, PA: Lippincott Williams & Wilkins; 2006.)

with Morton neuroma often exhibits an antalgic gait in an effort to reduce weight bearing during walking.

Plain radiographs are indicated in all patients who present with Morton neuroma. Based on the patient's clinical presentation, additional testing may be indicated, including complete blood cell count, sedimentation rate, and antinuclear antibody testing. MRI or ultrasound of the Morton neuroma is indicated to help confirm the diagnosis if fracture, effusion, tendinopathy, crystal arthropathy, joint mice, synovitis, foreign body, bursitis, or ligamentous injury is suspected (Figs. 22.6 and 22.7).

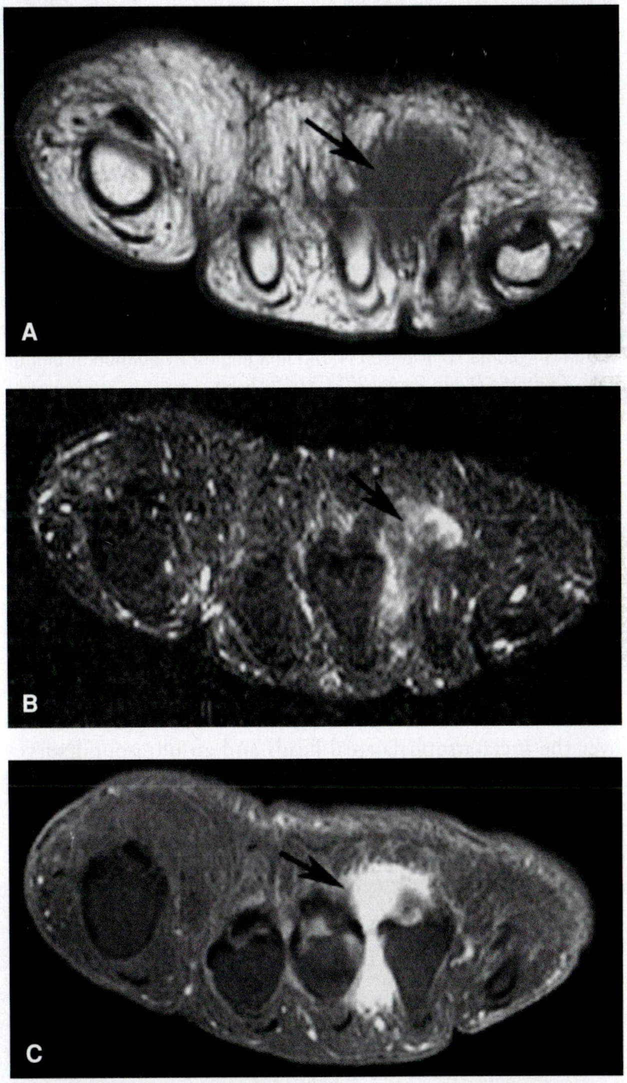

FIGURE 22.6 Axial T1-weighted **(A)**, T2-weighted **(B)**, and post-contrast enhanced fat-suppressed T1-weighted **(C)** images demonstrate a Morton neuroma between the third and fourth metatarsals that extends dorsally (*arrow*). Note the mixed signal intensity on the T2-weighted image **(B)** and intense enhancement **(C)**. (From Berquist TH. *Imaging of the Foot and Ankle*. 3rd ed. Philadelphia, PA: Lippincott Williams & Wilkins; 2011:426.)

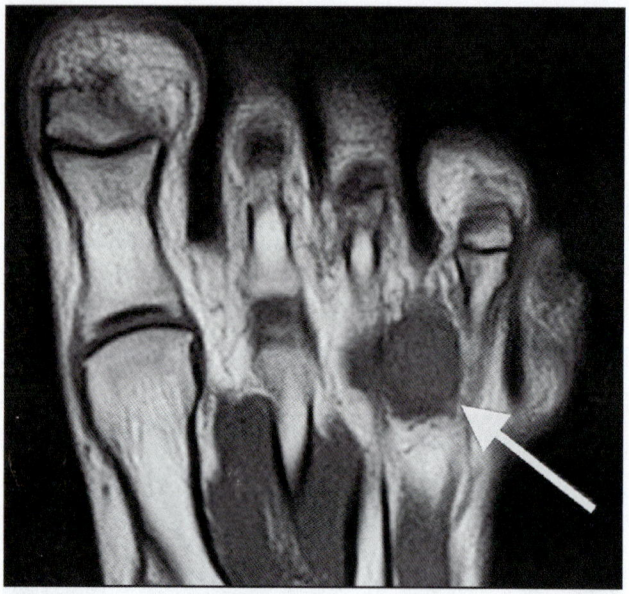

FIGURE 22.7 A 40-year-old woman presented with pain between the third and fourth metatarsal heads. This coronal, T1-weighted MR image of the forefoot demonstrates a dumbbell-shaped soft tissue mass in the third distal intermetatarsal space that is isointense to muscle (*arrow*). This lesion is classic for a Morton neuroma. (From Verma S, Feldman J, Mohsen N. MR imaging for evaluation of plantar pain. *Contemp Diagn Radiol* 2014;37(10):1–5.)

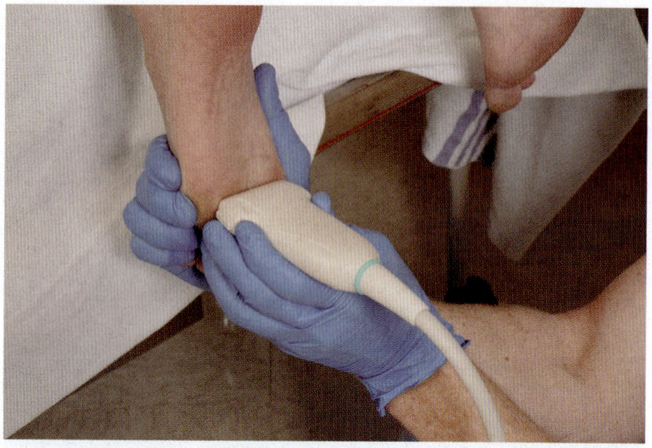

FIGURE 22.8 Correct transverse position for ultrasound transducer for ultrasound evaluation for Morton neuroma while performing Mulder maneuver.

ULTRASOUND TECHNIQUE

To perform ultrasound evaluation for Morton neuroma, the patient is placed in the prone position with the affected foot hanging comfortably over the edge of the examination table. With the patient in the above position, a high-frequency small linear ultrasound transducer is placed in a transverse position over the metatarsophalangeal heads and an ultrasound survey scan is taken (Fig. 22.8). The intermetatarsal space is identified between the heads of the metatarsals and the homogeneous appearing intermetatarsal soft tissue is searched for the appearance of a rounded hyperechoic Morton neuroma (Fig. 22.9). Dynamic scanning while performing the Mulder maneuver may help identify the neuroma as it is forced from between the metatarsal heads (Fig. 22.10). When the intermetatarsal space is identified, it is evaluated for the presence of Morton and intermetatarsal bursitis (Figs. 22.11 to 22.14). The adjacent metatarsals are then evaluated for fracture and/or other bony abnormalities (Fig. 22.15).

CLINICAL PEARLS

Toe pathology—including tendinopathy, occult fractures, osteoarthritis, rheumatoid arthritis, crystal arthropathies, avascular necrosis bursitis, synovitis, and impingement

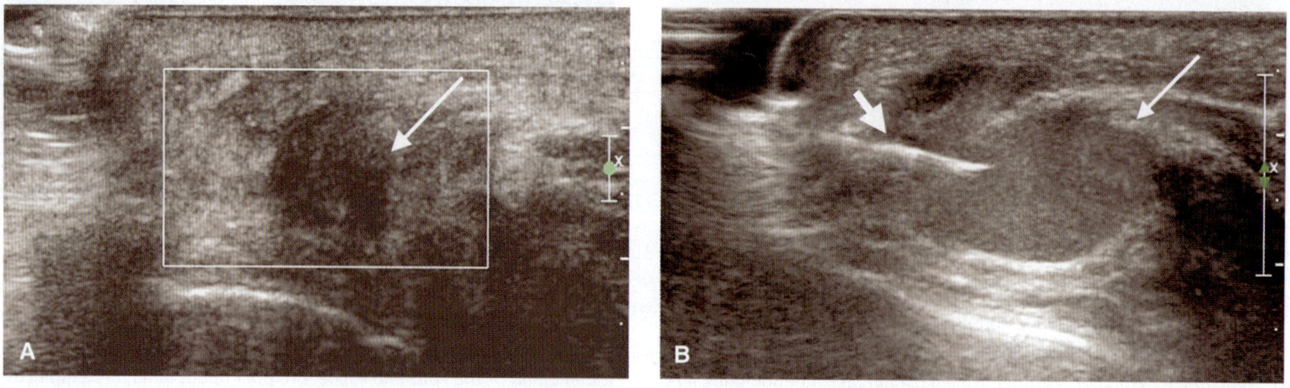

FIGURE 22.9 Morton neuroma. **A:** Long-axis scan of plantar aspect of foot shows hypoechoic Morton neuroma (*arrow*) between third and fourth metatarsal heads. **B:** The neuroma (*long arrow*) is now echogenic following insertion of a needle (*short arrow*) and injection of a therapeutic mixture of long-acting steroid and local anesthetic. (From Adler RA. Ultrasound-guided interventions. In: Beggs I, ed. *Musculoskeletal Ultrasound*. Philadelphia, PA: Lippincott Williams & Wilkins; 2014:311.)

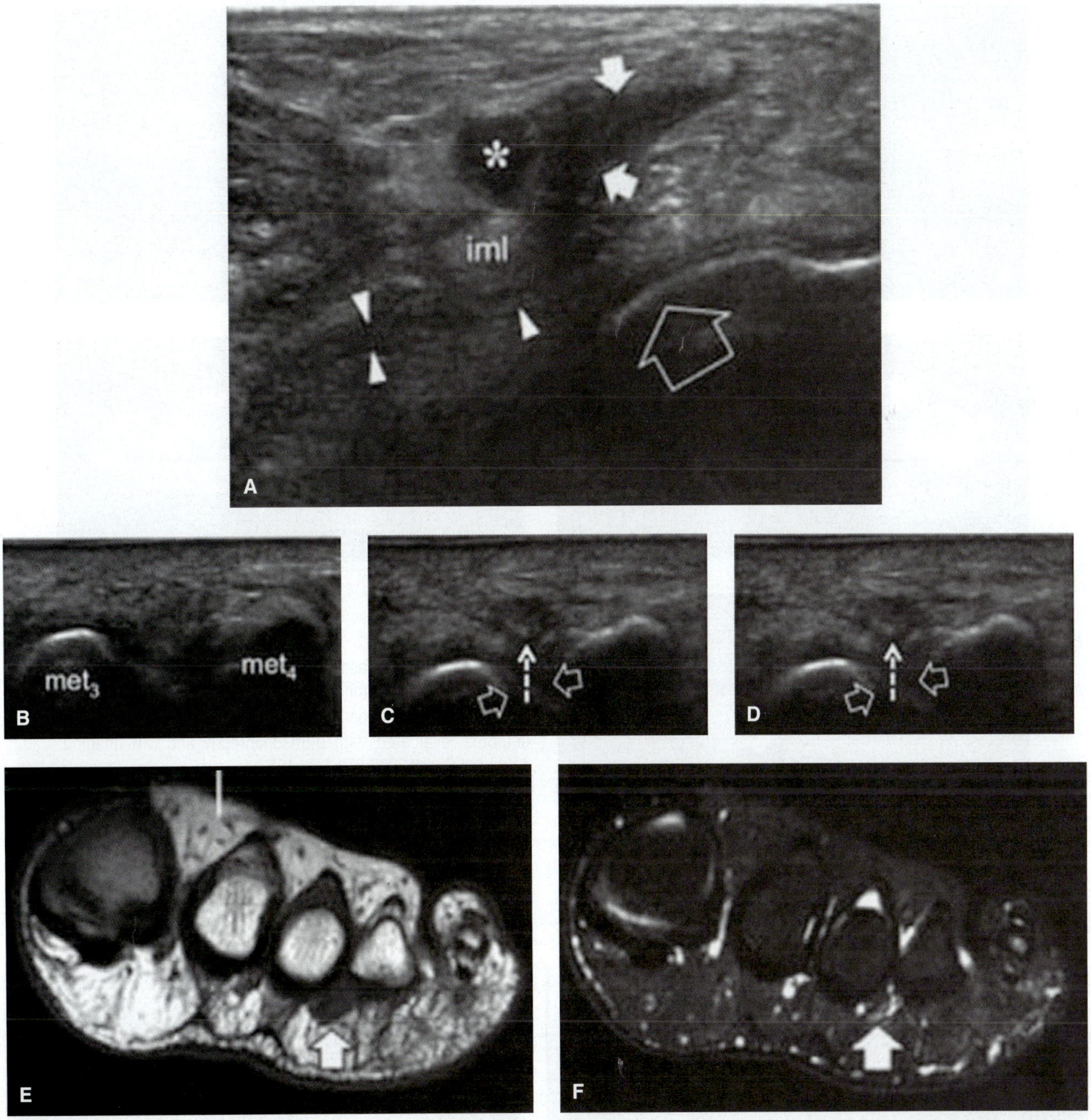

FIGURE 22.10 Morton neuroma. **A:** Longitudinal ultrasound image of the third web space obtained with a dorsal approach while pressing with the thumb (*open arrow*) from the plantar aspect of the foot shows the interdigital nerve (*arrowheads*) as it passes underneath the intermetatarsal ligament (IML) before deflecting dorsally and continuing in a fusiform hypoechoic Morton neuroma (*white arrows*). A fluid-filled intermetatarsal bursa (*asterisk*) can be appreciated dorsal to the neuroma. Sonographic Mulder test. Transverse ultrasound images of the third web space obtained in a resting state **(B)** and while squeezing the third (met$_3$) and fourth (met$_4$) metatarsals together **(C)**. With this maneuver, the metatarsal gets closer (*open arrows*) and a mushroom-like hypoechoic neuroma is seen popping up (*dashed arrow*) from the intermetatarsal space. Short-axis T1-weighted **(D)** and fat-suppressed T2-weighted **(E,F)** magnetic resonance images of the forefoot demonstrate a hypointense neuroma (*arrows*) of the interdigital nerve to the third web space. (From Matinoli C, Court-Payen M, Michaud J, et al. Imaging of neuropathies about the ankle and foot. *Semin Musculoskelet Radiol* 2010;14(3):344–356.)

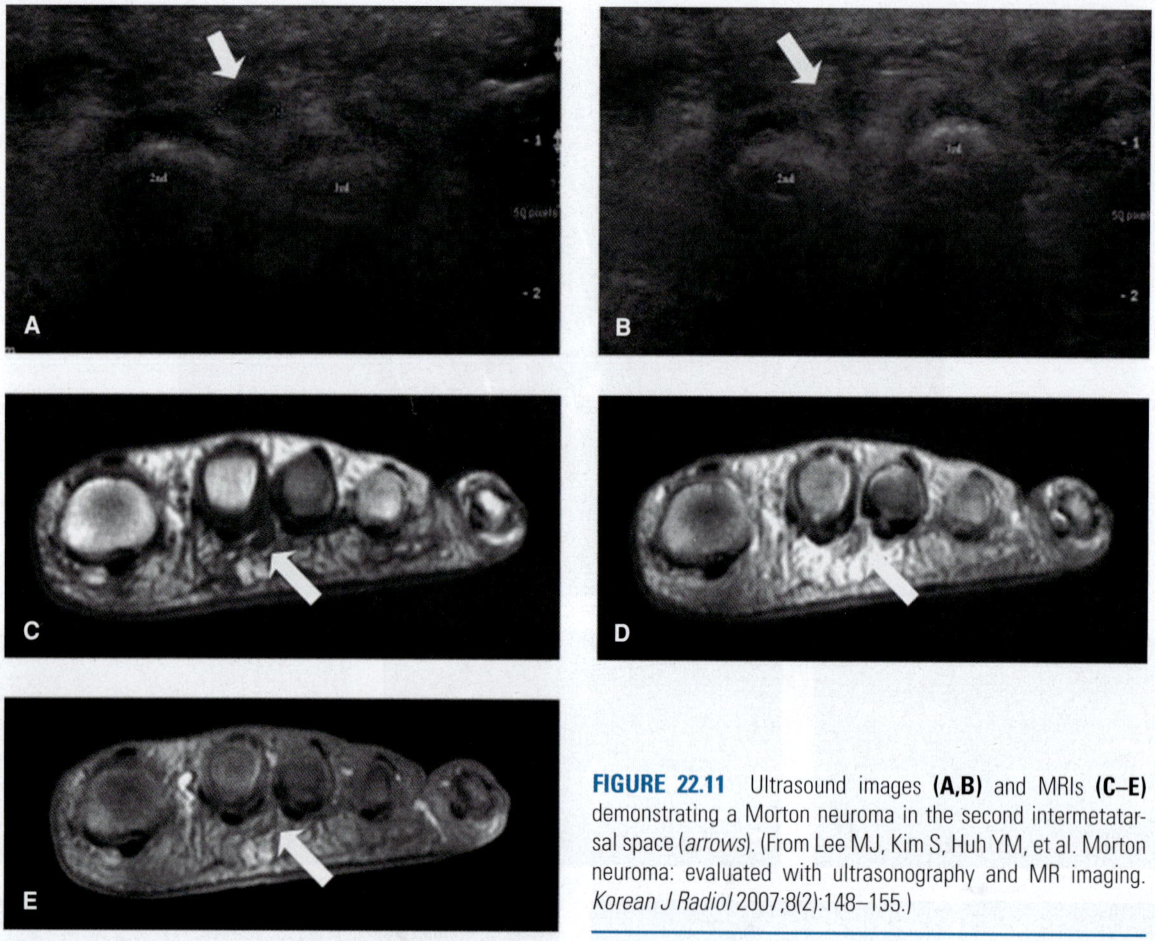

FIGURE 22.11 Ultrasound images **(A,B)** and MRIs **(C–E)** demonstrating a Morton neuroma in the second intermetatarsal space (*arrows*). (From Lee MJ, Kim S, Huh YM, et al. Morton neuroma: evaluated with ultrasonography and MR imaging. *Korean J Radiol* 2007;8(2):148–155.)

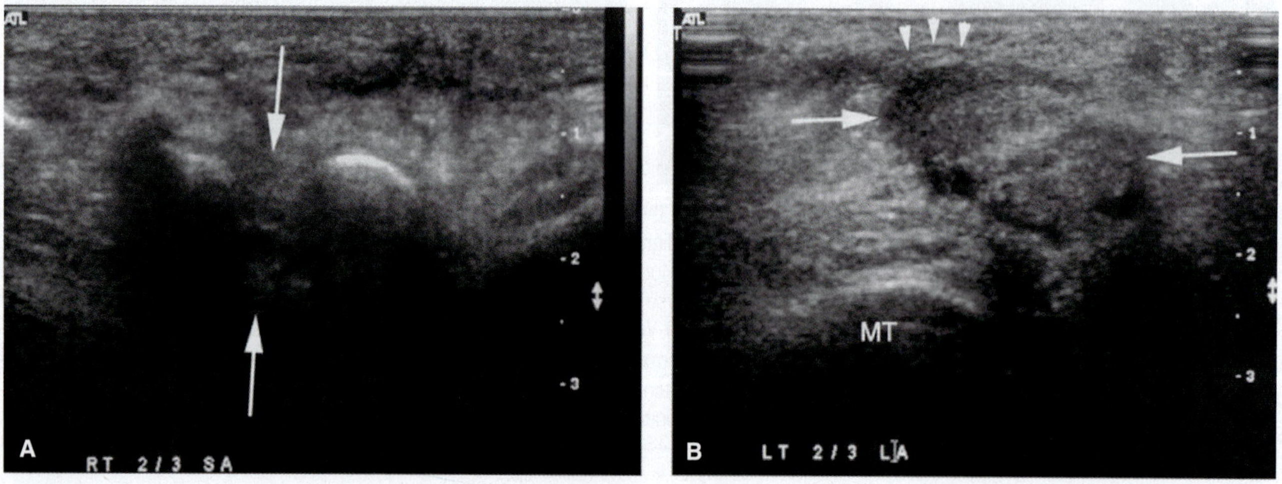

FIGURE 22.12 **A:** Short-axis sonogram shows a Morton neuroma as a heterogeneous mass (*arrows*) between the heads of the second and third metatarsals on this sonogram obtained from the plantar surface of the foot. **B:** Long-axis sonogram of plantar surface in same patient demonstrates the neuroma (*arrows*) plantar to the metatarsal head (MT) and the interdigital artery (*arrowheads*) stretched over the neuroma. (From Thain LM, Downey DB. Sonography of peripheral nerves: technique, anatomy, and pathology. *Ultrasound Q* 2002;18(4):225–245.)

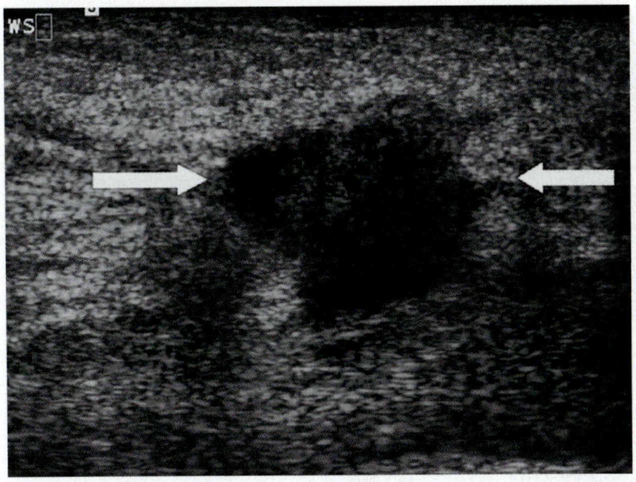

FIGURE 22.13 Morton neuroma. A longitudinal gray scale image of a left third web space shows a hypoechoic mass (*white arrows*) with irregular and partially demarcated margins. (From Hwang S, Adler RS. Sonographic evaluation of the musculoskeletal soft tissue masses. *Ultrasound Q* 2005;21(4):259–270; Fig. 7.)

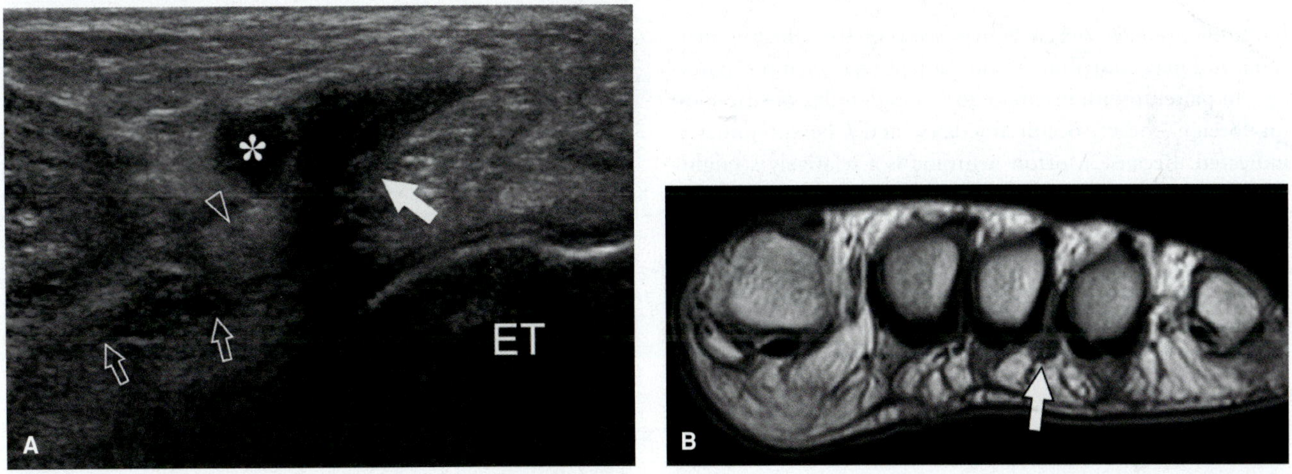

FIGURE 22.14 Morton neuroma. **A:** Longitudinal ultrasound image of the third web space obtained with a dorsal approach while pressing with the thumb (ET) from the plantar aspect of the foot shows the interdigital nerve (*void arrows*) as it passes underneath the intermetatarsal ligament (*arrowhead*) before deflecting dorsally and continuing in a fusiform hypoechoic Morton neuroma (*white arrow*). A fluid-filled intermetatarsal bursa (*asterisk*) is dorsal to the neuroma. **B:** Correlative axial TSE T1-weighted magnetic resonance image confirms the presence of a small neuroma (*arrow*) in the third web space. (From Martinoli C, Tagliafico A, Beggs I. Nerves. In: Beggs I, ed. *Musculoskeletal Ultrasound*. Philadelphia, PA: Lippincott Williams & Wilkins; 2014:311.)

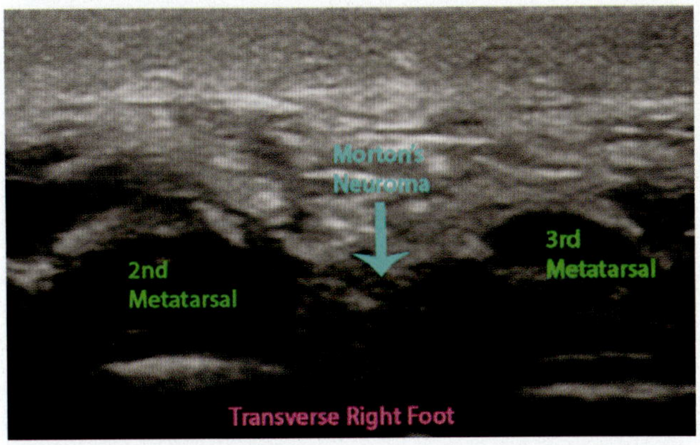

FIGURE 22.15 Transverse ultrasound image demonstrating a large Morton neuroma between the second and third metatarsals.

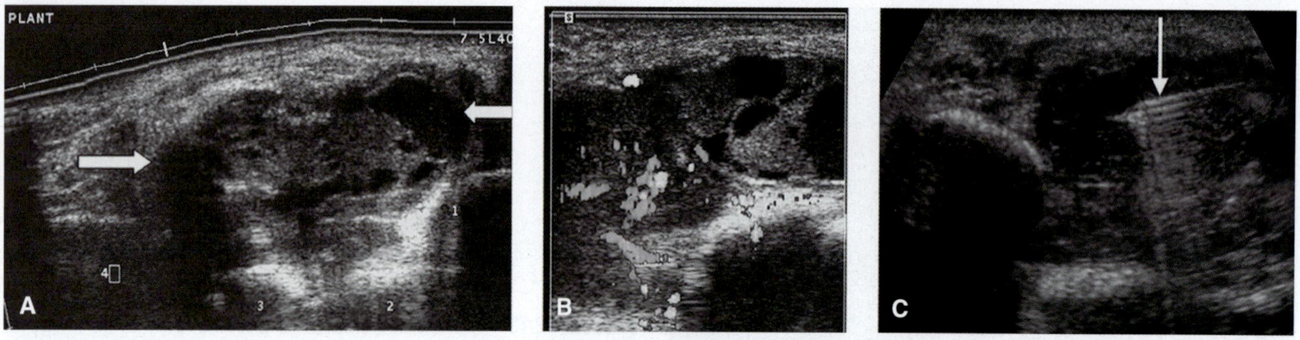

FIGURE 22.16 Synovial sarcoma. Patient with a history of excised Morton neuroma, underwent a sonographically guided biopsy of a recurrent mass in a plantar aspect of the foot. **A:** A coronal gray scale image of the plantar aspect of the foot demonstrates a complex solid mass (*arrows*) with mixed echogenicity with cystic areas. The metatarsals are numbered from 1 to 4. **B:** On power Doppler, the mass demonstrates increased vascular flow. **C:** A needle (*white arrow*) is placed in the solid component of the mass during the biopsy. (From Hwang S, Adler RS. Sonographic evaluation of the musculoskeletal soft tissue masses. *Ultrasound Q* 2005;21(4):259–270.)

syndromes—may coexist with disease of the Morton neuroma and may contribute to the patient's pain symptomatology. In patients with insensate feet, a high index of suspicion for foreign bodies, occult fractures, and Charcot joints is indicated. Because Morton neuroma is a relatively straightforward clinical diagnosis, there is a tendency to proceed with treatment without adequate evaluation and follow-up. It should be remembered that other pathologic conditions may mimic the clinical presentation of Morton neuroma and care must be taken to correctly identify the cause of the patient's symptoms (Fig. 22.16). In this setting ultrasound guidance for biopsy will simplify the procedure and improve the results.

Suggested Readings

Betts RP, Bygrave CJ, Jones S, et al. Ultrasonic diagnosis of Morton's neuroma: a guide to problems, pointers, pitfalls and prognosis. *Foot* 2003;13(2):92–99.

George VA, Khan AM, Hutchinson CE, et al. Morton's neuroma: the role of MR scanning in diagnostic assistance. *Foot* 2005;15(1):14–16.

Kay D, Bennett GL. Morton's neuroma. *Foot Ankle Clin North Am* 2003;8(1):49–59.

Waldman SD. Injection technique for Morton's neuroma. In: *Atlas of Pain Management Injection Techniques.* 3rd ed. Philadelphia, PA: Saunders; 2012:473–474.

CHAPTER 23

Intermetatarsal Bursitis

ANATOMIC CONSIDERATIONS

In a manner analogous to that of the digital nerves of the hand, the digital nerves of the foot travel through the intrametatarsal space to innervate each toe. The plantar digital nerves, which are derived from the posterior tibial nerve, provide sensory innervation to the major portion of the plantar surface (Fig. 23.1). These nerves are subject to entrapment and resultant development of perineural fibrosis and degeneration resulting in the clinical syndrome known as Morton neuroma (Fig. 23.2). The dorsal aspect of the foot is innervated by terminal branches of the deep and superficial peroneal nerves. The

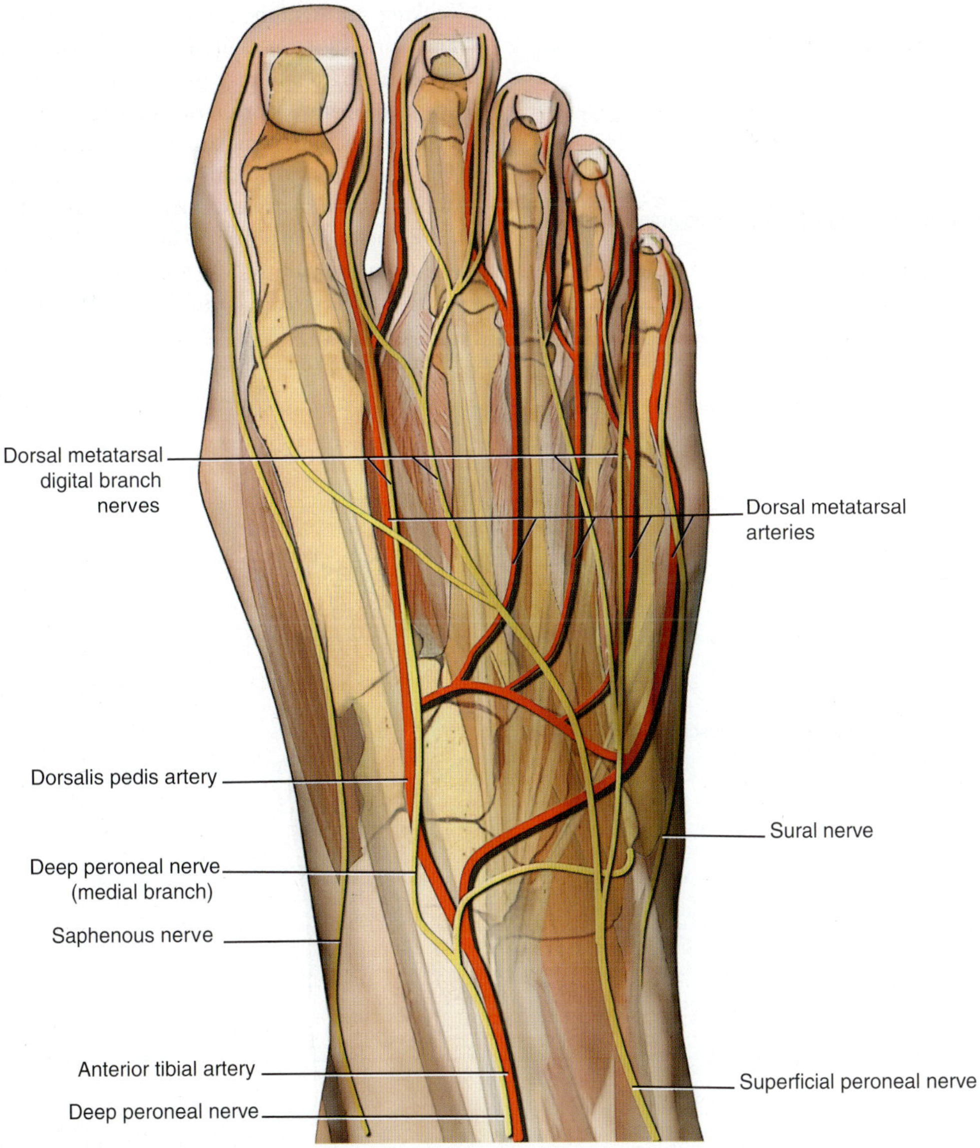

FIGURE 23.1 Anatomy of the metatarsophalangeal and digital nerves.

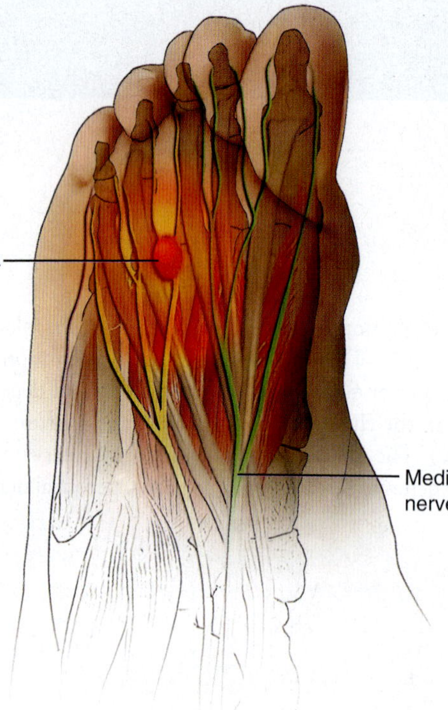

FIGURE 23.2 Patients suffering from Morton neuroma present with the complaint of pain in the plantar surface with associated dysesthesias radiating into the adjacent toes.

overlap of the innervation of these nerves may be considerable. The intermetatarsal bursa lies between the metatarsophalangeal joints in a position that is just dorsal to the interdigital nerves (Fig. 23.3). The bursae extend approximately 1 cm beyond the distal border of the ligament in the web spaces between the second and third and third and fourth digits (Fig. 23.4).

CLINICAL CORRELATES

Intermetatarsal bursitis refers to a constellation of symptoms including pain and tenderness over the affected intermetatarsal spaces which radiate distally into the toes especially if the adjacent interdigital nerve is inflamed. The pain of intermetatarsal bursitis is exacerbated by weight bearing and wearing high heels or shoes which are too narrow. Obesity may also predispose to this condition. The patient suffering from intermetatarsal bursitis is often unable to stand on tiptoes or walk up stairs. Walking and standing for long periods makes the pain worse. The pain of intermetatarsal bursitis is constant and is characterized as sharp and may interfere with sleep. Coexistent neuritis, neuropathy, Morton neuroma formation, stress fractures, metatarsalgia, and synovitis may confuse the clinical picture (Fig. 23.5). As the bursitis worsens, the affected intermetatarsal bursae tend to expand surrounding the adjacent interdigital nerves making the patient's clinical presentation indistinguishable from the pain of Morton neuroma. If the inflammation of the intermetatarsal bursae becomes chronic, calcification of

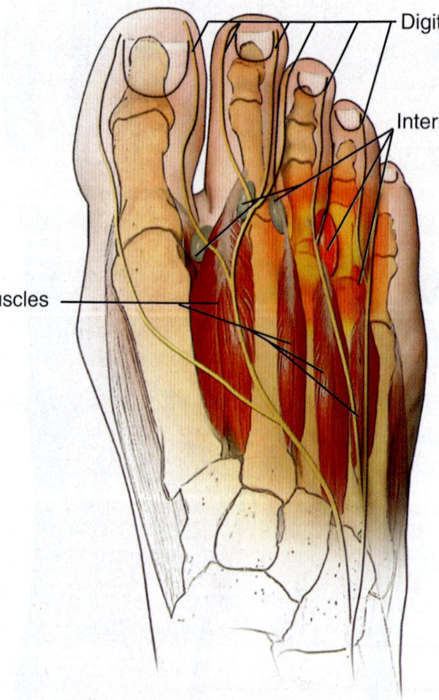

FIGURE 23.3 Anatomy of the intermetatarsal bursa.

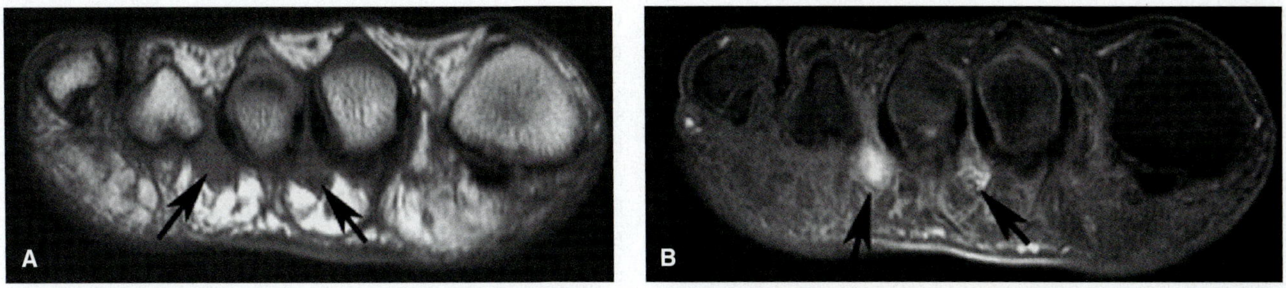

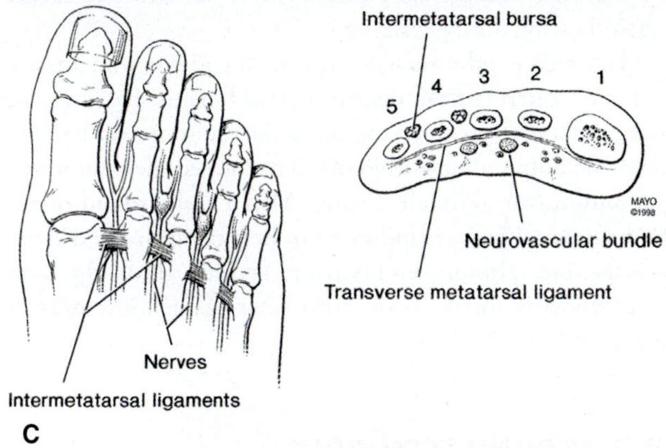

FIGURE 23.4 Morton neuroma. Axial T1-weighted **(A)** and postcontrast fat-suppressed T1-weighted **(B)** images demonstrating neuromas between the second and third and third and fourth metatarsal bases. **C:** Illustration of the location of Morton neuromas and intermetatarsal bursae with relation to the transverse metatarsal ligament. (From Berquist TH. *Imaging of the Foot and Ankle.* 3rd ed. Philadelphia, PA: Lippincott Williams & Wilkins; 2011:200.)

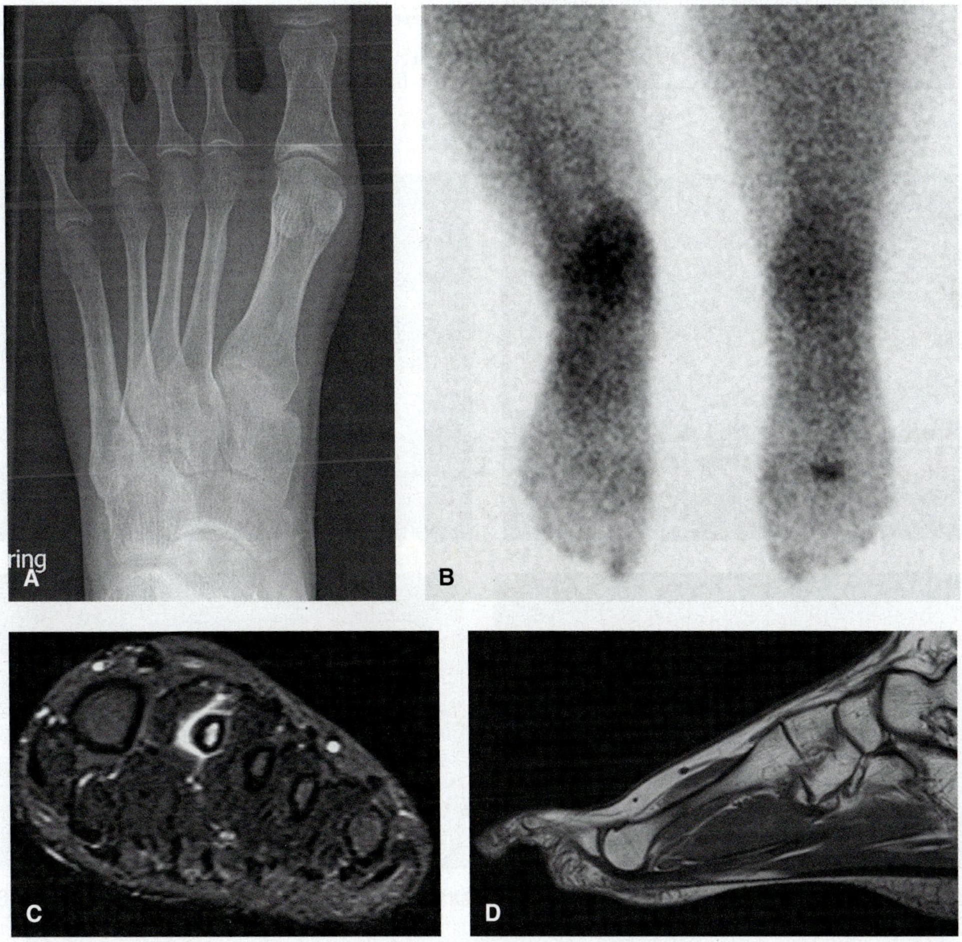

FIGURE 23.5 **A:** Radiograph shows subtle cortical thickening to the second metatarsal shaft consistent with a stress fracture. **B:** Bone scintigram confirms this to be consistent with a fracture. STIR **(C)** and T1-weighted **(D)** MR images confirm the associated edema and cortical thickening. (From Pope TL Jr, Harris JH Jr, eds. *Harris & Harris' The Radiology of Emergency Medicine.* 5th ed. Philadelphia, PA: Lippincott Williams & Wilkins; 2013:961.)

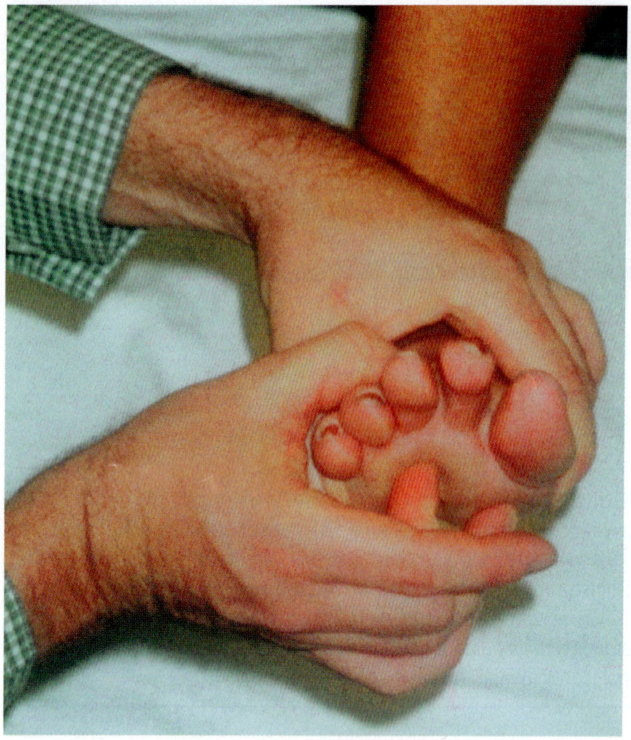

FIGURE 23.6 Mulder maneuver is accomplished by firmly squeezing the two metatarsal heads together with one hand while placing firm pressure on the interdigital space with the other hand.

the bursae and fibrosis of the surrounding interdigital space may occur.

On physical examination, pain can be reproduced by squeezing the affected web space between the index finger and thumb. If the interdigital nerve is involved or if a Morton neuroma has developed, a positive Mulder sign can be elicited by firmly squeezing the two metatarsal heads together with one hand while placing firm pressure on the interdigital space with the other hand (Fig. 23.6). The patient with intermetatarsal bursitis often exhibits an antalgic gait in an effort to reduce weight bearing during walking.

Plain radiographs are indicated in all patients who are suspected of suffering from intermetatarsal bursitis. Based on the patient's clinical presentation, additional testing may be indicated, including complete blood cell count, sedimentation rate, and antinuclear antibody testing. MRI or ultrasound of the intermetatarsal bursa is indicated to help confirm the diagnosis if fracture, effusion, tendinopathy, crystal arthropathy, joint mice, synovitis, foreign body, bursitis, or ligamentous injury is suspected (Figs. 23.7 and 23.8).

ULTRASOUND TECHNIQUE

To perform ultrasound evaluation for intermetatarsal bursitis, the patient is placed in the prone position with the affected foot hanging comfortably over the edge of the examination

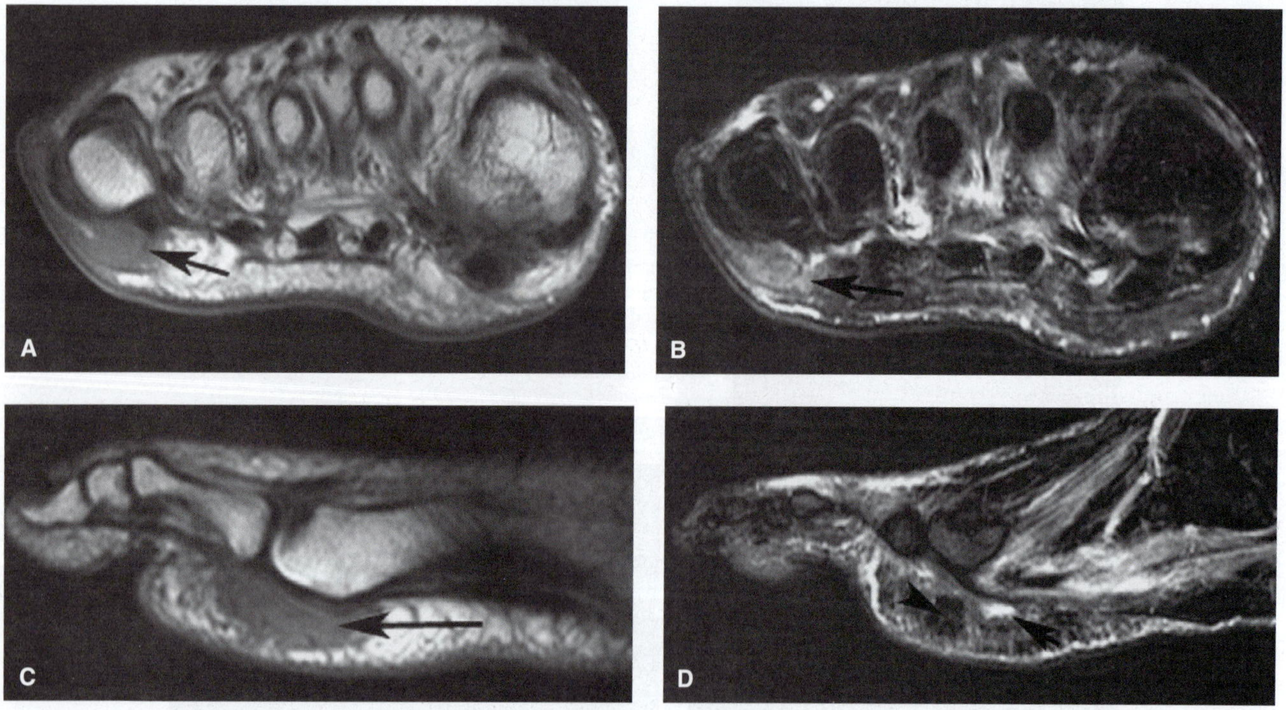

FIGURE 23.7 Abnormal signal intensity with bursa beneath the fifth metatarsal head. Axial T1-weighted **(A)** and T2-weighted **(B)** images demonstrate an elliptical area of abnormal signal intensity beneath the fifth metatarsal head (*arrow*). Sagittal T1- **(C)** and T2- **(D)** weighted images show the abnormal soft tissue collection with a small adventitious bursa (*arrow* in **D**) and area of low-signal intensity on T2-weighted image D (*arrowhead*) due to fibrous tissue. (From Berquist TH. *Imaging of the Foot and Ankle*. 3rd ed. Philadelphia, PA: Lippincott Williams & Wilkins; 2011:196.)

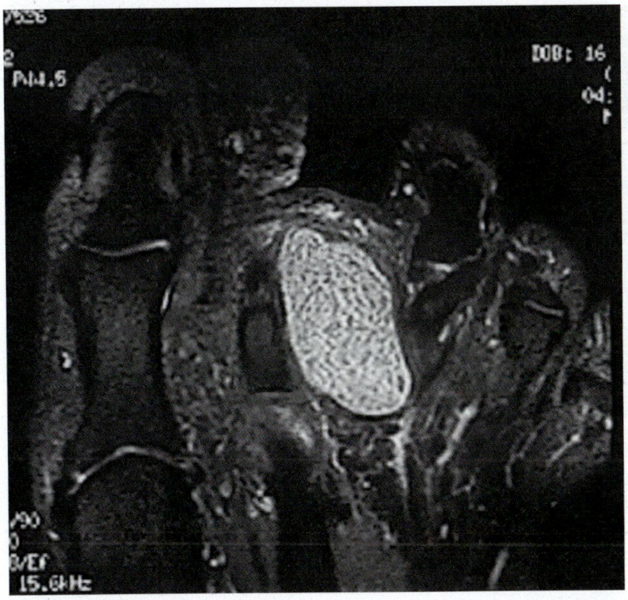

FIGURE 23.8 Intermetatarsal bursitis. Axial fat-suppressed T2 MR image showing a distended bursa in the 3/4 web space. The multiple tiny low signal foci within the bright fluid represent "rice bodies"-fibrinous debris. This was the first presentation in a patient subsequently diagnosed with rheumatoid arthritis. (From Schatz J, Soper J, McCormack S, et al. Imaging of tumors in the ankle and foot. *Top Magn Reson Imaging* 2010;21(1):37–50.)

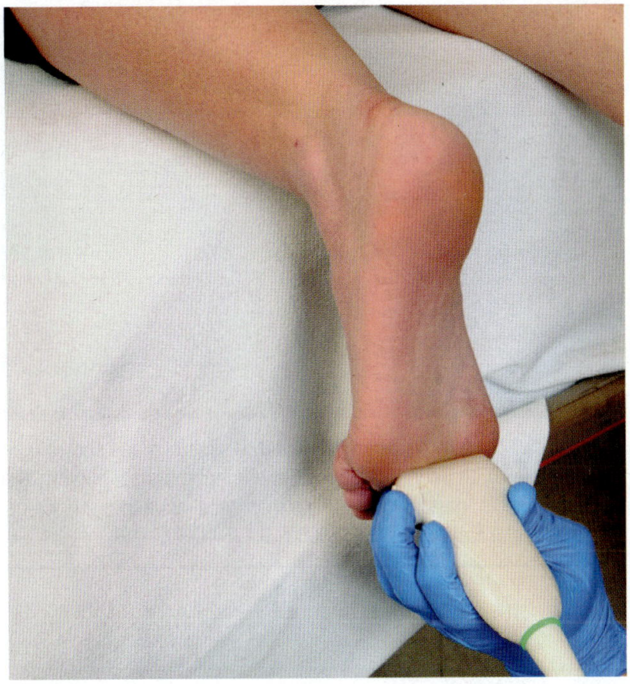

FIGURE 23.9 Correct transverse position for ultrasound transducer for ultrasound evaluation for intermetatarsal bursa.

table. With the patient in the above position, a high-frequency small linear ultrasound transducer is placed in a transverse position over the metatarsophalangeal heads and an ultrasound survey scan is taken (Fig. 23.9). The intermetatarsal space is identified between the heads of the metatarsals and the homogeneous appearing intermetatarsal soft tissue is searched for the appearance of a rounded hypoechoic intermetatarsal bursa (Fig. 23.10). Dynamic scanning while performing the Mulder maneuver may help identify the inflamed and enlarged bursa as it is forced from between the metatarsal heads (Fig. 23.11). When the intermetatarsal space is identified, the space is evaluated for the presence of Morton neuroma, intermetatarsal bursitis, and other abnormal mass (Figs. 23.12 to 23.14). Color Doppler may help identify inflammatory changes (Fig. 23.15).

CLINICAL PEARLS

Toe pathology—including tendinopathy, occult fractures, osteoarthritis, rheumatoid arthritis, crystal arthropathies, avascular necrosis bursitis, synovitis, and impingement syndromes—may coexist with disease of intermetatarsal bursitis and may contribute to the patient's pain symptoms. It should be remembered that there are many causes of metatarsalgia and the judicious use of multiple imaging modalities will help clarify the diagnosis in difficult cases (Fig. 23.16).

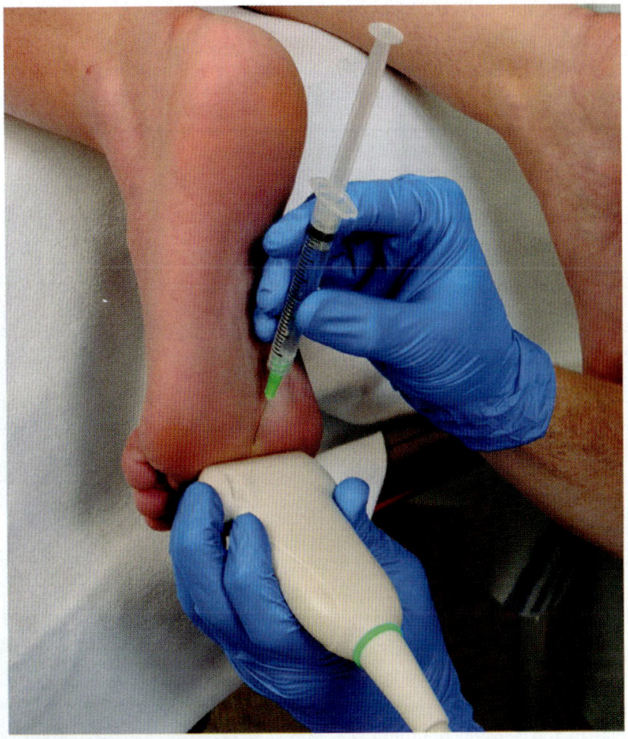

FIGURE 23.10 Dynamic scanning while performing the Mulder maneuver may help identify the inflamed and enlarged bursa as it is forced from between the metatarsal heads.

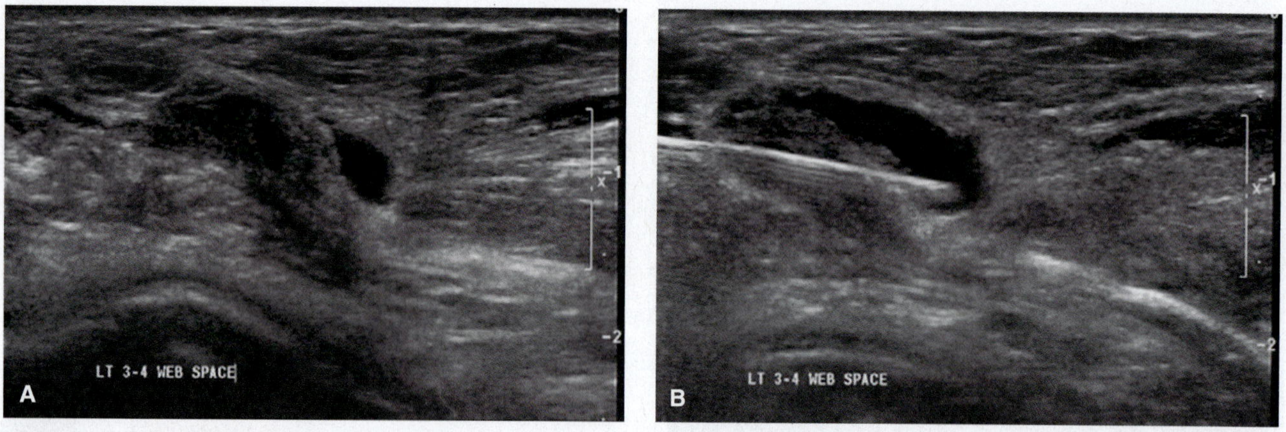

FIGURE 23.11 **A:** Ultrasound image in the sagittal plane showing a hypoechoic swelling in the third web space compatible with a Morton neuroma complex with perineural fibrosis and intermetatarsal bursitis. **B:** Ultrasound-guided injection of the third web space showing position of the 25-gauge needle, passing through the thickened nerve into the intermetatarsal bursa. (From Lucas PE. Imaging-guided interventions in the ankle and foot. *Techn Foot Ankle Surg* 2008;7(3):176–187.)

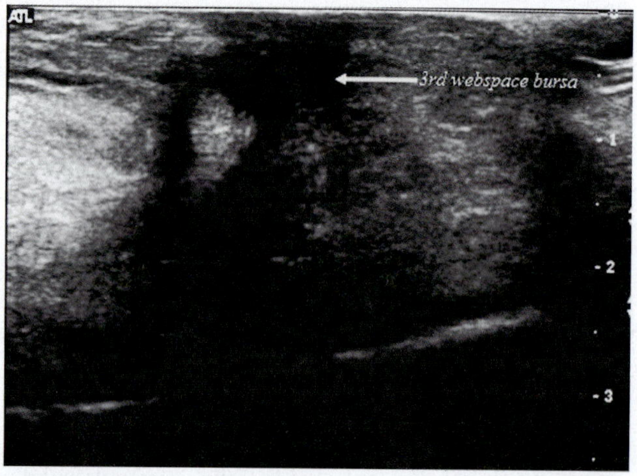

FIGURE 23.12 Longitudinal ultrasound image of the third web space demonstrates an irregular hypoechoic collection that was compressible, consistent with an intermetatarsal bursa. (From Adler R, Sofka CM, Positano RG. *Atlas of Foot and Ankle Sonography*. Philadelphia, PA: Lippincott Williams & Wilkins; 2004:19.)

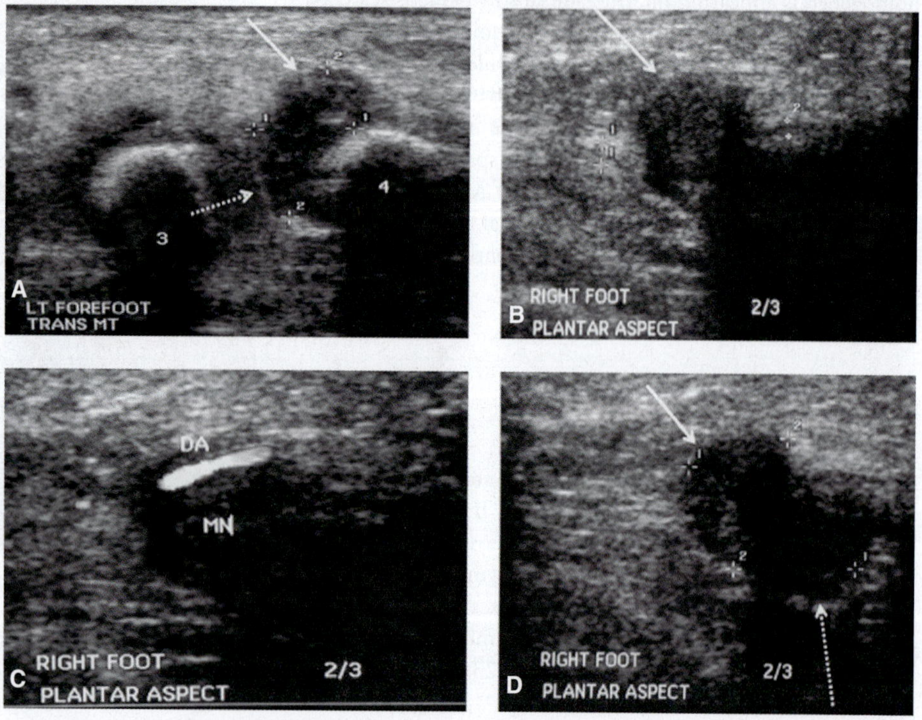

FIGURE 23.13 **A:** Transverse plantar view of a three to four superficial Morton neuroma (*arrow*) and a deeper intermetatarsal bursae (*dotted arrow*). Longitudinal plantar views of the same lesions showing the interdigital nerve on either side of the swollen neuroma **(B)**, the digital artery passing superficial to the Morton neuroma **(C)**, and the underlying intermetatarsal bursae (*dotted arrow;* **D**). (From Simmons DN. Imaging of the painful forefoot. *Techn Foot Ankle Surg* 2008;7(4):238–249.)

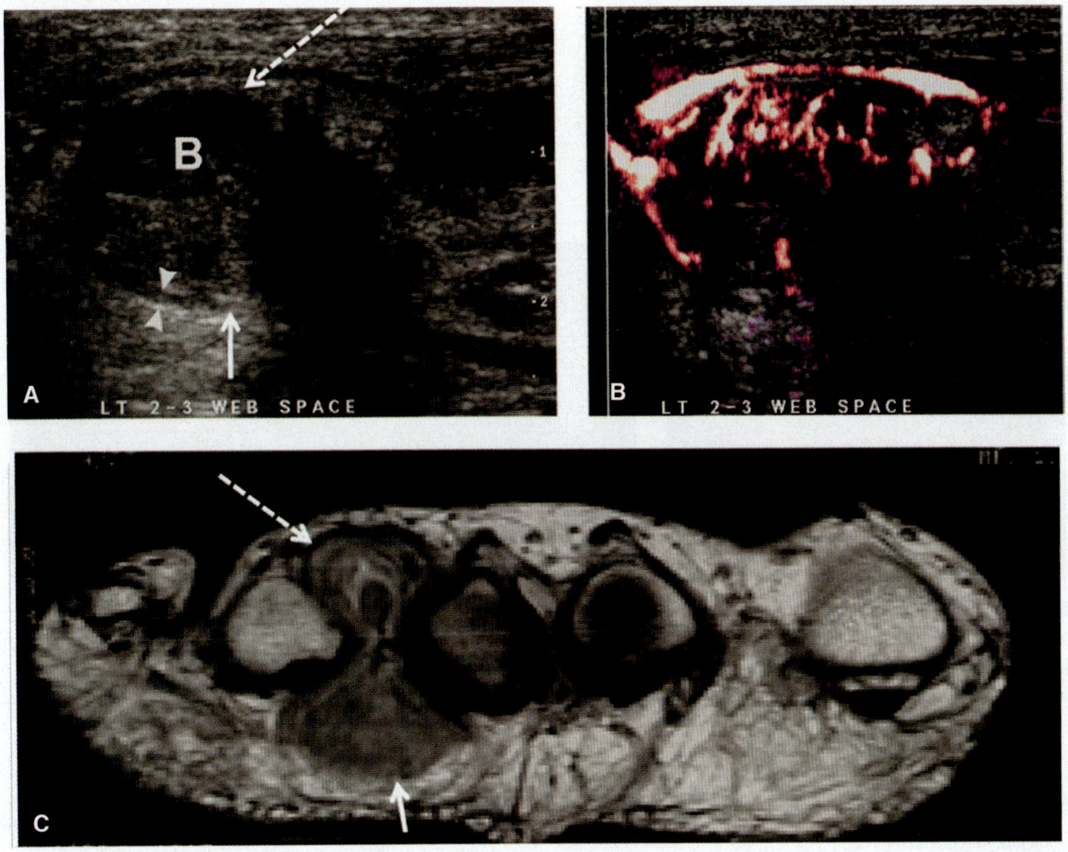

FIGURE 23.14 **A:** Dorsal longitudinal ultrasound image of swollen intermetatarsal bursa (*dotted arrow*) and adjacent Morton neuroma. *Arrowheads* indicate the digital nerve. **B:** Color Doppler scanning image showing the marked hypervascularity of the margins of the bursa. **C:** Magnetic resonance scan indicates swollen intermetatarsal bursa (*dotted arrow*) and Morton neuroma (*solid arrow*). (From Simmons DN. Imaging of the painful forefoot. *Techn Foot Ankle Surg* 2008;7(4):238–249.)

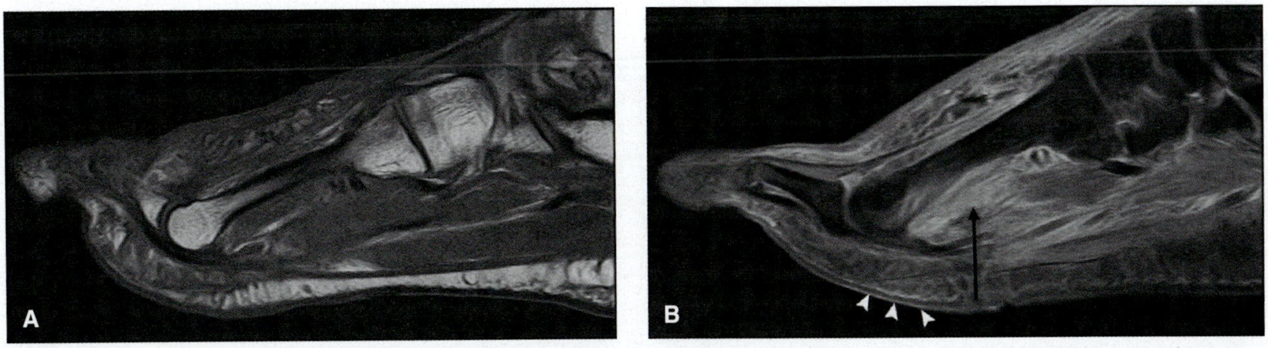

FIGURE 23.15 Cellulitis and myositis. Precontrast, sagittal, T1-weighted **(A)** and postcontrast, sagittal, fat-saturated **(B)** MR images of the forefoot show enhancement of the skin (*arrowheads*) and muscle (*arrow*), consistent with cellulitis and myositis. (From Verma S, Feldman J, Mohsen N. MR imaging for evaluation of plantar pain. *Contemp Diagn Radiol* 2014;37(10):1–5.)

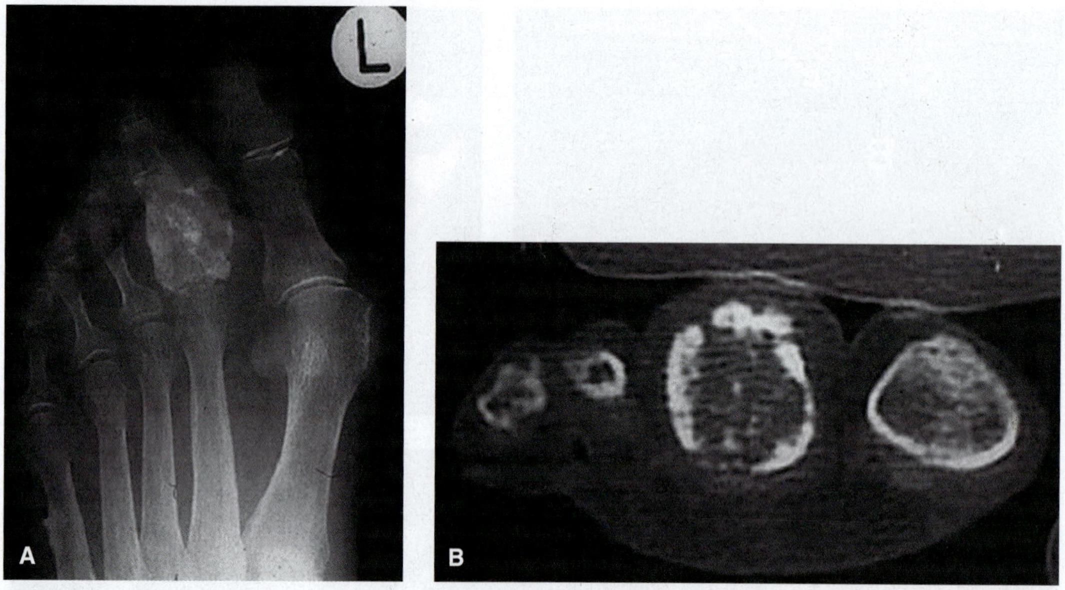

FIGURE 23.16 Chondrosarcoma. **A:** Calcified lesion in the proximal phalanx of the second toe is expanded and extends into the soft tissues. **B:** The coronal CT scan demonstrating the cortical disruption, soft tissue extension, and chondroid calcification of a chondrosarcoma. (From Schatz J, Soper J, McCormack S, et al. Imaging of tumors in the ankle and foot. *Top Magn Reson Imaging* 2010;21(1):37–50.)

Suggested Readings

Franson J, Baravarian B. Intermetatarsal compression neuritis. *Clin Podiatr Med Surg* 2006;23(3):569–578.

Lento PH, Strakowski JA. The use of ultrasound in guiding musculoskeletal interventional procedures. *Phys Med Rehabil Clin N Am* 2010;21(3):559–583.

Waldman SD. Injection technique for intrametatarsal bursa. In: *Atlas of Pain Management Injection Techniques.* 3rd ed. Philadelphia, PA: Saunders; 2012:476–479.

Wessely MA. MR imaging of the ankle and foot: a review of the normal imaging appearance with an illustration of common disorders. *Clin Chiro* 2007;10(2):101–111.

CHAPTER 24

Sesamoiditis

ANATOMIC CONSIDERATIONS

The sesamoid bones are small, rounded structures that are embedded in the flexor tendons of the foot and usually are in close proximity to the joints. Sesamoid bones of the first metatarsal occur in almost all patients, with sesamoid bones being present in the flexor tendons of the second and fifth metatarsals in a significant number of patients (Figs. 24.1 and 24.2). These sesamoid bones serve to decrease friction and pressure of the flexor tendon as it passes in proximity to a joint.

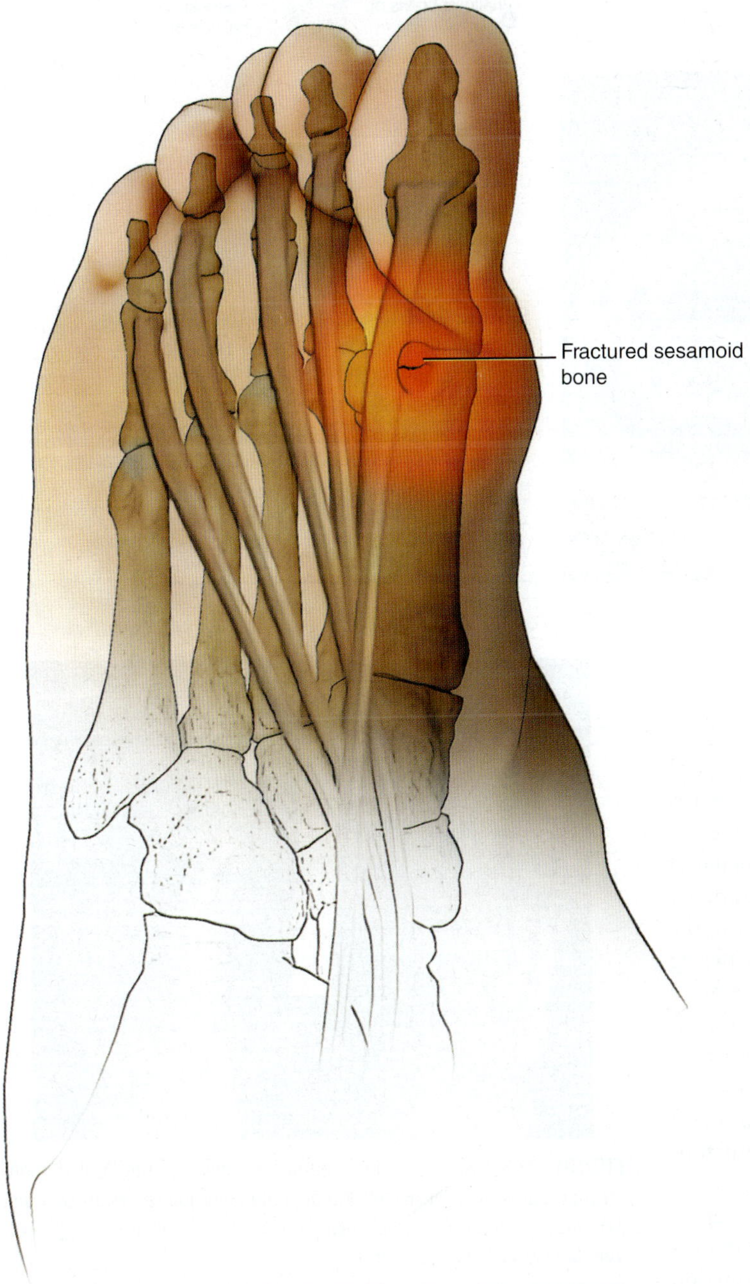

FIGURE 24.1 Sesamoiditis most commonly affects the first sesamoid bone of the first metatarsal head, although the sesamoid bones of the second and fifth metatarsal heads also are subject to the development of sesamoiditis.

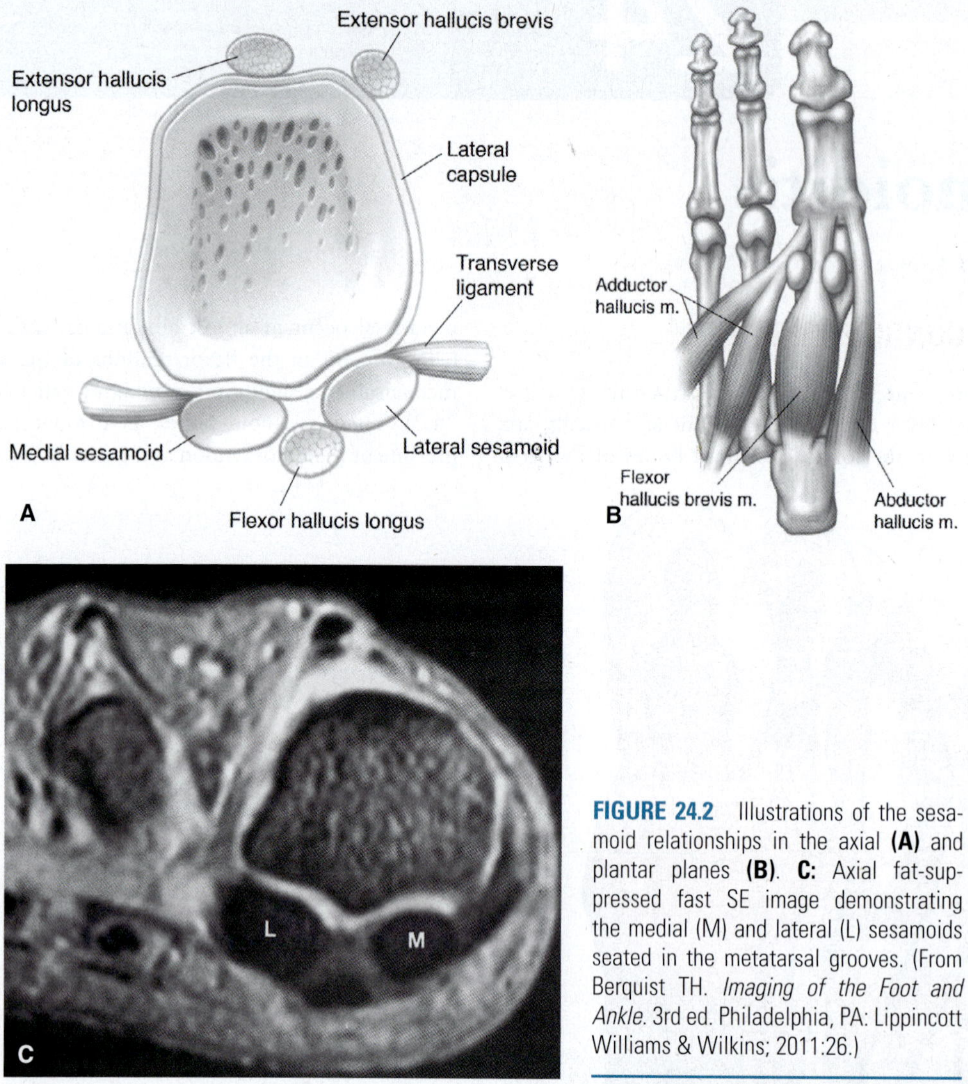

FIGURE 24.2 Illustrations of the sesamoid relationships in the axial **(A)** and plantar planes **(B)**. **C:** Axial fat-suppressed fast SE image demonstrating the medial (M) and lateral (L) sesamoids seated in the metatarsal grooves. (From Berquist TH. *Imaging of the Foot and Ankle*. 3rd ed. Philadelphia, PA: Lippincott Williams & Wilkins; 2011:26.)

CLINICAL CORRELATES

Sesamoiditis is one of the most common pain syndromes of the forefoot. Caused by inflammation of the sesamoid bones, sesamoiditis is characterized by tenderness and pain over the metatarsal heads. The first sesamoid bone of the first metatarsal head is most commonly affected, although the sesamoid bones of the second and fifth metatarsal heads also are subject to the development of sesamoiditis (Fig. 24.3). The patient suffering from sesamoiditis frequently complains that it feels like he or she is walking with a stone in his or her shoe. The pain of sesamoiditis worsens with prolonged standing or walking for long distances and is exacerbated by improperly fitting or padded shoes. Sesamoiditis is most often associated with pushing-off injuries during football or repetitive microtrauma from running or dancing.

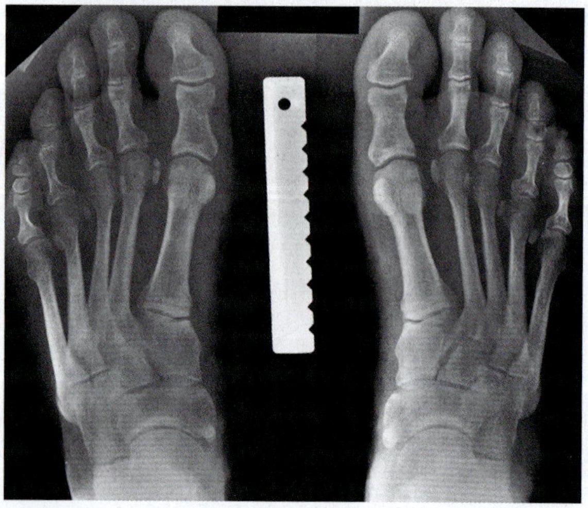

FIGURE 24.3 Standing posteroanterior views of the feet demonstrating sesamoids at all metatarsophalangeal joints. (From Berquist TH. *Imaging of the Foot and Ankle*. 3rd ed. Philadelphia, PA: Lippincott Williams & Wilkins; 2011:26.)

On physical examination, the pain of sesamoiditis can be reproduced by pressure on the affected sesamoid bone. Metatarsalgia is frequently confused with sesamoiditis. In contradistinction

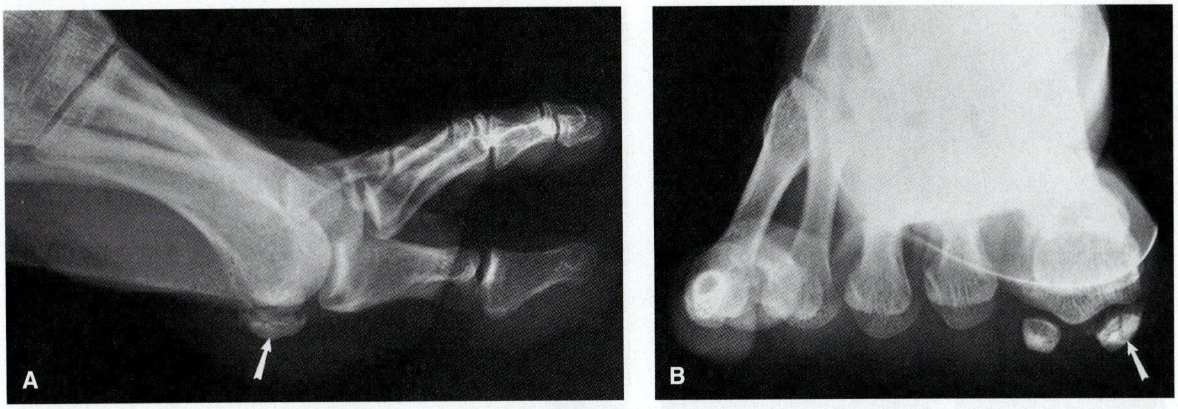

FIGURE 24.4 Lateral **(A)** and sesamoid **(B)** views demonstrating sclerosis and fragmentation of the medial sesamoid (*arrow*) due to fracture with avascular necrosis. (From Berquist TH. *Imaging of the Foot and Ankle.* 3rd ed. Philadelphia, PA: Lippincott Williams & Wilkins; 2011:194.)

to metatarsalgia where the tender area of palpation remains over the metatarsal heads, with sesamoiditis, the tender area moves with the flexor tendon when the patient is asked to actively flex his or her toe. The patient with sesamoiditis often exhibits an antalgic gait in an effort to reduce weight bearing during walking. With acute trauma to the sesamoid, ecchymosis over the plantar surface of the foot may be present and on occasion fracture of the sesamoid bone may occur (Figs. 24.4 and 24.5).

Plain radiographs are indicated in all patients who present with sesamoiditis (Fig. 24.6). Based on the patient's clinical presentation, additional testing may be indicated, including complete blood cell count, sedimentation rate, and antinuclear antibody testing. MRI or ultrasound of the intermetatarsal bursa is indicated to help confirm the diagnosis if fracture, effusion, tendinopathy, crystal arthropathy, joint mice, synovitis, foreign body, bursitis, or ligamentous injury is suspected (Figs. 24.7 and 24.8).

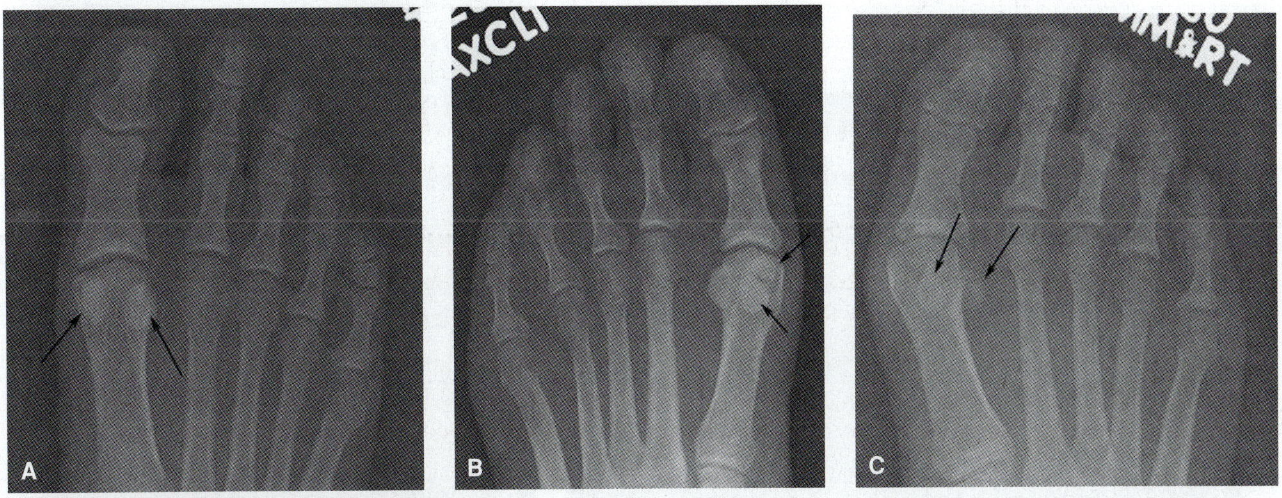

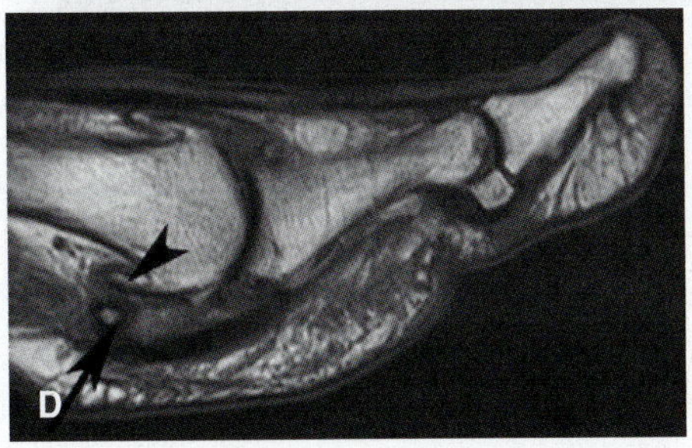

FIGURE 24.5 **A:** Radiograph demonstrating medial and lateral sesamoids (*arrows*) formed from single ossification centers. **B:** Radiograph demonstrating a bipartite medial sesamoid (*arrows*) with the lateral sesamoid formed from a single ossification center. **C:** Hallux valgus with rotation of the sesamoids laterally out of the normal metatarsal grooves. **D:** T1-weighted MR image demonstrating fragmentation of the sesamoid (*arrow*) and degenerative changes in the first metatarsophalangeal joint with osteophyte formation (*arrowhead*). (From Berquist TH. *Imaging of the Foot and Ankle.* 3rd ed. Philadelphia, PA: Lippincott Williams & Wilkins; 2011:193.)

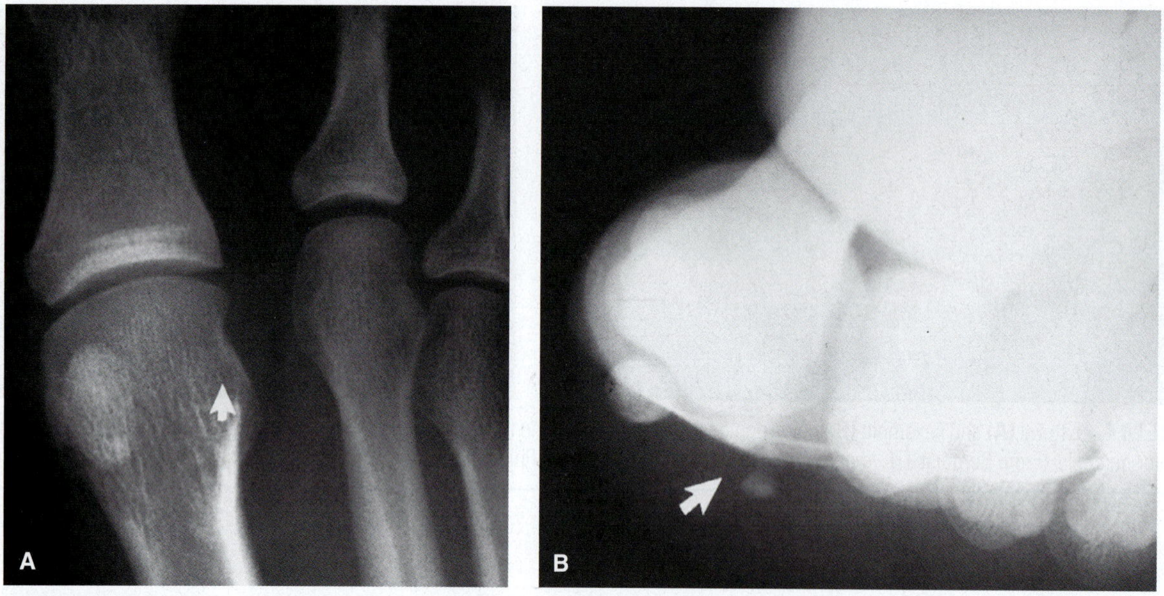

FIGURE 24.6 A long-distance runner with chronic pain under the first metatarsal head. **A:** Anteroposterior radiograph shows an absent lateral sesamoid (*arrow*). **B:** Sesamoid view shows only a small remnant (*arrow*) of the lateral sesamoid resulting from avascular necrosis and bone resorption. (From Berquist TH. *Imaging of the Foot and Ankle*. 3rd ed. Philadelphia, PA: Lippincott Williams & Wilkins; 2011:193.)

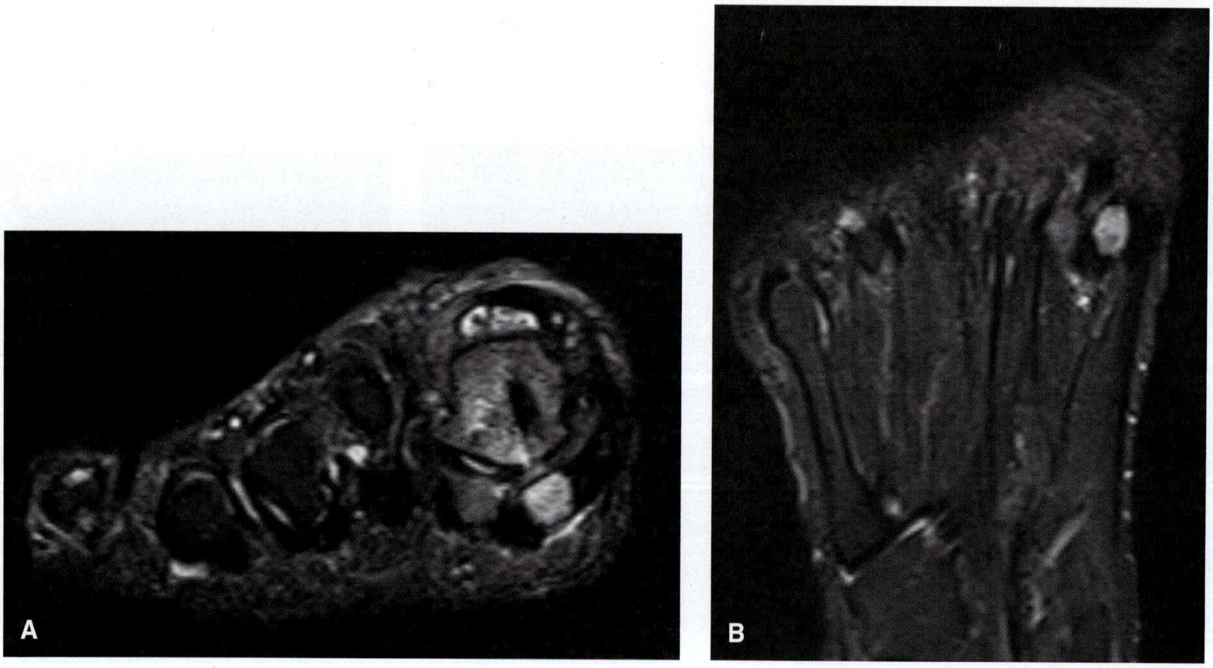

FIGURE 24.7 Axial **(A)** and coronal **(B)** STIR images of the sesamoids showing marked edema to the tibial sesamoid consistent with sesamoiditis. (From Pope TL Jr, Harris JH Jr, eds. *Harris & Harris' The Radiology of Emergency Medicine*. 5th ed. Philadelphia, PA: Lippincott Williams & Wilkins; 2013:962.)

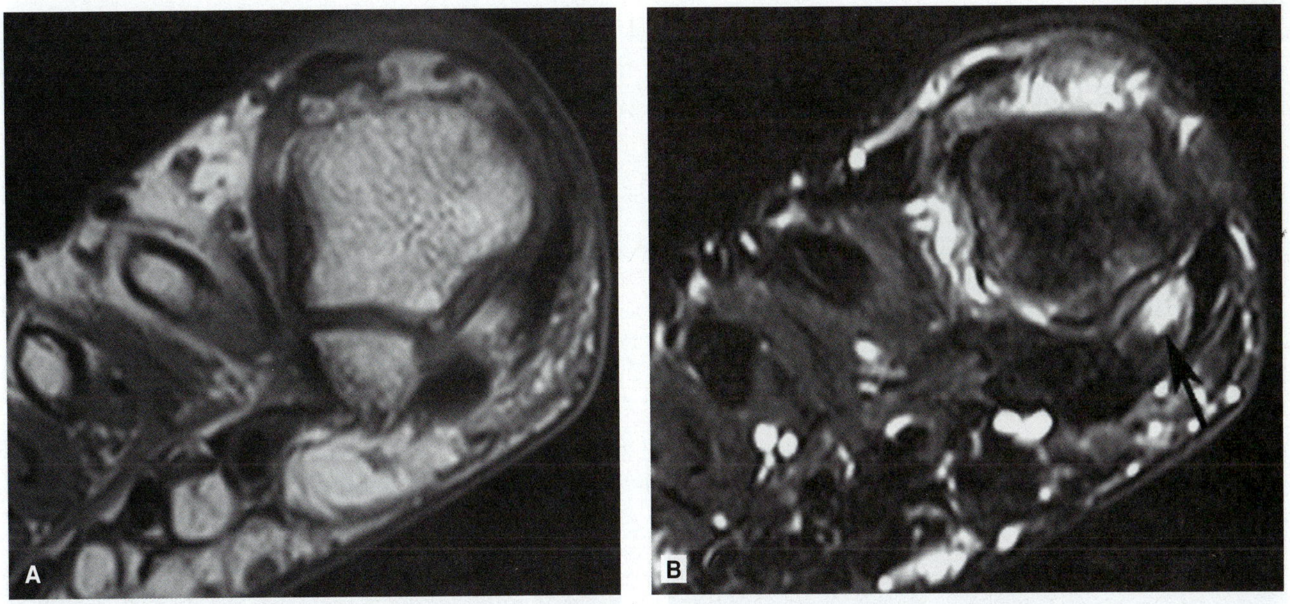

FIGURE 24.8 Marrow edema and fracture of the medial sesamoid. Axial T1-weighted **(A)** and T2-weighted **(B)** images demonstrate marrow edema and a subtle fracture (*arrow*) in the medial sesamoid. There is also synovitis in the joint. (From Berquist TH. *Imaging of the Foot and Ankle*. 3rd ed. Philadelphia, PA: Lippincott Williams & Wilkins; 2011:195.)

ULTRASOUND TECHNIQUE

To perform ultrasound evaluation of the sesamoid bones of the foot, the patient is then placed in the supine position with the patient's arms folded comfortably across the chest. With the patient in the above position, a high-frequency small linear ultrasound transducer is placed in a longitudinal plane over the painful metatarsophalangeal head and an ultrasound survey scan is taken (Fig. 24.9).

The hypoechoic joint space is identified between the head of the metatarsal and the base of the proximal phalanges and the curvilinear sesamoid bone with its acoustic shadow are identified (Fig. 24.10). When the sesamoid bone is identified, the sesamoid is evaluated for erosion, fragmentation, and fracture (Figs. 24.11 and 24.12).

CLINICAL PEARLS

Toe pathology—including tendinopathy, occult fractures, osteoarthritis, rheumatoid arthritis, crystal arthropathies, avascular necrosis bursitis, synovitis, and impingement syndromes—may coexist with sesamoiditis and may contribute to the patient's pain symptoms. The judicious use of multiple imaging modalities will help clarify the diagnosis in difficult patients (Fig. 24.13).

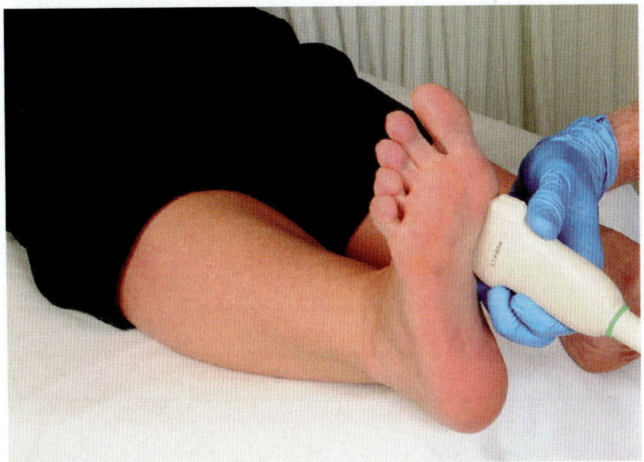

FIGURE 24.9 Correct longitudinal position for ultrasound transducer for ultrasound evaluation of the sesamoid bones of the feet.

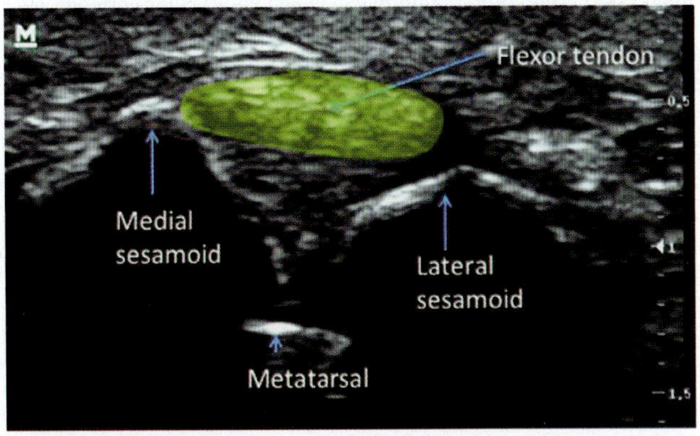

FIGURE 24.10 The lateral and medial sesamoids overlying the metatarsals (*blue ovals*). Lateral is to the right in this image.

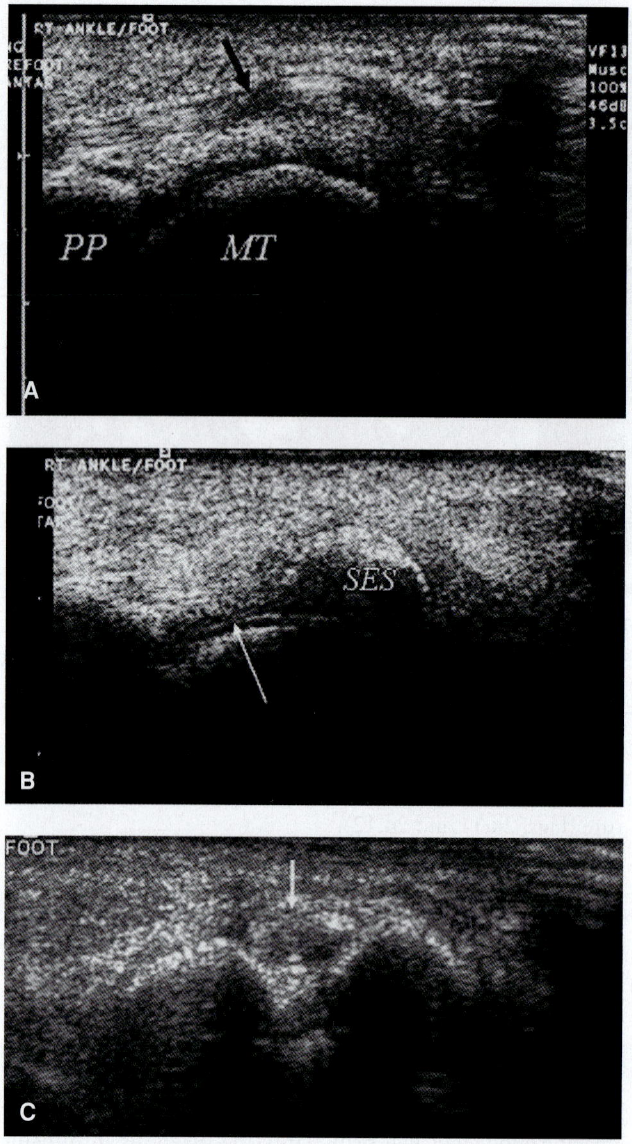

FIGURE 24.11 Longitudinal images of the plantar aspect of the first metatarsophalangeal (MTP) joint at two slightly offset parasagittal planes. **A:** The flexor hallucis longus tendon (*arrow*) and the first metatarsal and proximal phalanx (MT and PP, respectively) are indicated. **B:** Moving the transducer slightly more medial reveals the medial sesamoid (SES). The normal uniformly hypoechoic articular cartilage over the first metatarsal head can also be seen (*long thin white arrow*). **C:** Transverse ultrasound image of the sesamoids showing normal curvilinear sesamoids demonstrating posterior acoustic shadowing. The flexor hallucis longus tendon can be seen in the cross section (*arrow*). (From Adler R, Sofka CM, Positano RG. *Atlas of Foot and Ankle Sonography*. Philadelphia, PA: Lippincott Williams & Wilkins; 2004:26.)

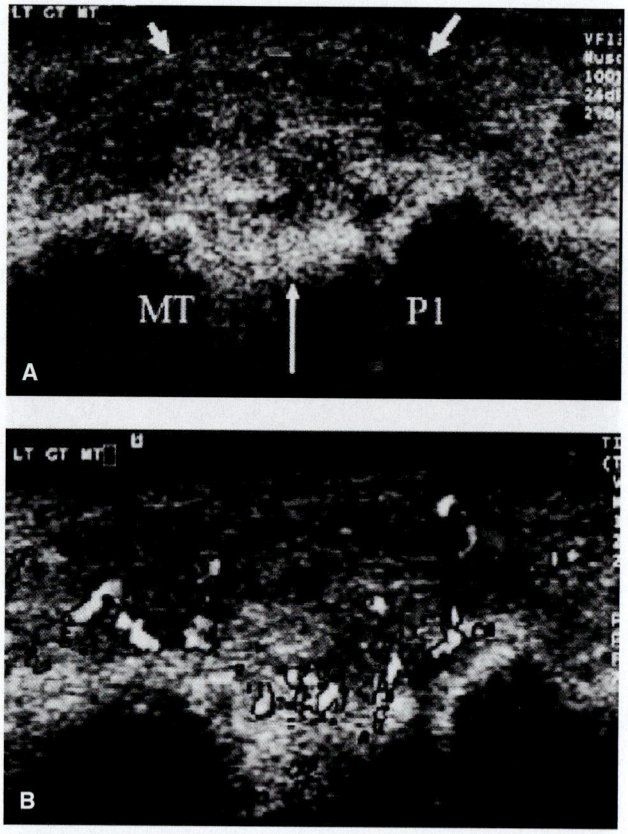

FIGURE 24.12 **A:** Longitudinal ultrasound image over the medial joint line of the first metatarsophalangeal (MTP) joint depicts cortical irregularity (*long arrow*) of the first metatarsal head (MT). A well-defined heterogeneous soft tissue mass (*short arrows*) abuts the cortical surface of the metatarsal head. **B:** Power Doppler imaging of the same area displays abnormal vascularity within the mass as well as adjacent to the cortical surface of the MTP joint. These features reflect the inflammatory nature of this tophaceous deposit. (From Adler R, Sofka CM, Positano RG. *Atlas of Foot and Ankle Sonography*. Philadelphia, PA: Lippincott Williams & Wilkins; 2004:28.)

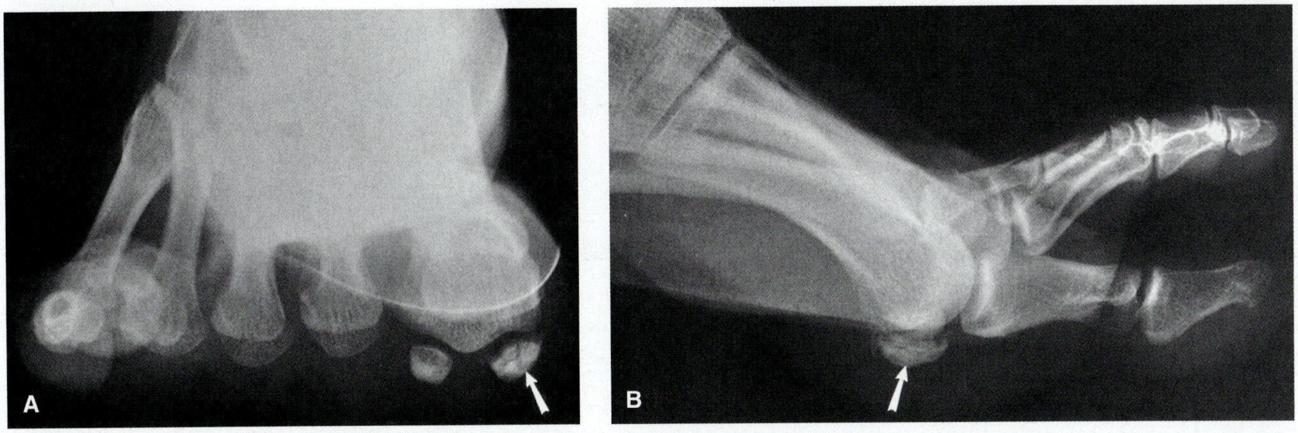

FIGURE 24.13 Sesamoid view **(A)** and lateral **(B)** radiographs demonstrate sclerosis and fragmentation of the medial sesamoid (*arrow*). (From Berquist TH. Foot, ankle, and calf. In: Berquist TH, ed. *MRI of the Musculoskeletal System*. 6th ed. Philadelphia, PA: Lippincott Williams & Wilkins; 2013:563.)

Suggested Readings

Anwar R, Anjum SN, Nicholl JE. Sesamoids of the foot *Curr Orthop* 2005;19(1):40–48.

Cohen BE. Hallux sesamoid disorders. *Foot Ankle Clin* 2009;14(1):91–104.

Lento PH, Strakowski JA. The use of ultrasound in guiding musculoskeletal interventional procedures. *Phys Med Rehabil Clin N Am* 2010;21(3):559–583.

Sanders TG, Rathur SK. Imaging of painful conditions of the hallucal sesamoid complex and plantar capsular structures of the first metatarsophalangeal joint. *Radiol Clin North Am* 2008;46(6):1079–1092.

Waldman SD. Injection technique for sesamoiditis. In: *Atlas of Pain Management Injection Techniques.* 3rd ed. Philadelphia, PA: Saunders; 2012:476–479.

Wessely MA. MR imaging of the ankle and foot: a review of the normal imaging appearance with an illustration of common disorders. *Clin Chiro* 2007; 10(2):101–111.

INDEX

Note: Page numbers followed by the letter "f" refer to figures and those followed by the letter "t" refer to tables